Biologics in Allergic/ Immunologic Conditions

Editor

FLAVIA C.L. HOYTE

IMMUNOLOGY AND ALLERGY CLINICS OF NORTH AMERICA

www.immunology.theclinics.com

Consulting Editor
ROHIT KATIAL

November 2024 • Volume 44 • Number 4

ELSEVIER

1600 John F. Kennedy Boulevard • Suite 1800 • Philadelphia, Pennsylvania, 19103-2899

http://www.theclinics.com

IMMUNOLOGY AND ALLERGY CLINICS OF NORTH AMERICA Volume 44, Number 4

November 2024 ISSN 0889-8561, ISBN-13: 978-0-443-29736-6

Editor: Taylor Hayes

Developmental Editor: Nitesh Barthwal

Immunology and Allergy Clinics of North America (ISSN 0889–8561) is published quarterly by Elsevier Inc., 360 Park Avenue South, New York, NY 10010-1710. Months of issue are February, May, August, and November. Periodicals postage paid at New York, NY and additional mailing offices. Subscription prices are $375.00 per year for US individuals, $100.00 per year for US students and residents, $458.00 per year for Canadian individuals, $100.00 per year for Canadian students, $484.00 per year for international individuals, $220.00 per year for international students. For institutional access pricing please contact Customer Service via the contact information below. To receive student/resident rate, orders must be accompanied by name of affiliated institution, date of term, and the *signature* of program/residency coordinator on institution letterhead. Orders will be billed at individual rate until proof of status is received. Foreign air speed delivery is included in all *Clinics* subscription prices. All prices are subject to change without notice. Orders, claims, and journal inquiries: Please visit our Support Hub page https://service.elsevier.com for assistance.

Reprints. For copies of 100 or more, of articles in this publication, please contact the Commercial Reprints Department, Elsevier Inc., 360 Park Avenue South, New York, New York 10010-1710. Tel. 212-633-3874, Fax: 212-633-3820, E-mail: reprints@elsevier.com.

Immunology and Allergy Clinics of North America is covered in MEDLINE/PubMed (Index Medicus), Current Contents/Life Sciences, Science Citation Index, ISI/BIOMED, Chemical Abstracts, and EMBASE/Excerpta Medica.

Contributors

CONSULTING EDITOR

ROHIT KATIAL, MD, FAAAAI, FACAAI, FACP
Professor of Medicine, Associate Vice President of Education, Director, Center for Clinical Immunology, Irene J. & Dr. Abraham E. Goldminz, Chair in Immunology and Respiratory Medicine, Division of Allergy and Clinical Immunology, Department of Medicine, National Jewish Health and University of Colorado, Denver, Colorado, USA

EDITOR

FLAVIA C.L. HOYTE, MD
Professor of Medicine, Division of Allergy and Clinical Immunology, National Jewish Health, Denver, Colorado, USA

AUTHORS

MUHAMMAD ADRISH, MD, MBA
Associate Professor, Department of Pulmonary and Critical Care, Baylor College of Medicine, Houston, Texas, USA

MICHELE BEAUDOIN, MD
Resident Physician, Department of Pediatrics, NYU Grossman School of Medicine, Hassenfeld Children's Hospital, New York, New York, USA

JONATHAN A. BERNSTEIN, MD
Professor of Medicine, Allergist-Immunologist, Division of Rheumatology, Allergy and Immunology, University of Cincinnati, Cincinnati, Ohio, USA

JOSHUA S. BERNSTEIN, MD
Assistant Professor, Allergist-Immunologist, Division of Rheumatology, Allergy and Immunology, University of Cincinnati, Cincinnati, Ohio, USA

MARK BOGUNIEWICZ, MD
Professor, Division of Allergy-Immunology, Department of Pediatrics, National Jewish Health, University of Colorado School of Medicine, Denver, Colorado, USA

JACOB T. BOYD, MD, PhD
Resident Physician, Department of Otolaryngology–Head and Neck Surgery, University of Colorado Anschutz School of Medicine, Aurora, Colorado, USA

KANWALJIT K. BRAR, MD
Associate Professor, Division of Allergy and Immunology, Department of Pediatrics, NYU Grossman School of Medicine, Hassenfeld Children's Hospital, New York, New York, USA

CHLOE CITRON, MD
Resident Physician, Department of Pediatrics, NYU Grossman School of Medicine, Hassenfeld Children's Hospital, New York, New York, USA

BRINDA DESAI, MD
Clinical Instructor and Research Fellow, Department of Medicine, University of California San Diego, La Jolla, California, USA

MAULI DESAI, MD
Associate Professor, Division of Allergy and Immunology, Department of Medicine, Albert Einstein College of Medicine, Montefiore Medical Center, Bronx, New York, USA

EJIOFOR EZEKWE, MD, PhD
Clinical Fellow, Human Eosinophil Section, Laboratory of Parasitic Diseases, National Institute of Allergy and Infectious Diseases, National Institutes of Health, Bethesda, Maryland, USA

ADAM HAINES, MD
Fellow, Division of Allergy & Immunology, Department of Pediatrics, Albert Einstein College of Medicine, Montefiore Medical Center, Bronx, New York, USA

YASMIN HASSOUN, MD
Assistant Professor, Division of Allergy and Immunology, Department of Pediatrics, Cincinnati Children's Hospital Medical Center, University of Cincinnati College of Medicine, Cincinnati, Ohio, USA

FLAVIA C.L. HOYTE, MD
Professor of Medicine, Division of Allergy and Clinical Immunology, National Jewish Health, Denver, Colorado, USA

JENNY HUANG, MD
Allergist, Division of Allergy, Asthma, and Immunology, Scripps Clinic, San Diego, California, USA

ELLIOT ISRAEL, MD
Gloria and Anthony Simboli Distinguished Professor of Medicine, Division of Pulmonary and Critical Care Medicine and Division of Allergy and Immunology, Brigham and Women's Hospital, Harvard Medical School, Boston, Massachusetts, USA

ROHIT KATIAL, MD, FAAAAI, FACAAI, FACP
Professor of Medicine, Associate Vice President of Education, Director, Center for Clinical Immunology, Irene J. & Dr. Abraham E. Goldminz, Chair in Immunology and Respiratory Medicine, Division of Allergy and Clinical Immunology, Department of Medicine, National Jewish Health and University of Colorado, Denver, Colorado, USA

ASHOKE R. KHANWALKAR, MD
Assistant Professor, Department of Otolaryngology–Head and Neck Surgery, University of Colorado Anschutz School of Medicine, Aurora, Colorado, USA

AMY D. KLION, MD
Senior Investigator, Head, Human Eosinophil Section, Deputy Chief, Laboratory of Parasitic Diseases, National Institute of Allergy and Infectious Diseases, National Institutes of Health, Bethesda, Maryland, USA

DAVID M. LANG, MD
Professor of Medicine, Department of Allergy and Clinical Immunology, Cleveland Clinic, Cleveland, Ohio, USA

GABRIEL LAVOIE, MD, FRCPC
Clinical and Research Fellow, Respiratory Medicine Unit and Oxford Respiratory NIHR BRC, Nuffield Department of Clinical Medicine, University of Oxford, John Radcliffe Hospital, Oxford, United Kingdom

NJIRA L. LUGOGO, MD, MSc
Professor, Department of Medicine, University of Michigan, Ann Arbor, Michigan, USA

RACHA ABI MELHEM, MD
Resident Physician, Department of Internal Medicine, Staten Island University Hospital, Bayonne, New Jersey, USA

ARJUN MOHAN, MD
Associate Professor, Department of Medicine, University of Michigan, Ann Arbor, Michigan, USA

MICHAEL NEVID, MD
Assistant Professor, Division of Allergy-Immunology, Department of Pediatrics, National Jewish Health, University of Colorado School of Medicine, Denver, Colorado, USA

JOHN J. OPPENHEIMER, MD
Clinical Professor, Division of Allergy and Immunology, Department of Medicine, UMDNJ-Rutgers, Newark, New Jersey, USA

IAN D. PAVORD, DM, FRCP, FMedSci
Professor of Respiratory Medicine, Respiratory Medicine Unit and Oxford Respiratory NIHR BRC, Nuffield Department of Clinical Medicine, University of Oxford, John Radcliffe Hospital, Oxford, United Kingdom

LUKE M. PITTMAN, MD
Program Director, National Capital Consortium Allergy and Immunology Fellowship, Department of Medicine, Allergy and Immunology Service, Walter Reed National Military Medical Center, Bethesda, Maryland, USA

ORLANDO RIVERA II, MD
Allergy and Immunology Fellow, Division of Allergy and Immunology, National Jewish Health, University of Colorado, Denver, Colorado, USA

JUSTIN D. SALCICCIOLI, MBBS, MA
Instructor of Medicine, Division of Pulmonary and Critical Care Medicine, Brigham and Women's Hospital, Harvard Medical School, Boston, Massachusetts, USA

ANDREW L. WESKAMP, DO
Allergy and Immunology Fellow, National Capital Consortium Allergy and Immunology Fellowship, Department of Medicine, Allergy and Immunology Service, Walter Reed National Military Medical Center, Bethesda, Maryland, USA

ANDREW A. WHITE, MD
Director, Aspirin Exacerbated Respiratory Disease Clinic; Division of Allergy, Asthma, and Immunology, Scripps Clinic, San Diego, California, USA

Contents

Atopic dermatitis (AD) is a common chronic pruritic inflammatory skin disease that affects all ages and is recognized as a global health problem. Pathophysiology is complex with skin barrier abnormalities, immune dysregulation, and microbial dysbiosis all implicated. Markers of immune and inflammatory activation in the circulation provide a rationale for systemic therapy. Type 2 immune polarization is central, though other cytokine pathways including Th22 and Th17/IL-23 have been described, suggesting additional therapeutic targets in a subset of patients. Dupilumab and tralokinumab are monoclonal antibodies currently approved for moderate-to-severe AD with lebrikizumab and nemolizumab in late stages of development.

Antihistamine refractory chronic spontaneous urticaria (CSU) has a prevalence of up to 50%. Anti-immunoglobulin E (IgE) therapies have revolutionized management of CSU, yet refractory cases persist, suggesting a role for biologic agents that impact alternative routes of mast cell stimulation independent of cross-linking at FcεR1. This review addresses anti-IgE and Th2-targeted therapies in the management of CSU. In addition, we explore novel treatments targeting alternative pathways of mast cell activation including MAS-related G protein-coupled receptor-X2 and sialic acid-binding immunoglobulin-like lectin-6, inhibiting intracellular signaling via Bruton's tyrosine kinase, and disrupting KIT activation by SCF.

Eosinophilic gastrointestinal diseases (EGIDs) encompass a group of disorders characterized by an abnormal accumulation of eosinophils in various parts of the gastrointestinal tract. EGIDs present with a wide range of symptoms such as abdominal pain, vomiting, diarrhea, difficulty swallowing, and food impaction. Monoclonal antibodies, targeting inflammatory cytokines or eosinophils, are the next emerging therapy for EGIDs. The only Food and Drug Administration-approved monoclonal antibody is dupilumab, and it has been approved for the treatment of eosinophilic esophagitis (EoE). In this article, the authors will discuss biologics that have been used in the treatment of eosinophilic gastrointestinal diseases.

Hypereosinophilic syndrome (HES) and eosinophilic granulomatosis with polyangiitis (EGPA) are complex disorders defined by blood and tissue eosinophilia and heterogeneous clinical manifestations. Historically, the mainstay of therapy for both conditions has been systemic glucocorticoids. However, recent availability of biologics that directly or indirectly target eosinophils has provided new avenues to pursue improved outcomes with decreased toxicity. In this article, we summarize the evidence supporting the use of specific biologics in HES and/or EGPA and provide a framework for their clinical use in patients.

Immunoglobuin E (IgE)-mediated food allergies greatly impact patients and their families, causing financial and emotional stress, and placing them at risk for lifethreatening reactions. Until recently, food allergies have been treated with allergen avoidance and emergency treatment of allergic reactions. Omalizumab was recently approved in adults and children greater than one year who are allergic to one or more foods for the prevention of serious allergic reactions in the setting of accidental exposure. Omalizumab also shows promise when combined with oral immunotherapy for possible allergen ingestion. Other classes of biologics and small molecule inhibitors have also demonstrated potential for use in preventing and treating food allergy.

Chronic rhinosinusitis (CRS) is categorized phenotypically into CRS with and without nasal polyps (CRSwNP, CRSsNP). Endotyping categorizes the disease based on immune cell activity and inflammatory mechanisms into Type 1, Type 2, and Type 3. The Type 2 endotype is the most researched and associated with asthma, atopic disease, and severe CRSwNP. For patients with poorly controlled CRSwNP, there are 3 approved biologic treatments: omalizumab, dupilumab, and mepolizumab. Many other biologics are being tested in Type 2, non-Type 2, and mixed endotypes in CRSwNP and CRSsNP. These studies will play a significant role in shaping the future of CRS management.

Biologic medications have dramatically altered the landscape for treatment of allergic conditions including aspirin-exacerbated respiratory disease (AERD) and allergic bronchopulmonary aspergillosis (ABPA). Biologics should be considered for patients who are refractory to first line therapies for ABPA. Biologics should be discussed with patients with AERD. Variable responses to different biologics indicate that there may be various endotypes of AERD and ABPA, similar to asthma. Alternative biologics may be considered in patients who fail to respond to initial treatment.

The development of multiple targeted biologic therapies over the past two decades has revolutionized the management of asthma. Currently, there are 6 monoclonal antibodies that target specific inflammatory mediators involved in the pathophysiology of asthma, and together, they provide the opportunity for personalized treatment options beyond bronchodilators and inhaled or systemic glucocorticoids in severe and difficult-to-control cases of asthma. These agents are the anti-IgE antibody omalizumab, the anti-IL-5 antibodies mepolizumab and reslizumab, the IL-5 receptor alpha antagonist benralizumab, the IL-4 receptor alpha antagonist dupilumab, and the anti-thymic stromal lymphopoietin antibody tezepelumab.

Our modern understanding of asthma mainly concerns identification of inflammatory endotype to guide management. The distinction mostly concerns identification of type-2 inflammation, for which different biomarkers have been well characterized. Blood eosinophils corroborate activity in the interleukin (IL)-5 axis while fraction of exhaled nitric oxide is indicative of the IL-4/IL-13 axis, giving us an indication of activity in these distinct but complementary pathways. These biomarkers predict disease activity, with increased risk of exacerbations when elevated, and a further, multiplicative increase when both are elevated. Serum immunoglobulin E is also implicated in this pathway, and can represent allergen-related stimulation.

Establishing a universal definition for asthma remission has the potential to improve asthma outcomes and advance research. However, there is still no consensus definition despite broad multidisciplinary efforts to achieve this goal. This study explores the evolving concept of asthma remission, emphasizing the potential of biologics to achieve this state. We will discuss various proposed definitions of asthma remission, international guidelines, and studies evaluating the effectiveness of biologics at achieving clinical remission. We highlight the need for a consensus definition of asthma remission to standardize treatment goals and improve patient outcomes.

Mauli Desai, Adam Haines, and John J. Oppenheimer

Presently, there are 6 biologic agents available for the treatment of asthma. Each of these agents has undergone robust clinical trials in their approval programs. Such studies rely upon very rigid entry criteria that may not translate to real-world efficacy. Thus, exploring the efficacy of these agents in a larger, more heterogeneous, population brings a sense of comfort regarding their efficacy in the real-world. This review explores the available literature regarding the use of biologics in the real world, with a focus on markers of likely response to therapy.

Brinda Desai, Muhammad Adrish, Arjun Mohan, and Njira L. Lugogo

Advances in our understanding of asthma pathophysiology have led to the advent of multiple targeted asthma therapies such as biologics. However, partial response to biologics occurs, indicating residual disease activity in some patients. Hence, there exists a need for new therapies that focus on novel pathways, alongside perhaps evaluation of combination biologic therapies and modulators of downstream cytokine activation. Therefore, although our current focus is on biologics; it is critical to take a more holistic approach including consideration for nonbiologic therapies that have the potential to significantly advance asthma care.

IMMUNOLOGY AND ALLERGY CLINICS OF NORTH AMERICA

SERIES OF RELATED INTEREST

Medical Clinics
https://www.medical.theclinics.com/

THE CLINICS ARE AVAILABLE ONLINE!
Access your subscription at:
www.theclinics.com

Foreword

Biologics: A New Era in Allergy and Immunology

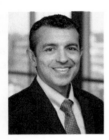

Rohit Katial, MD, FAAAAI, FACAAI, FACP
Consulting Editor

The landscape of allergy and immunology has undergone a transformative evolution with the advent of biologic therapies. These targeted agents have revolutionized our approach to managing a spectrum of conditions, offering hope and improving quality of life to countless patients. This issue of *Immunology and Allergy Clinics of North America* is dedicated to exploring the current and emerging role of biologics for the allergist and immunologist.

Dr Flavia C.L. Hoyte has assembled an exceptional group of world-renowned experts, who delve into the intricacies of biologic therapies across a wide range of allergic and immunologic diseases, from atopic dermatitis and chronic urticaria to eosinophilic gastrointestinal diseases, hypereosinophilic syndrome, eosinophilic granulomatosis with polyangiitis, food allergies, chronic rhinosinusitis, aspirin-exacerbated respiratory disease, allergic bronchopulmonary aspergillosis, and asthma including remission. This issue provides a comprehensive overview of the latest advancements and clinical applications across this myriad of conditions.

As the Consulting Editor, I am privileged to have contributed to this invaluable resource. The articles within this issue not only highlight the efficacy and safety of groundbreaking treatments but also address critical aspects, such as the role of biomarkers, real-world evidence, and the exciting pipeline of emerging biologics.

I am confident that this issue will serve as an indispensable reference for clinicians, researchers, and health care providers alike. By fostering a deeper understanding of biologic therapies, we can collectively optimize patient care and drive future innovations in the field of allergy and immunology.

Immunol Allergy Clin N Am 44 (2024) xiii–xiv
https://doi.org/10.1016/j.iac.2024.08.006
0889-8561/24/© 2024 Published by Elsevier Inc.

immunology.theclinics.com

I extend my sincere gratitude to Dr Flavia C.L. Hoyte for her exceptional leadership and to the esteemed contributors for their invaluable expertise. I truly hope you will find this not only an invaluable update on the topic but also a reference for the future.

Rohit Katial, MD, FAAAAI, FACAAI, FACP
Division of Allergy & Clinical Immunology
Department of Medicine
National Jewish Health and University of Colorado
1400 Jackson Street
Denver, CO 80206, USA

E-mail address:
KatialR@NJHealth.org

Preface

Biologics: A New Era in Allergy and Immunology

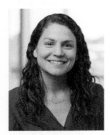

Flavia C.L. Hoyte, MD
Editor

The last decade has witnessed a revolutionary transformation in the field of allergy and immunology, largely driven by the advent and rapid development of biologic therapies. This issue of *Immunology and Allergy Clinics of North America* aims to encapsulate these advancements and their profound impact on patient care across a spectrum of allergic and immunologic conditions. It serves as a comprehensive resource for physicians, researchers, and health care professionals dedicated to leveraging these breakthroughs to enhance patient outcomes.

The primary purpose of this issue is to provide an in-depth exploration of the transformative role of biologics in allergy and immunology. Each article, authored by leading experts, offers insights into the mechanisms, clinical applications, and future directions of these therapies. The first seven articles cover a broad spectrum of conditions, from atopic dermatitis and urticaria to eosinophilic gastrointestinal diseases, hypereosinophilic syndrome, eosinophilic granulomatosis with polyangiitis, food allergies, chronic rhinosinusitis with nasal polyps, aspirin-exacerbated respiratory disease, and allergic bronchopulmonary aspergillosis. The last five articles cover various aspects of biologic therapy for asthma, the first condition in the field of allergy and immunology to be treated with biologics. These later articles review in comprehensive fashion the randomized placebo controlled trial and real-world trial data supporting the use of currently approved biologics for asthma, the role of biomarkers in determining choice of biologic and predicting response to therapy, the ability of biologics to help achieve asthma remission, and several emerging biologic therapies for asthma.

This issue is the result of the collective efforts of numerous experts who have generously shared their knowledge, experience, and time. I extend my deepest gratitude to all the authors for their invaluable contributions. Special thanks to the editorial team for their dedication and hard work in bringing this project to fruition.

Immunol Allergy Clin N Am 44 (2024) xv–xvi
https://doi.org/10.1016/j.iac.2024.08.005
0889-8561/24/© 2024 Published by Elsevier Inc.

immunology.theclinics.com

"Biologics in Allergy and Immunology" is intended to be a reference for current and future practitioners in the field. The development of biologics has been rapid, and the horizon holds several promising therapies for allergic and immunologic conditions. These advancements bring exciting possibilities for our field and renewed hope for our patients. The integration of biologics, personalized medicine, and advanced diagnostics represents the future of allergy and immunology, ensuring that patients receive the most effective and targeted treatments available. As you read through the articles, I hope you find the information both enlightening and useful in your clinical practice.

DISCLOSURES

AstraZeneca: Advisory, speaking; GSK: Advisory; Genentech: Advisory; Teva: Advisory; Sanofi: Advisory.

Flavia C.L. Hoyte, MD
Division of Allergy and
Clinical Immunology
National Jewish Health
1400 Jackson Street
Denver, CO 80206, USA

E-mail address:
HoyteF@NJHealth.org

Current and Emerging Biologics for Atopic Dermatitis

Michael Nevid, MD[a], Mark Boguniewicz, MD[b],*

KEYWORDS

- Atopic dermatitis • Eczema • Biologics • Monoclonal antibody • Dupilumab
- Tralokinumab • Lebrikizumab • Nemolizumab

KEY POINTS

- Atopic dermatitis is a common chronic inflammatory skin disease characterized by skin barrier dysfunction, immune dysregulation, and microbial dysbiosis.
- Inflammatory cytokines and their receptors have become specific targets of biologics.
- Dupilumab, which targets IL-4 receptor alpha, has shown robust clinical efficacy and is approved for moderate-to-severe atopic dermatitis down to 6 months of age in the United States
- Tralokinumab, a selective IL-13 inhibitor, was recently approved down to 12 years for moderate-to-severe atopic dermatitis in the United States
- Emerging biologics include lebrikizumab, which also targets IL-13, and nemolizumab, which targets IL-31 receptor A.

INTRODUCTION

While topical therapy has been a mainstay of treatment for atopic dermatitis (AD), biologic therapy with monoclonal antibodies (mAb) represents a targeted approach to the treatment of this common inflammatory skin disease.[1] Evaluating how biologics best fit into the treatment armamentarium for AD requires an understanding not only of the pathology of the disease, but also of the prevalence and burden of the disease, along with associated co-morbidities and limitations of current therapy. At the present time, patients classified as having moderate or severe AD are candidates for biologic therapy. However, as we define biomarkers specific for the disease and unique endophenotypes, targeted therapy with more precise biologics may lead to a personalized approach to treating AD.

---

[a] Division of Allergy-Immunology, Department of Pediatrics, National Jewish Health and University of Colorado School of Medicine, 1400 Jackson Street, J312, Denver, CO 80206, USA;
[b] Division of Allergy-Immunology, Department of Pediatrics, National Jewish Health and University of Colorado School of Medicine, 1400 Jackson Street, J310, Denver, CO 80206, USA
* Corresponding author.
E-mail address: boguniewiczm@njhealth.org

Immunol Allergy Clin N Am 44 (2024) 577–594
https://doi.org/10.1016/j.iac.2024.08.001   **immunology.theclinics.com**
0889-8561/24/© 2024 Elsevier Inc. All rights reserved, including those for text and data mining, AI training, and similar technologies.

OVERVIEW OF ATOPIC DERMATITIS

The prevalence of AD and importance as a global health problem in developed and developing countries have been reviewed.[2] AD can be a life-long disease, and a subset of patients present with adult-onset disease. In all ages, AD has a profound impact on the quality of life (QoL) of patients and families. While a majority of patients or caregivers report that pruritus is the most bothersome symptom, sleep disturbance can also be a major problem impacting the ability of patients and their families to function in a school, work, or social environment. In a study of adults with moderate-to-severe AD participating in a trial of a biologic therapy, 85% reported problems with itch frequency, 41.5% reported itching ≥18 hours/day, 55% reported AD-related sleep disturbance ≥ 5 days/week, and 21.8% had clinically relevant anxiety or depression assessed by Hospital Anxiety and Depression Scale scores.[3] The economic burden of the disease translates to billions of dollars of cost to patients, caregivers, as well as society. A comprehensive report on the burden of AD for the National Eczema Association found a conservative estimate of the annual costs of AD in the United States to be greater than $5 billion.[4] Thus, any pharmacoeconomic evaluation of new therapies for AD needs to take into consideration diverse factors including associated co-morbidities.

PATHOPHYSIOLOGY OF ATOPIC DERMATITIS AND IMPLICATIONS FOR TARGETED THERAPY

AD is characterized by skin barrier abnormalities, immune dysregulation, and microbial dysbiosis.[5] Both innate immune cells including type 2 innate lymphoid cells, dendritic cells, eosinophils, mast cells, and basophils, as well as adaptive immune cells such as T cells and B cells participate in the complex immune network that contributes to cutaneous inflammation in AD. Type 2 cytokines including IL-4, IL-5, and IL-13 appear to be central to the pathophysiology of AD,[6,7] although Th22 and Th17 may also be involved in a subset of AD patients which has therapeutic implications,[8] Of note, non-lesional skin in patients with AD is characterized by both immune abnormalities as well as broad terminal differentiation defects, implying a role for systemic immune activation.[9] A number of studies point to the systemic nature of the disease.[10,11] The role of IL-4 and IL-13 in the induction and perpetuation of type 2 immune responses that have been implicated in atopic diseases besides AD, including asthma and chronic sinusitis with nasal polyposis, have been reviewed.[12] The efficacy of a biologic targeting key cytokines in treating these atopic diseases highlights common pathogenic pathways and supports the pivotal role of IL-4 and IL-13 in the pathogenesis of these atopic diseases. However, insights into disease pathophysiology may not always translate into clinically meaningful therapies in AD, as evidenced by failure of biologics targeting thymic stromal lymphopoietin, a key cytokine thought to orchestrate allergic inflammation. As AD is often the first step in the atopic march leading to the development of asthma and allergic disorders,[13,14] it is tempting to speculate that treatment of AD may be not only disease modifying, but could also alter the atopic march.[15]

CURRENTLY APPROVED BIOLOGICS FOR MODERATE-TO-SEVERE ATOPIC DERMATITIS
Dupilumab in Adults

Dupilumab is a fully human monoclonal antibody directed against the IL-4 receptor α subunit that blocks signaling of both IL-4 and IL-13 (**Fig. 1**). In 2 randomized, placebo-controlled, phase 3 trials of identical design (SOLO 1 and SOLO 2), 671

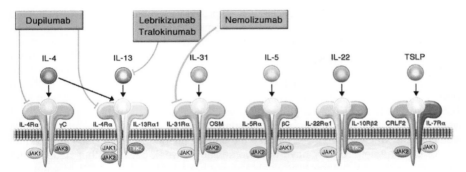

Fig. 1. Cell surface receptors which are targets of biologics approved for or under investigation for the treatment of atopic dermatitis. (*From* Chovatiya R, Paller AS. JAK inhibitors in the treatment of atopic dermatitis. J Allergy Clin Immunol. 2021 Oct;148(4):927-940.)

and 708 adult patients with moderate-to-severe AD inadequately controlled on topical treatment were assigned in a 1:1:1 ratio to monotherapy with subcutaneous dupilumab 300 mg weekly, 300 mg every other week alternating with placebo, or placebo weekly.[16] Patients on dupilumab were given an initial 600 mg loading dose. The primary outcome was the proportion of patients who had both an investigator's global assessment (IGA) of 0 or 1 (clear or almost clear, respectively) and a reduction of 2 points or more in that score from baseline at week 16. In SOLO 1, the primary outcome was achieved in 38% of the patients who received dupilumab every other week and in 37% who received dupilumab weekly, as compared with 10% who received placebo (P<.001 for both comparisons with placebo). The results in SOLO 2 were similar, with the primary outcome occurring in 36% of the patients who received dupilumab every other week and in 36% who received dupilumab weekly, as compared with 8% who received placebo (P<.001 for both comparisons). Improvement of at least 75% in Eczema Area and Severity Index (EASI) (EASI-75) from baseline to week 16 was reported in significantly more patients who received either dupilumab regimen versus those who received placebo (P<.001 for all comparisons). In these trials, the 2 dosing regimens (300 mg weekly or every other week) showed similar efficacy and safety. Dupilumab was also associated with improvement in other clinical end points, including reduction in pruritus and symptoms of anxiety or depression as well as improvement in QoL. Injection-site reactions and conjunctivitis were more frequent in the dupilumab-treated patients than in the placebo groups. While the conjunctivitis has not been fully explained, it was for the most part self-limited, and only 1 patient in the SOLO trials discontinued study treatment. Of interest, this AE was not reported in the asthma or chronic sinusitis with nasal polyposis trials with dupilumab. It is also worth recognizing that median AD disease duration in the patients enrolled in these pivotal trials was ~26 years, median affected body surface area was >50%, and median EASI ~ 30 (≥21.1 = severe AD). In this context, the bar for dupilumab *monotherapy* at 16 weeks (primary outcome by IGA of clear/almost clear) was set ambitiously high. In addition, it is important for clinicians to understand that patients with severe AD (IGA of 4) who improved to mild (IGA of 2) would not have met the primary outcome of the study, and yet for many of these patients with longstanding, debilitating disease, such a change would be associated with significant improvement in their QoL and would be clinically meaningful outside the confines of a study protocol.

A 52-week study (LIBERTY AD CHRONOS) provided results of long-term safety and efficacy in managing AD.[17] Patients were randomized to either 300 mg dupilumab subcutaneously weekly or every other week or placebo and, in addition, patients could use concomitant topical corticosteroids (TCS) (or topical calcineurin inhibitor if TCS was not advisable) as needed based on disease activity. At week 16, more patients who received dupilumab plus TCS achieved the coprimary endpoints of IGA 0/1 (39% on weekly injections and 39% on every other week treatment vs 12% on placebo plus TCS; $P<0.0001$) and EASI-75 (64%, 69% vs 23%; $P<0.0001$), with similar results at week 52. Although there was some overlap, patients meeting these endpoints at week 16 and week 52 were necessarily the same patients as some patients rated as IGA of 0/1 at week 16 may have had worsening at week 52, but other patients not meeting the primary outcome at week 16 may have had an IGA of 0/1 at week 52. No unexpected AEs were reported, with injection-site reactions and conjunctivitis again occurring more often in patients treated with dupilumab plus TCS versus those on placebo plus TCS. Long-term open extension studies continue to add to the safety profile of this biologic, most recently reporting 4 year safety data.[18] Other studies adding to the safety profile included a randomized, double-blinded, placebo-controlled study in adults with AD that showed that dupilumab did not adversely affect antibody responses to vaccines including Tdap and quadrivalent meningococcal polysaccharide.[19] In addition, a blinded, placebo-controlled trial demonstrated that patients treated with dupilumab had decreased *Staphylococcus aureus* colonization and increased microbial diversity that correlated with clinical improvement of AD and decrease in biomarkers of type 2 immunity.[20] Dupilumab received FDA approval in March 2017 for treatment of adult patients with moderate-to-severe AD whose disease is not adequately controlled with topical prescription therapies or when those therapies are not advisable.

Dupilumab in Adolescents and Children

A phase 3 randomized double-blind, parallel-group monotherapy trial was conducted in the United States and Canada in 251 adolescent patients aged 12 to 17 years with moderate-to-severe AD.[21] Patients were stratified by severity and body weight to 16-weeks of treatment with 1 of 4 regimens: dupilumab 400 mg loading dose, 200 mg every 2 weeks (q2w) (baseline weight <60 kg); dupilumab 600 mg loading dose, 300 mg q2w (baseline weight ≥60 kg); dupilumab 600 mg loading dose, 300 mg every 4 weeks (q4w); or placebo (all patients received injections q2w to maintain study blinding). A significantly higher proportion of patients treated with both dupilumab regimens achieved EASI-75 and IGA 0 or 1 at week 16 versus placebo-treated patients. Efficacy of the q2w regimen was generally superior to the q4w regimen. The incidence of conjunctivitis in the dupilumab-treated patients was similar to that seen in the adult AD trials. Self-reported comorbid type 2 diseases in this population included asthma (53.6%), food allergies (60.8%), and allergic rhinitis (65.6%). In a post-hoc subgroup analysis of patients whose IGA was >1 at week 16, 80.5% of the patients receiving dupilumab q2w versus 23.5% on placebo experienced clinically meaningful improvements in AD signs, symptoms, or quality of life at week 16.[22] Clinically meaningful improvement in 1 or more of 3 domains of signs, symptoms, and quality of life was defined as an improvement of ≥ 50% in EASI, ≥ 3 points in Peak Pruritus Numerical Rating Scale (PP NRS), or ≥ 6 points in the Children's Dermatology Life Quality Index(CDLQI) from baseline. These data, similar to the adult AD experience, point to the limitations of using IGA as a primary outcome in AD since it under-estimates overall benefit of dupilumab.[23]

Dupilumab with TCS was further studied in children 6 to 11 years with severe AD. In a double-blind phase 3 trial, 367 patients were randomized 1:1:1 to 300 mg dupilumab q4w, dupilumab q2w (100 mg q2w, baseline weight <30 kg; 200 mg q2w, baseline weight ≥30 kg), or placebo with concomitant medium-potency TCS.[24] At 16 weeks, both the q4w and q2w dupilumab plus TCS regimens resulted in clinically meaningful and statistically significant improvement in signs, symptoms, and quality of life versus placebo plus TCS in all prespecified endpoints. For q4w, q2w, and placebo, 32.8%, 29.5%, and 11.4% of the patients, respectively, achieved IGA scores of 0 or 1; 69.7%, 67.2%, and 26.8% achieved EASI-75; and 50.8%, 58.3%, and 12.3% achieved ≥4-point reduction in worst itch score. Optimal dupilumab doses for efficacy and safety were 300 mg q4w in children <30 kg and 200 mg q2w in children ≥30 kg. Conjunctivitis and injection-site reactions were more common with dupilumab plus TCS than with placebo plus TCS.

LIBERTY AD PRE-SCHOOL was a phase 2/3 trial of children aged 6 months to <6 years with moderate-to-severe AD. In the phase 2 trial, dupilumab pharmacokinetics and safety were evaluated in 40 patients with severe AD.[25] This included an initial cohort of children aged ≥2 to <6 years followed by a younger cohort aged ≥6 months to <2 years. Pharmacokinetic sampling, safety monitoring, and efficacy assessments were performed during the 4-week period after a single subcutaneous injection of dupilumab, in 2 sequential dosing groups (3 mg/kg, then 6 mg/kg). Treatment with low-to-medium potency TCS was allowed. Within each age cohort, pharmacokinetic exposures after a single injection of dupilumab increased in a greater than dose-proportional manner. At week 3, treatment with 3 and 6 mg/kg dupilumab reduced scores of mean EASI by 44.6% and 49.7% (older cohort) and 42.7% and 38.8% (younger cohort), and mean PP NRS scores by 22.9% and 44.7% (older cohort) and 11.1% and 18.2% (younger cohort), respectively. At week 4, improvements in most efficacy outcomes diminished in both age groups, particularly with the lower dose. The safety profile was comparable to that seen in adults, adolescents, and children. Single-dose dupilumab was generally well-tolerated and substantially reduced clinical signs/symptoms of AD. Slightly better responses were seen in older than younger children. The pharmacokinetics of dupilumab were non-linear, consistent with previous studies in adults and adolescents. In the phase 3 part of this trial, patients were randomly assigned to subcutaneous placebo or dupilumab (weight ≥5 kg to <15 kg: 200 mg; ≥15 kg to <30 kg: 300 mg) q4w plus low-potency TCS (hydrocortisone acetate 1% cream) for 16 weeks.[26] The primary endpoint at week 16 was the proportion of patients with an IGA 0 or 1 (clear or almost clear). The key secondary endpoint (coprimary endpoint for the European Union [EU] and EU reference market) at week 16 was the proportion of patients with EASI-75. A total of 162 patients were randomly assigned to receive dupilumab (n=83) or placebo (n=79) plus TCS. Baseline demographics showed that 77% of the children were severe (IGA 4, EASI 34, SCORAD 72). Self-reported atopic comorbidities included 68% food allergies, 44% allergic rhinitis, 41% asthma, and 4% allergic conjunctivitis. Of note, prior systemic therapy for AD included corticosteroids in 19%, cyclosporin A (CsA) 11%, methotrexate 7%, azathioprine 1%, and mycophenolate 1%. Eleven patients were under 2 years of age, and 6 of those patients were treated with dupilumab. At week 16, significantly more patients in the dupilumab group than in the placebo group had IGA 0 to 1 (23 [28%] versus 3 [4%], difference 24% [95% CI 13–34]; $P<0.0001$) and EASI-75 (44 [53%]versus 8 [11%], difference 42% [95% CI 29–55]; $P<0.0001$). Overall prevalence of AE was similar in the dupilumab group (53 [64%] of 83 patients) and placebo group (58 [74%] of 78 patients). Conjunctivitis incidence was higher in the dupilumab group (4 [5%]) than the placebo group (0). No dupilumab-related AEswere serious or led to treatment discontinuation.

Data on immunization with live viral vaccines in patients on dupilumab is lacking. A recent case series of live-attenuated vaccine administration (MMR ± varicella) in 9 dupilumab-treated children aged 8 to 56 months reported no AE.[27] Based on a systematic review of the literature, an expert Delphi Panel recently concluded that vaccines including live vaccines can be administered to patients receiving dupilumab in a shared decision-making capacity.[28]

Current Dupilumab Dosing in Atopic Dermatitis

Dupilumab is approved in the United States for patients aged ≥6 months with moderate-to-severe AD uncontrolled by topical prescription medicines or when those medications are not advised. The approved dosing regimen in adults 18 years and older is a 600 mg loading dose subcutaneously followed by 300 mg subcutaneously every 2 weeks. In patients 6 months to 5 years and 6 years to 17 years, dosing is weight based. See **Tables 1** and **2** for pediatric dosing. Dupilumab can be administered by pre-filled syringe for patients of any age or by pre-filled autoinjector pen for patients 2 years or older. It can be self-administered and does not require any baseline or interval laboratory tests.

There are limited data on treatment regimens other than q2w dosing. In a study, patients who stopped dupilumab treatment before re-starting open label therapy showed quick re-capture of disease control and no adverse events.[29] It may be reasonable, although off-label, to taper dupilumab to a less frequent dosing regimen in a patient who has been clear/almost clear for at least 6 to 12 months, while monitoring for relapse.[30] Data from an ongoing open label 5-year trial (NCT02612454) in pediatric patients may provide practical insights. Of note, AD patients with co-morbidities including asthma and rhinosinusitis appear to respond to treatment with dupilumab as well as those without these concomitant diseases.[31] Real world data suggest dupilumab continuation at 6 and 12 months was 91.9% and 77.3%, respectively.[32] A 2-year interim analysis of the ongoing PROSE 5 year prospective observational study of patients 12 years and older found sustained disease control in patients with moderate-to-severe AD.[33] Additional real world data from registries will continue to yield valuable practical information. Also, studies in young children whose immune profile has been shown to be different from older patients may determine if early treatment with this biologic can be disease modifying.

AD patients starting treatment with dupilumab with a history of any preceding ocular signs or symptoms should be educated on recognizing early signs of ocular surface disease, which may include sensation of dryness or grittiness.[30] This can usually be adequately treated with lubricating tears while continuing on dupilumab. A comprehensive approach to ocular surface disease has been reviewed.[34] For some patients, reducing the frequency of injections has allowed for maintaining control of the skin disease while minimizing ocular surface disease symptoms. In addition, other AEs that have been reported with dupilumab post approval include facial redness that may be previously unrecognized allergic contact dermatitis, *Malassezia* yeast hypersensitivity, rosacea, or psoriasis.[30] Joint symptoms have also been described with increased activity of IL-17 in the face of blocked IL-4 as an explanation.[35]

Table 1
Dosing regimen for dupilumab in children 6 months to 5 Years

Weight	Initial Loading Dose	Maintenance Dose
5 to <15 kg	No loading dose	200 mg every 4 wks
15 to <30 kg	No loading dose	300 mg every 4 wks

Table 2
Dosing regimen for dupilumab in children 6 years to 17 years

Weight	Initial Loading Dose	Maintenance Dose
15 to <30 kg	600 mg	300 mg every 4 wks
30 to <60 kg	400 mg	200 mg every 2 wks
≥60 kg	600 mg	300 mg every 2 wks

Tralokinumab

Tralokinumab is a selective IL-13 inhibitor that has undergone clinical trials in AD. Tralokinumab was approved for use in moderate-to-severe AD in adults by the Food and Drug Administration (FDA) on December 28, 2021. Tralokinumab is a human IgG4 mAb binding to an epitope which overlaps with IL-13Rα1 and IL-13Rα2 thereby preventing IL-13 from binding and exerting its biological effects (see **Fig. 1**).[36,37] In double-blinded placebo- controlled phase 3 clinical trials of adults with moderate-to-severe AD (ECZTRA 1 and ECZTRA 2), tralokinumab met primary endpoints of IGA score of 0 or 1 and ≥75% improvement in EASI (EASI-75) at week 16.[38] Patients were initially given a 600 mg loading dose followed by 300 mg of tralokinumab or placebo every 2 weeks for 16 weeks. Patients were instructed to use emollients but not TCS. Patients requiring rescue TCS were considered non-responders. Patients treated with tralokinumab and meeting primary endpoints were then re-randomized to either every 2-week dosing of tralokinumab, every 4 week dosing, or placebo for a 36-week maintenance period. Of note, at week 52, over 50% of patients receiving tralokinumab every 2 weeks maintained eczema control without the need for rescue topical medication. Furthermore, between 21% and 47% of patients re-randomized to control after 16 weeks of receiving tralokinumab maintained response without need for rescue treatment at 52 weeks, thus suggesting the possibility of induction of disease remission for these patients. In these studies, tralokinumab was reported to be well-tolerated with similar AE frequency and severity as placebo except for conjunctivitis, which was seen in a greater frequency in the treatment group. However, conjunctivitis remained overall infrequent with <10% of the patients in the initial treatment group reporting it and <9% of the patients reporting it in the maintenance group. Most cases were mild and self-limiting, although 1 case led to discontinuation of the biologic. In an attempt to more closely simulate clinical practice, another phase 3 trial (ECZTRA 3) was performed in adults with moderate-to-severe AD.[39] This study had a similar design to ECZTRA 1 and ECZTRA 2; however, patients were instructed to use TCS, and the maintenance treatment period occurred over 16 weeks without a placebo control group. At week 16, primary endpoints were met in significantly greater proportion of patients treated with tralokinumab as compared to controls. This effect was maintained during the next 16 weeks of the study in both the every 2 week and every 4 week tralokinumab-treated cohorts.

Tralokinumab has also been studied in adolescents aged 12 to 17 years with moderate-to-severe AD in the phase 3 placebo-controlled ECZTRA 6 trial.[40] Primary endpoints in this study including IGA score 0 or 1 and EASI-75 without rescue were also met at week 16 in a greater proportion of tralokinumab-treated patients (either tralokinumab 150 mg or 300 mg every other week) as compared with controls. In this age group, the drug was noted to be well tolerated with a majority of AE in the mild-to-moderate range. The most common AE reported were upper respiratory infection, AD exacerbation, injection-site reaction, asthma, and headache. Of note, conjunctivitis was infrequently reported with occurrence in only 2 patients in the treatment arm. On December 15th 2023, the FDA expanded tralokinumab's approval to include children aged 12 to 17 with moderate-to-severe AD.

Although data regarding vaccine response to live vaccinations among tralokinumab-treated patients are lacking, there is evidence that the drug does not appear to negatively impact response to other vaccinations including tetanus, diphtheria, pertussis vaccine (Tdap) and meningococcal vaccines.[41]

In summary of earlier-mentioned clinical trials evaluating tralokinumab, the biologic has shown consistent therapeutic benefits with improvement in eczema control measures (IGA and EASI) over 16 weeks in adolescents and adults with moderate-to-severe AD. Sustained benefits of treatment were noted with extension trials up to 52 weeks. Conjunctivitis was noted as a side effect, although reported to be relatively infrequent and often of mild severity. In a systematic analysis of 5 placebo-controlled phase 2/3 trials of tralokinumab, conjunctivitis was noted to be more frequently observed in patients treated with tralokinumab as compared to controls (7.5% incidence in tralokinumab as compared to 3.2% in placebo).[42] Most events were described as mild-to-moderate, and only 2 patients had to discontinue tralokinumab because of conjunctivitis.

Current Tralokinumab Dosing in Atopic Dermatitis

The current recommended dosing for tralokinumab in patients 18 years and older is 600 mg for an initial loading dose followed by 300 mg every other week. In addition, for patients 18 and older, there is an option of switching to every 4 week dosing of 300 mg after 16 weeks in patients who are under 100 kg and achieving clear or almost clear skin. The pediatric dosing for patients 12 to 17 years of age includes a 300 mg initial loading dose followed by 150 mg every other week. Tralokinumab is administered subcutaneously via a 150 mg/mL pre-filled syringe. Similar to dupilumab, tralokinumab may be administered at home and no pre-treatment or monitoring laboratory studies are required. It is recommended that all age-appropriate vaccines are administered prior to initiation of tralokinumab, and live vaccines are to be avoided during treatment with tralokinumab. As noted above, common AEs in clinical studies included upper respiratory infections, conjunctivitis, and injection site reactions.[38–40] Eosinophilia was also reported in these studies although the overall safety profile of patients with eosinophilia was not different from the total cohort safety profile.

BIOLOGICS IN LATE STAGES OF DEVELOPMENT
Lebrikizumab

Lebrikizumab is another biologic specifically targeting IL-13. It is a high-affinity IgG4 mAb which binds soluble IL-13 and prevents its downstream signaling by preventing the heterodimerization of IL4Rα/IL-13-Rα1.[43] Two recent phase 3 randomized placebo-controlled trials (Advocate1 and Advocate2) were completed in adolescents and adults with moderate-to-severe eczema. Patients treated with lebrikizumab met the primary outcome of IGA score of 0 or 1 with a greater than 2-point decrease in IGA score at a significantly improved rate as compared with controls at week 16.[44] The trials consisted of an induction period in which patients were given either a placebo or a loading dose of 500 mg at baseline and week 2 and then 250 mg every 2 weeks. At 16 weeks, patients with a noted response to lebrikizumab were subsequently randomized to receive lebrikizumab every 2 weeks, every 4 weeks, or placebo for additional 36 weeks. Those patients without a response were given open label lebrikizumab every 2 weeks. Of note, patients were prohibited from applying any topical treatments.

In trial 1, 43.1% of the patients in the treatment group met primary outcome as compared with 12.7% of controls (*P*<.001). In trial 2, 33.2% of the treatment group met primary outcome as compared with 10.8% in controls (*P*<.001). Secondary endpoints including EASI-75 and EASI-90 response rates were also noted in higher proportions of the lebrikizumab-treated patients compared with controls at week 16. Significant reduction in itch scores (Pruritus NRS) and the Sleep-Loss Scale was also noted in the treatment groups as compared with controls. The most significant AE seen at a higher rate in lebrikizumab-treated patients as compared with controls was conjunctivitis (7.4% of treatment group vs 2.8% of controls in the first trial and 7.5% vs 2.1% in the second trial). Overall, AE were mild and did not lead to discontinuation of the medication. AD exacerbation was seen at a lower frequency in lebrikizumab-treated patients as compared with controls. Of note, these AEs were noted at the end of the 16-week induction period. Results from the maintenance period of this study have yet to be published and a longer term extension study (ADjoin; NCT04392154) is currently ongoing.

Another recent phase 3 clinical trial called the ADhere trial enrolled patients in Europe and North America with moderate-to-severe AD to receive lebrikizumab in combination with TCS[45] Patients were randomized to receive lebrikizumab every 2 weeks with an initial loading dose of 500 mg followed by 250 mg every 2 weeks thereafter in combination with topical steroids or placebo in combination with topical corticosteroids. A total of 211 patients were recruited. Primary endpoints including IGA score of 0 or 1 and a 2-point reduction from baseline was achieved in 41.2% of those receiving lebrikizumab with topical corticosteroids as compared to 22.1% in those receiving placebo and topical corticosteroids (*P*=.01). A significantly greater percentage of patients receiving lebrikizumab achieved EASI-75 (69.5% vs 42.2%, *P*<.001). In terms of safety, there were severe treatment emergent adverse events (TEAEs) in less than 2% of controls and lebrikizumab-treated patients. Conjunctivitis, headache, herpes infection, hypertension, and injection site reactions were reported more frequently in lebrikizumab-treated patients as compared with controls.

Although tralokinumab and lebrikizumab both target the same cytokine (IL-13), a subtle distinction in their mechanism of action may have therapeutic implications. Tralokinumab blocks signaling through both IL-13Rα1 and IL-13Rα2, whereas lebrikizumab does not affect binding of IL-13 to IL-13Rα2. IL-13 Rα2 is a decoy receptor and may further mitigate the effects of IL-13.[46] Perhaps this biological mechanism may allow lebrikizumab to allow for further inhibition of IL-13-mediated disease, although this remains theoretic at present moment. In November 2023, lebrikizumab was approved in the European Union for the treatment of moderate-to-severe AD in adults and adolescents 12 years and older with a body weight of at least 40 kg who are candidates for systemic therapy.It was subsequently approved in the United Kingdom in December 2023 and in Japan in January 2024 for the same indication.

Nemolizumab

Another cytokine as a target for biologics in the treatment of AD is IL-31. Evidence in humans and mouse models supports the role of IL-31 in itch in AD patients. Injecting IL-31 into mice increased itching, which was mitigated by an anti-IL-31 antibody.[47] In human studies, the IL-31A receptor was found to be upregulated in AD patients versus controls and cutaneous lymphoid antigen-staining T cells of AD patients had higher IL-31 mRNA expression.[48]

Nemolizumab is a humanized mAb targeting IL-31 receptor A and is currently under investigation. A phase 1 study found a significant difference in visual analog scale

(VAS) for pruritus in patients treated with a single dose of nemolizumab as compared with controls.[49] This study enrolled both healthy individuals and AD patients with moderate or greater severity despite use of TCS. Overall, this study found nemolizumab was well tolerated by both healthy individuals and AD patients with only mild and self-limiting AE. In AD patients, the most common AE was exacerbation of AD. AD patients had a decrease in pruritus VAS noted at 1 week post-biologic which persisted through 8 weeks of the study period. Sleep efficiency was also improved in AD patients receiving the drug as compared with controls.

Phase 2 trials of patients with moderate-to-severe AD similarly found improved pruritus VAS scores as compared to controls. Ruzicka and colleagues[50] performed a double-blinded placebo-controlled trial of 264 moderate to severe AD patients treated with nemolizumab 0.1 mg/kg, 0.5 mg/kg, or 2 mg/kg or placebo every 4 weeks or 2 mg/kg every 8 weeks. Patients were allowed to use topical emollients. Patients without significant improvement or with eczema on examination were given TCS as rescue therapy. Primary endpoints of percentage improvement in VAS at week 12 were met for all doses studied and were reported as significantly different in those receiving nemolizumab as compared with controls. Secondary endpoints including changes in EASI score from baseline and change in body surface area affected by AD were decreased in nemolizumab-treated patients. Of note, 18% of the study participants dropped out of the study before completion with 14 of these patients discontinuing due to AE. The most common AE was exacerbation of AD, and peripheral edema was another AE in patients receiving the drug as compared to placebo.

Another 24-week phase 2b placebo-controlled double-blinded study of nemolizumab in moderate-to-severe AD patients was conducted in North America, Europe, and Australia.[51] The primary endpoint was percent change from baseline EASI score at week 24. A total of 226 patients were recruited and received a loading dose of 20, 60, or 90 mg on day 1 followed by 10, 30, or 90 mg every 4 weeks. Patients were continued on low or mid potency TCS. At week 24, all treatment doses showed greater improvement in EASI score as compared with placebo controls. The 30 mg nemolizumab dose appeared to have the strongest effect (-68.8% vs -52.1%, least-square mean reduction for placebo; $P=.016$). Increased proportions of patients achieving EASI-50, EASI-75, and EASI-90 were seen in the nemolizumab cohorts versus placebo controls. A significant and early change in average daily PP NRS scores was noted as early as week 1 for all 3 doses of nemolizumab compared to controls. In terms of safety, overall similar numbers of TEAEs were noted in controls and nemolizumab cohorts. Some of the most common TEAEs included nasopharyngitis seen in 21.4% of controls and 26.6% of treatment groups and AD exacerbations which were seen in 16.1% of controls and 10.1% of those treated with nemolizumab. Of note, asthma events were seen at a higher rate in the treatment arm, with 11.2% of the patients experiencing this event as compared with 1.8% of the controls.

In a long-term extension study, the effects of nemolizumab persisted to 64 weeks.[52] No new safety concerns were identified in the study. The most common AEs were nasopharyngitis, exacerbation of AD, and increased blood creatine phosphokinase. In a double-blinded placebo-controlled phase 3 trial of patients in Japan, investigators found a significant difference in VAS for pruritus in those receiving 60 mg of nemolizumab versus control.[53] Patients recruited to this study had shown suboptimal control of their AD-associated pruritus while on medium potency TCS or calcineurin inhibitors, which were continued throughout the study. Overall, at week 16, a -42.8% change in VAS score was noted in nemolizumab-treated patients as compared to a -21.4% change in placebo controls ($P<.001$). Although secondary endpoints including percent change in EASI score and percent change in DLQI score suggested differences in treatment versus control groups, no clinical inferences were made due to the lack of adjustments for multiple comparisons. Subsequently, 2 long-term phase 3 studies were completed evaluating efficacy of nemolizumab 60 mg every 4 weeks in a 52-week open label long-term extension studies.[54] Patients in these studies continued TCS or topical calcineurin inhibitors. These studies reported improvement in VAS scores and EASI scores in patients receiving nemolizumab. TEAEs were reported to be predominantly of mild severity. The most common TEAEs included nasopharyngitis and AD. Of note, these studies did not provide a control group as they were open label long-term extensions studies.

In summary of the clinical trials outlined earlier, nemolizumab has been shown to decrease pruritus with a tolerable AE profile in patients treated with TCS or calcineurin inhibitors. Thus, nemolizumab's role in future therapeutic regimens may be as an adjunctive agent to control pruritus in those on other maintenance therapies. Nemolizumab was approved in Japan in March 2022 for use in adults and children over the age of 13 years for the treatment of itch associated with AD, though only when existing treatment is insufficiently effective.

BIOLOGICS TARGETING OX40/OX40 LIGAND

Another target of biologics under investigation for AD patients has been the OX40/OX40 ligand interaction. OX40 ligand is upregulated on antigen-presenting cells and its binding to OX40 promotes Th2 inflammation.[55] The involvement in the OX40/OX40 ligand interaction in Th2 inflammation was demonstrated by use of an OX40 ligand inhibitor which decreased production of Th2 cytokines.[56] This in vitro finding was supported by the clinical finding that AD patients have increased numbers of OX40 ligand–expressing dendritic cells and increases in OX40 expression in skin.[57]

A human anti-OX40 mAb (KHK4083) has been developed and through antibody-dependent cellular cytotoxicity depletes activated T cells. A phase 1 study in Japan assessed the safety profile of this biologic in moderate-to-severe AD patients.[58] Twenty-two patients were recruited into the open label study which reported no serious AE. Most prevalent AEs were pyrexia and chills. Improvements in clinical scores including EASI and IGA were sustained through week 22, 18 weeks after the last injection.

A phase 2a study of the humanized mAb against OX40 (GBR830) found greater improvement in EASI scores in treatment groups as compared to control.[59] This study also found sustained improvement in EASI scores after discontinuation of the drug. Skin biopsies from patients treated with GBR830 showed reductions in baseline epidermal thickness and downregulation of both Th1 and Th2 biomarkers. The most common AE was headache, which was not significantly different in the control versus treatment group. There was 1 severe TEAE (coronary artery occlusion), which was determined not to be due to the drug given pre-existing comorbid risk factors.

More recently, a double-blinded placebo-controlled phase 2b study was conducted at multiple sites enrolling 274 patients with moderate-to-severe AD to receive subcutaneous rocatinlimab (KHK4083/AMG451) at different doses and frequencies versus placebo.[60] This study found reductions in EASI scores in all rocatinlimab groups. Treatment was reported to be well tolerated with most common AE including pyrexia, nasopharyngitis, chills, and headache. Several studies accessing rocatinlimab in AD are currently registered on Clinicaltrials.gov.

Another biologic targeting OX40/OX40 L is the anti-OX40 L mAb KY1005 (amlitelimab). This biologic has undergone a phase 1 trial in 64 healthy subjects, with no serious AE observed.[61] One suspected pseudoallergy response was noted during the study. In addition to generating pharmacokinetic data, amlitelimab was found to mitigate cutaneous blood perfusion changes and erythema of keyhole limpet hemocyanin administration, demonstrating potential as an immunomodulatory agent. A phase 2a trial of 89 patients with moderate-to-severe AD found that amlitelimab was generally well tolerated without significant AE and led to clinically significant changes in EASI scores after 16 weeks as compared to placebo.[62] In summary of the studies assessing anti-OX40/OX-40L antibodies, while these biologics appear to have promising efficacy and safety profiles, more robust phase 3 clinical trials are needed to further evaluate the efficacy and safety of these drugs as well as long-term extension studies to determine if the effect and safety are maintained over time.

Choice of Biologic in the Clinical Setting

Although there have been robust clinic trial data supporting the use of biologics in patients with moderate-to-severe AD, there have been relatively few publications outlining methods for choice of biologics for individual patients. There is a lack of head-to-head trials of individual biologics and thus there is limited knowledge of which biologic may be most effective for specific patients. Currently, dupilumab and tralokinumab are the 2 biologics that are FDA approved for AD. However, it is likely that several of the earlier-mentioned biologics may be approved in the near future. Currently, practitioners may consider comorbid indications of dupilumab including asthma, chronic rhinosinusitis with nasal polyposis, and eosinophilic esophagitis when chosing a biologic. Age may also play a role as dupilumab is currently the only biologic approved in pediatric patients under 12 years of age and is now approved down to 6 months of age. A recent systematic review and meta-analysis of 149 clinical trials in patients with moderate-to-severe AD found that in 5 of 6 clinical outcomes, the oral Janus kinase inhibitor upadacitinib was most effective; however, this medication was also noted to have the highest AE profile.[63] Biologics including dupilumab, tralokinumab, and lebrikizumab were noted to be of intermediate efficacy, however, all 3 were reported to have a lower AE profile.

A challenge for future treatment of AD is to identify which patients may respond best to specific biologics in terms of both efficacy and AE. Currently, case reports or case series present clinical descriptions of differential responses.[64] In the future, data gleaned from endotyping AD patients (eg, the National Institute of Health [NIH] Longitudinal Endotyping of Atopic Dermatitis Through Transcriptomic Skin Analysis) may provide directions for a "personalized medicine" approach.

CURRENT GUIDELINES

The recent 2023 Joint Task Force AD Guidelines include recommendations derived from a systematic review and meta-analysis of systemic therapies.[63] In patients with moderate-to-severe disease refractory to mid to high potency topical agents, the panel recommended adding dupilumab or tralokinumab. Strength of recommendation was strong in favor of both of these biologics based on high certainty evidence.[65] In addition, updated guidelines from the AAD for management of AD in adults also endorse use of currently approved biologics for adults with moderate-to-severe AD.[66]

SUMMARY

AD is a common chronic inflammatory skin disease of children, as well as adults. While the pathophysiology is complex, immune dysregulation primarily of the type 2 axis remains central to the disease. The association of AD with atopic co-morbidities such as asthma suggests the possibility not only of targeting multiple diseases with 1 biologic, but possibly interrupting the march from AD to asthma and allergic disorders. Currently, dupilumab, a fully human monoclonal antibody targeting the IL-4 Rα subunit and tralokinumab, targeting IL-13 has been approved for treatment of patients with moderate-to-severe AD whose disease is not adequately controlled with topical prescription therapies or when those therapies are not advisable. Dupilumab is approved down to 6 months of age, while tralokinumab is approved for patients 12 years and older. Other biologics in late stage of development for AD include lebrikizumab directed at IL-13 and nemolizumab targeting the IL-31 receptor A. Long-term safety and efficacy trials, head-to-head comparative trials, and real world experience will help answer a number of clinically relevant questions regarding optimal treatment regimens with these biologics. Trials of early intervention in younger patients could address the potential for disease-modifying effects. In addition, advances in our understanding of disease mechanisms may lead to identification of unique endophenotypes that could allow clinicians to identify which patients would be the best candidates for specific therapies as we evolve toward a personalized approach to treatment of AD.

CLINICS CARE POINTS

- Per recent 2023 Joint Task Force AD Guidelines, dupilumab or tralokinumab is recommended for patients with moderate-to-severe disease refractory to high-potency topical agents
- Dupilumab has additional indications for several other atopic diseases, including asthma
- Conjunctivitis is a common adverse effect of dupilumab and tralokinumab seen in atopic dermatitis patients; however, it is often of mild severity and in most cases can be managed with lubricating eye drops while continuing on the biologic

DISCLOSURE

M. Nevid has no conflicts to disclose. M. Boguniewicz has been involved in clinical research for Regeneron and Sanofi-Genzyme and served as a consultant for Amgen, Eli Lilly, LEO Pharma, Regeneron, and Sanofi-Genzyme.

REFERENCES

1. Boguniewicz M, Leung DY. Targeted therapy for allergic diseases: at the intersection of cutting-edge science and clinical practice. J Allergy Clin Immunol 2015; 135(2):354–6. https://doi.org/10.1016/j.jaci.2014.12.1907.
2. Boguniewicz M. Biologics for atopic dermatitis. Immunol Allergy Clin North Am 2020;40(4):593–607. https://doi.org/10.1016/j.iac.2020.06.004.
3. Simpson EL, Bieber T, Eckert L, et al. Patient burden of moderate to severe atopic dermatitis (AD): Insights from a phase 2b clinical trial of dupilumab in adults. J Am Acad Dermatol 2016;74(3):491–8. https://doi.org/10.1016/j.jaad.2015.10.043.
4. Drucker AM, Wang AR, Li WQ, et al. The Burden of Atopic Dermatitis: Summary of a Report for the National Eczema Association. J Invest Dermatol 2017;137(1): 26–30. https://doi.org/10.1016/j.jid.2016.07.012.
5. Boguniewicz M, Leung DY. Atopic dermatitis: a disease of altered skin barrier and immune dysregulation. Research Support, N.I.H., Extramural Review. Immunol Rev 2011;242(1):233–46. https://doi.org/10.1111/j.1600-065X.2011.01027.x.

6. Hamid Q, Boguniewicz M, Leung DY. Differential in situ cytokine gene expression in acute versus chronic atopic dermatitis. J Clin Invest 1994;94(2):870–6. https://doi.org/10.1172/JCI117408.

7. Hamid Q, Naseer T, Minshall EM, et al. In vivo expression of IL-12 and IL-13 in atopic dermatitis. J Allergy Clin Immunol 1996;98(1):225–31. https://doi.org/10.1016/s0091-6749(96)70246-4.

8. Gittler JK, Shemer A, Suarez-Farinas M, et al. Progressive activation of T(H)2/T(H)22 cytokines and selective epidermal proteins characterizes acute and chronic atopic dermatitis. J Allergy Clin Immunol 2012;130(6):1344–54. https://doi.org/10.1016/j.jaci.2012.07.012.

9. Suarez-Farinas M, Tintle SJ, Shemer A, et al. Nonlesional atopic dermatitis skin is characterized by broad terminal differentiation defects and variable immune abnormalities. J Allergy Clin Immunol 2011;127(4):954–64. https://doi.org/10.1016/j.jaci.2010.12.1124, e1-4.

10. Brunner PM, Silverberg JI, Guttman-Yassky E, et al. Increasing comorbidities suggest that atopic dermatitis is a systemic disorder. J Invest Dermatol 2017;137(1):18–25. https://doi.org/10.1016/j.jid.2016.08.022.

11. Gandhi NA, Bennett BL, Graham NM, et al. Targeting key proximal drivers of type 2 inflammation in disease. Nat Rev Drug Discov 2016;15(1):35–50. https://doi.org/10.1038/nrd4624.

12. Gandhi NA, Pirozzi G, Graham NMH. Commonality of the IL-4/IL-13 pathway in atopic diseases. Expert Rev Clin Immunol 2017;13(5):425–37. https://doi.org/10.1080/1744666X.2017.1298443.

13. Schneider L, Hanifin J, Boguniewicz M, et al. Study of the atopic march: development of atopic comorbidities. Pediatr Dermatol 2016;33(4):388–98. https://doi.org/10.1111/pde.12867.

14. Davidson WF, Leung DYM, Beck LA, et al. Report from the National Institute of Allergy and Infectious Diseases workshop on "Atopic dermatitis and the atopic march: Mechanisms and interventions". J Allergy Clin Immunol 2019;143(3):894–913. https://doi.org/10.1016/j.jaci.2019.01.003.

15. Geba GP, Li D, Xu M, et al. Attenuating the atopic march: Meta-analysis of the dupilumab atopic dermatitis database for incident allergic events. J Allergy Clin Immunol 2023;151(3):756–66. https://doi.org/10.1016/j.jaci.2022.08.026.

16. Simpson EL, Bieber T, Guttman-Yassky E, et al. Two phase 3 trials of dupilumab versus placebo in atopic dermatitis. N Engl J Med 2016;375(24):2335–48. https://doi.org/10.1056/NEJMoa1610020.

17. Blauvelt A, de Bruin-Weller M, Gooderham M, et al. Long-term management of moderate-to-severe atopic dermatitis with dupilumab and concomitant topical corticosteroids (LIBERTY AD CHRONOS): a 1-year, randomised, double-blinded, placebo-controlled, phase 3 trial. Lancet 2017;389(10086):2287–303. https://doi.org/10.1016/s0140-6736(17)31191-1.

18. Beck LA, Deleuran M, Bissonnette R, et al. Dupilumab provides acceptable safety and sustained efficacy for up to 4 years in an open-label study of adults with moderate-to-severe atopic dermatitis. Am J Clin Dermatol 2022;23(3):393–408. https://doi.org/10.1007/s40257-022-00685-0.

19. Blauvelt A, Simpson EL, Tyring SK, et al. Dupilumab does not affect correlates of vaccine-induced immunity: A randomized, placebo-controlled trial in adults with moderate-to-severe atopic dermatitis. J Am Acad Dermatol 2019;80(1):158–167 e1. https://doi.org/10.1016/j.jaad.2018.07.048.

20. Callewaert C, Nakatsuji T, Knight R, et al. IL-4Ralpha blockade by dupilumab decreases staphylococcus aureus colonization and increases microbial diversity in

atopic dermatitis. J Invest Dermatol 2020;140(1):191–202 e7. https://doi.org/10.1016/j.jid.2019.05.024.

21. Simpson EL, Paller AS, Siegfried EC, et al. Efficacy and safety of dupilumab in adolescents with uncontrolled moderate to severe atopic dermatitis: a phase 3 randomized clinical trial. JAMA Dermatol 2020;156(1):44–56. https://doi.org/10.1001/jamadermatol.2019.3336.

22. Paller AS, Bansal A, Simpson EL, et al. Clinically meaningful responses to dupilumab in adolescents with uncontrolled moderate-to-severe atopic dermatitis: post-hoc analyses from a randomized clinical trial. Am J Clin Dermatol 2020; 21(1):119–31. https://doi.org/10.1007/s40257-019-00478-y.

23. Silverberg JI, Simpson EL, Ardeleanu M, et al. Dupilumab provides important clinical benefits to patients with atopic dermatitis who do not achieve clear or almost clear skin according to the Investigator's Global Assessment: a pooled analysis of data from two phase III trials. Br J Dermatol 2019;181(1):80–7. https://doi.org/10.1111/bjd.17791.

24. Paller AS, Siegfried EC, Thaci D, et al. Efficacy and safety of dupilumab with concomitant topical corticosteroids in children 6 to 11 years old with severe atopic dermatitis: A randomized, double-blinded, placebo-controlled phase 3 trial. J Am Acad Dermatol 2020;83(5):1282–93. https://doi.org/10.1016/j.jaad.2020.06.054.

25. Paller AS, Siegfried EC, Simpson EL, et al. A phase 2, open-label study of single-dose dupilumab in children aged 6 months to <6 years with severe uncontrolled atopic dermatitis: pharmacokinetics, safety and efficacy. J Eur Acad Dermatol Venereol : JEADV 2021;35(2):464–75. https://doi.org/10.1111/jdv.16928.

26. Paller AS, Simpson EL, Siegfried EC, et al. Dupilumab in children aged 6 months to younger than 6 years with uncontrolled atopic dermatitis: a randomised, double-blind, placebo-controlled, phase 3 trial. Lancet 2022;400(10356): 908–19. https://doi.org/10.1016/S0140-6736(22)01539-2.

27. Siegfried EC, Wine Lee L, Spergel JM, et al. A case series of live attenuated vaccine administration in dupilumab-treated children with atopic dermatitis. Pediatr Dermatol 2024;41(2):204–9. https://doi.org/10.1111/pde.15518.

28. Lieberman JA, Chu DK, Ahmed T, et al. A systematic review and expert Delphi Consensus recommendation on the use of vaccines in patients receiving dupilumab: a position paper of the American College of Allergy, Asthma and Immunology. Ann Allergy Asthma Immunol 2024. https://doi.org/10.1016/j.anai.2024.05.014.

29. Deleuran M, Thaci D, Beck LA, et al. Dupilumab shows long-term safety and efficacy in patients with moderate to severe atopic dermatitis enrolled in a phase 3 open-label extension study. J Am Acad Dermatol 2020;82(2):377–88. https://doi.org/10.1016/j.jaad.2019.07.074.

30. Boguniewicz M, Fonacier L, Guttman-Yassky E, et al. Atopic dermatitis yardstick update. Ann Allergy Asthma Immunol 2023;130(6):811–20. https://doi.org/10.1016/j.anai.2023.03.010.

31. Boguniewicz M, Beck LA, Sher L, et al. Dupilumab improves asthma and sinonasal outcomes in adults with moderate to severe atopic dermatitis. J Allergy Clin Immunol Pract 2021;9(3):1212–1223 e6. https://doi.org/10.1016/j.jaip.2020.12.059.

32. Silverberg JI, Guttman-Yassky E, Gadkari A, et al. Real-world persistence with dupilumab among adults with atopic dermatitis. Ann Allergy Asthma Immunol 2021;126(1):40–5. https://doi.org/10.1016/j.anai.2020.07.026.

33. Simpson EL, Lockshin B, Lee LW, et al. Real-world effectiveness of dupilumab in adult and adolescent patients with atopic dermatitis: 2-year interim data from the PROSE registry. Dermatol Ther (Heidelb) 2024;14(1):261–70. https://doi.org/10.1007/s13555-023-01061-4.

34. Wu D, Daniel BS, Lai AJX, et al. Dupilumab-associated ocular manifestations: A review of clinical presentations and management. Surv Ophthalmol 2022;67(5):1419–42. https://doi.org/10.1016/j.survophthal.2022.02.002.

35. Woodbury MJ, Smith JS, Merola JF. Dupilumab-associated arthritis: a dermatology-rheumatology perspective. Am J Clin Dermatol 2023;24(6):859–64. https://doi.org/10.1007/s40257-023-00804-5.

36. Popovic B, Breed J, Rees DG, et al. Structural characterisation reveals mechanism of IL-13-neutralising monoclonal antibody tralokinumab as inhibition of binding to IL-13Ralpha1 and IL-13Ralpha2. J Mol Biol 2017;429(2):208–19. https://doi.org/10.1016/j.jmb.2016.12.005.

37. Simpson EL, Guttman-Yassky E, Eichenfield LF, et al. Tralokinumab therapy for moderate-to-severe atopic dermatitis: Clinical outcomes with targeted IL-13 inhibition. Allergy 2023;78(11):2875–91. https://doi.org/10.1111/all.15811.

38. Wollenberg A, Blauvelt A, Guttman-Yassky E, et al. Tralokinumab for moderate-to-severe atopic dermatitis: results from two 52-week, randomized, double-blind, multicentre, placebo-controlled phase III trials (ECZTRA 1 and ECZTRA 2). Br J Dermatol 2021;184(3):437–49. https://doi.org/10.1111/bjd.19574.

39. Silverberg JI, Toth D, Bieber T, et al. Tralokinumab plus topical corticosteroids for the treatment of moderate-to-severe atopic dermatitis: results from the double-blind, randomized, multicentre, placebo-controlled phase III ECZTRA 3 trial. Br J Dermatol 2021;184(3):450–63. https://doi.org/10.1111/bjd.19573.

40. Paller AS, Flohr C, Cork M, et al. Efficacy and safety of tralokinumab in adolescents with moderate to severe atopic dermatitis: the phase 3 ECZTRA 6 randomized clinical trial. JAMA Dermatol 2023;159(6):596–605. https://doi.org/10.1001/jamadermatol.2023.0627.

41. Merola JF, Bagel J, Almgren P, et al. Tralokinumab does not impact vaccine-induced immune responses: Results from a 30-week, randomized, placebo-controlled trial in adults with moderate-to-severe atopic dermatitis. J Am Acad Dermatol 2021;85(1):71–8. https://doi.org/10.1016/j.jaad.2021.03.032.

42. Wollenberg A, Beck LA, de Bruin Weller M, et al. Conjunctivitis in adult patients with moderate-to-severe atopic dermatitis: results from five tralokinumab clinical trials. Br J Dermatol 2022;186(3):453–65. https://doi.org/10.1111/bjd.20810.

43. Ultsch M, Bevers J, Nakamura G, et al. Structural basis of signaling blockade by anti-IL-13 antibody Lebrikizumab. J Mol Biol 2013;425(8):1330–9. https://doi.org/10.1016/j.jmb.2013.01.024.

44. Silverberg JI, Guttman-Yassky E, Thaci D, et al. Two phase 3 trials of lebrikizumab for moderate-to-severe atopic dermatitis. N Engl J Med 2023;388(12):1080–91. https://doi.org/10.1056/NEJMoa2206714.

45. Simpson EL, Gooderham M, Wollenberg A, et al. Efficacy and safety of lebrikizumab in combination with topical corticosteroids in adolescents and adults with moderate-to-severe atopic dermatitis: a randomized clinical trial (ADhere). JAMA Dermatol 2023;159(2):182–91. https://doi.org/10.1001/jamadermatol.2022.5534.

46. Bernardo D, Bieber T, Torres T. Lebrikizumab for the treatment of moderate-to-severe atopic dermatitis. Am J Clin Dermatol 2023;24(5):753–64. https://doi.org/10.1007/s40257-023-00793-5.

47. Kasutani K, Fujii E, Ohyama S, et al. Anti-IL-31 receptor antibody is shown to be a potential therapeutic option for treating itch and dermatitis in mice. Br J Pharmacol 2014;171(22):5049–58. https://doi.org/10.1111/bph.12823.

48. Bilsborough J, Leung DY, Maurer M, et al. IL-31 is associated with cutaneous lymphocyte antigen-positive skin homing T cells in patients with atopic dermatitis. J Allergy Clin Immunol 2006;117(2):418–25. https://doi.org/10.1016/j.jaci.2005. 10.046.

49. Nemoto O, Furue M, Nakagawa H, et al. The first trial of CIM331, a humanized antihuman interleukin-31 receptor A antibody, in healthy volunteers and patients with atopic dermatitis to evaluate safety, tolerability and pharmacokinetics of a single dose in a randomized, double-blind, placebo-controlled study. Br J Dermatol 2016;174(2):296–304. https://doi.org/10.1111/bjd.14207.

50. Ruzicka T, Mihara R. Anti-interleukin-31 receptor a antibody for atopic dermatitis. N Engl J Med 2017;376(21):2093. https://doi.org/10.1056/NEJMc1704013.

51. Silverberg JI, Pinter A, Pulka G, et al. Phase 2B randomized study of nemolizumab in adults with moderate-to-severe atopic dermatitis and severe pruritus. J Allergy Clin Immunol 2020;145(1):173–82. https://doi.org/10.1016/j.jaci.2019. 08.013.

52. Kabashima K, Furue M, Hanifin JM, et al. Nemolizumab in patients with moderate-to-severe atopic dermatitis: Randomized, phase II, long-term extension study. J Allergy Clin Immunol 2018;142(4):1121–1130 e7. https://doi.org/10.1016/j.jaci. 2018.03.018.

53. Kabashima K, Matsumura T, Komazaki H, et al. Trial of nemolizumab and topical agents for atopic dermatitis with pruritus. N Engl J Med 2020;383(2):141–50. https://doi.org/10.1056/NEJMoa1917006.

54. Kabashima K, Matsumura T, Komazaki H, et al. Nemolizumab plus topical agents in patients with atopic dermatitis (AD) and moderate-to-severe pruritus provide improvement in pruritus and signs of AD for up to 68 weeks: results from two phase III, long-term studies. Br J Dermatol 2022;186(4):642–51. https://doi.org/ 10.1111/bjd.20873.

55. Wang YH, Liu YJ. OX40-OX40L interactions: a promising therapeutic target for allergic diseases? J Clin Invest 2007;117(12):3655–7. https://doi.org/10.1172/ JCI34182.

56. Ito T, Wang YH, Duramad O, et al. TSLP-activated dendritic cells induce an inflammatory T helper type 2 cell response through OX40 ligand. J Exp Med 2005;202(9):1213–23. https://doi.org/10.1084/jem.20051135.

57. Fujita H, Shemer A, Suarez-Farinas M, et al. Lesional dendritic cells in patients with chronic atopic dermatitis and psoriasis exhibit parallel ability to activate T-cell subsets. J Allergy Clin Immunol 2011;128(3):574–82. https://doi.org/10. 1016/j.jaci.2011.05.016, e1-12.

58. Nakagawa H, Iizuka H, Nemoto O, et al. Safety, tolerability and efficacy of repeated intravenous infusions of KHK4083, a fully human anti-OX40 monoclonal antibody, in Japanese patients with moderate to severe atopic dermatitis. J Dermatol Sci 2020;99(2):82–9. https://doi.org/10.1016/j.jdermsci.2020.06.005.

59. Guttman-Yassky E, Pavel AB, Zhou L, et al. GBR 830, an anti-OX40, improves skin gene signatures and clinical scores in patients with atopic dermatitis. J Allergy Clin Immunol 2019;144(2):482–493 e7. https://doi.org/10.1016/j.jaci. 2018.11.053.

60. Guttman-Yassky E, Simpson EL, Reich K, et al. An anti-OX40 antibody to treat moderate-to-severe atopic dermatitis: a multicentre, double-blind, placebo-

controlled phase 2b study. Lancet 2023;401(10372):204–14. https://doi.org/10.1016/s0140-6736(22)02037-2.

61. Saghari M, Gal P, Gilbert S, et al. OX40L inhibition suppresses KLH-driven immune responses in healthy volunteers: a randomized controlled trial demonstrating proof-of-pharmacology for KY1005. Clin Pharmacol Ther 2022;111(5):1121–32. https://doi.org/10.1002/cpt.2539.

62. Weidinger S, Bieber T, Cork MJ, et al. Safety and efficacy of amlitelimab, a fully human nondepleting, noncytotoxic anti-OX40 ligand monoclonal antibody, in atopic dermatitis: results of a phase IIa randomized placebo-controlled trial. Br J Dermatol 2023;189(5):531–9. https://doi.org/10.1093/bjd/ljad240.

63. Chu AWL, Wong MM, Rayner DG, et al. Systemic treatments for atopic dermatitis (eczema): Systematic review and network meta-analysis of randomized trials. J Allergy Clin Immunol 2023;152(6):1470–92. https://doi.org/10.1016/j.jaci.2023.08.029.

64. Mastorino L, Gelato F, Quaglino P, et al. Efficacy of tralokinumab after failure with upadacitinib and dupilumab in a patient affected by atopic dermatitis. J Dermatolog Treat 2023;34(1):2153578. https://doi.org/10.1080/09546634.2022.2153578.

65. Chu DK, Schneider L, et al. AAAAI/ACAAI joint task force atopic dermatitis guideline panel. atopic dermatitis (eczema) guidelines: 2023 American Academy of Allergy, Asthma and Immunology. Ann Allergy Asthma Immunol 2024;132:274–312. Atopic dermititis (eczema) guidelines: 2023 AAAAI/ACAAI JTF on Practice Parameters GRADE and Institute of Medicine-based recommendations.

66. Davis DMR, Drucker AM, Alikhan A, et al. Guidelines of care for the management of atopic dermatitis in adults with phototherapy and systemic therapies. J Am Acad Dermatol 2024;90(2):e43–56. https://doi.org/10.1016/j.jaad.2023.08.102.

Chronic Spontaneous Urticaria

Current and Emerging Biologic Agents

Joshua S. Bernstein, MD[a], Jonathan A. Bernstein, MD[a],
David M. Lang, MD[b],*

KEYWORDS

- Chronic spontaneous urticaria • Mast cell • Biologics • Omalizumab • Siglec-6
- BTK inhibitor • MRGPRX2 • C-kit • Dupilumab

KEY POINTS

- Our understanding of the mast cell is vital to treating chronic spontaneous urticaria.
- Although anti-immunoglobulin E (IgE) therapy has enabled many patients with antihistamine-resistant chronic spontaneous urticaria to achieve the goals of management, including patients with type I and type IIb endotypes, refractory cases remain—suggesting an important role for alternative pathways of mast cell stimulation independent of cross-linking at FcεR1 via IgE or immunoglobulin G antibodies.
- Novel therapeutic targets directed at treating CSU include targeting T helper 2 cells (Th2) inflammation, alarmins, alternative receptors on mast cells such as MAS-related G protein-coupled receptor-X2 and sialic acid-binding immunoglobulin-like lectin-6, inhibiting intracellular signaling via Bruton's tyrosine kinase, and disrupting KIT activation by SCF.

INTRODUCTION

Our understanding of the pathogenesis of chronic spontaneous urticaria (CSU) has improved dramatically in recent years.[1,2] However, despite advances in our understanding of CSU and availability of efficacious therapies, many patients with CSU continue to experience poor control and impaired quality of life.[2] An estimated 40% to 50% of patients with CSU do not achieve satisfactory control with antihistamine treatment alone, and also do not respond to H-1 antihistamine dose advancement, with/without H-2 antihistamine and/or antileukotriene agents.[2,3] Patients with CSU in this latter group are candidates for treatment with a biologic agent. The rationale for the development of biologic agents for treating CSU rests on the assumption

[a] Division of Rheumatology, Allergy and Immunology, University of Cincinnati, 234 Goodman Street, Cincinnati, OH 45219, USA; [b] Department of Allergy and Clinical Immunology, Cleveland Clinic, 9500 Euclid Avenue, A90, Cleveland, OH 44195, USA
* Corresponding author.
E-mail address: langd@ccf.org

Immunol Allergy Clin N Am 44 (2024) 595–613
https://doi.org/10.1016/j.iac.2024.07.001   immunology.theclinics.com

that T2 immune responses contribute substantially to disease activity in patients with refractory CSU.

ENDOTYPES

Two endotypes in antihistamine refractory CSU have been described (1): type I (autoallergic) CSU, characterized by immunoglobulin E (IgE) antibodies directed against self-antigens and type IIb (autoimmune) CSU, characterized by immunoglobulin G (IgG) autoantibodies against IgE or the high-affinity IgE receptor (FCeRI).[4] Both endotypes entail mast cell and basophil activation with the release of histamine and other inflammatory mediators (**Fig. 1**).[4]

At the present time, patients with CSU may be classified as

- Type I
- Type IIb
- Both type I and type IIb
- Neither type I nor type IIb.

THERAPIES IN MANAGEMENT OF CHRONIC SPONTANEOUS URTICARIA TARGETING IMMUNOGLOBULIN E
Omalizumab

At this time, omalizumab is the only Food and Drug Administration (FDA)-approved agent for antihistamine-resistant CSU. Omalizumab is a chimeric human–mouse recombinant

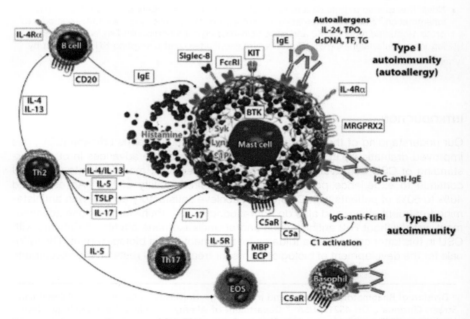

Fig. 1. *Endotypes of CSU and possible therapeutic targets.* Type I autoimmunity (autoallergy) occurs when mast cells are activated by IgE autoantibodies to autoallergens. Type IIb autoimmunity is characterized by mast cell activation from IgG-anti-IgE/IgG-anti-FcεRI. Th2 cytokines IL-4, IL-5, and IL-13 are responsible for stimulating IgE production. Type IIb autoimmunity activates complement, leading to histamine production. (*Figure from* Kolkhir, P., et al., Autoimmune chronic spontaneous urticaria. J Allergy Clin Immunol, 2022. 149(6): p. 1819-1831.)

antibody produced in a Chinese hamster ovary cell line that binds to the domain at which IgE binds to FCeRI on mast cells and basophils.[5] In randomized clinical trials (RCTs) of omalizumab in subjects with CSU, most adverse events were mild–moderate in severity and did not differ remarkably compared to placebo. Severe thrombocytopenia, eosinophilic conditions, serum sickness, and hair loss have been reported.[5] The rate of anaphylaxis observed in patients with moderate–severe allergic asthma receiving omalizumab is approximately 1 in 1000.[1,5] Malignancies were observed in RCTs in a small number of subjects with asthma receiving omalizumab and in subjects receiving placebo.[1,5] Of 4127 subjects randomized to omalizumab, 20 (0.5%) developed malignancy; of 2236 receiving placebo injections, 5 (0.2%) developed malignancy. A longitudinal study with a median follow-up of approximately 5 years compared safety of omalizumab in 5007 asthmatics receiving omalizumab with 2829 asthmatics not receiving omalizumab.[6] Rates of malignancy were similar: 12.3 per 1000 patient years for omalizumab, compared with 13.0 per 1000 patient years in asthmatics not receiving omalizumab. This implies omalizumab is not associated with an increased risk for malignancy. This study also found a higher rate of cardiovascular events in asthmatics receiving omalizumab (13.4 per 1000 patient years)—including myocardial infarction and cerebrovascular events—compared with nonomalizumab-treated asthmatics (8.1 per 1000 patient years). Although these results suggest omalizumab is associated with an increased risk of cardiovascular events, an analysis of 25 RCTs found no remarkable difference in cardiovascular event rates in 3342 omalizumab-treated asthmatics compared with 2895 asthmatic subjects with no omalizumab exposure.[5] Efforts to further understand possible risks for malignancy and for cardiovascular disease continue during postmarketing surveillance.

High-quality evidence from RCTs supports the therapeutic utility of omalizumab for patients with refractory CSU.[7–11] A meta-analysis identified 7 randomized, double-blind, placebo-controlled studies of omalizumab, including 1312 subjects with CSU, who received omalizumab at doses of 75, 150, 300, or 600 mg.[12] The 7 studies showed a low risk of bias; all used allocation concealment, and no evidence of publication bias was detected. Response was dose-dependent; the 300 mg dose was most efficacious. Rates of complete response were statistically significantly higher in subjects randomized to omalizumab compared to placebo (relative risk [RR] = 4.55, 95% confidence interval [CI] = 3.33–6.23, $P<.00001$). A more recent systematic review and network meta-analysis, which included 32 studies with 3641 adults and adolescents and examined 31 different systemic medications, concluded that omalizumab administered 300 mg every 4 weeks is the most effective currently available agent for CSU, shown to improve urticaria activity score over 7 days (UAS7), itch severity score over 7 days (ISS7), and number of hives score with high certainty of evidence; comparison with cyclosporine confirmed a safety advantage: odds ratio for occurrence of an adverse event with placebo as comparator was 1.09 with omalizumab (95% CI = 0.83, 1.42), 2.16 for cyclosporine at a dose of 3 to 5 mg/kg/d (95% CI = 0.77, 6.07).[13] Subjects enrolled in RCTs of omalizumab for CSU had a high disease burden, with a mean UAS7 of 31, and a history of prior corticosteroid treatment in approximately 50%.[14]

Table 1 describes the proportion of subjects who were free of hives and itching (UAS7 = 0) and who had clinically meaningful reduction in urticaria activity (UAS7 <6) in 5 RCTs in subjects randomized to omalizumab or placebo.[7–11] In these 5 RCTs, the primary outcome was the change in ISS7 compared with baseline; total study duration varied, but efficacy was assessed in each study at 12 weeks. A total of 614 subjects were randomized to 300 mg omalizumab every 4 weeks, while 361 received placebo. Subjects with UAS7 scores of 0 were 36% (222 out of 614) in subjects randomized to omalizumab and 6% (20 out of 361) in placebo-treated subjects. Subjects with UAS7

Table 1
Proportion of subjects in 5 randomized controlled trials evaluating the efficacy of omalizumab who became hive-free and who experienced clinically meaningful improvement

Author and Year	Study Duration[a]	Randomized Subjects		[b]UAS7 = 0		UAS7 < 6	
		Omalizumab 300 mg	Placebo	300 mg	Placebo	300 mg	Placebo
Maurer et al,[9] 2013	12 wk	79	79	35	4	52	15
Kaplan et al,[8] 2013	24 wk	252	83	85	4	132	10
Saini et al,[10] 2015	24 wk	81	80	29	7	42	9
Hide et al,[7] 2018	26 wk	35	36	11	1	19	6
Yuan et al,[11] 2022	20 wk	167	83	62	4	81	9
Total		614	361	222 (36%)	20 (6%)	326 (53%)	49 (13%)

[a] Efficacy analysis at week 12; total trial duration varied.
[b] UAS7 = Urticaria activity score over 7 d.

scores less than 6 were 53% (326 out of 614) in association with randomization to 300 mg omalizumab and 13% (49 out of 361) in subjects receiving placebo. This leads to a calculated number needed to treat of 3.3 for UAS7 scores of 0, and 2.5 for UAS7 less than 6, respectively—implying that for every 33 patients with antihistamine-resistant CSU treated with omalizumab at a dose of 300 mg every 4 weeks for 12 weeks, 10 will become "hive and itch free"; for every 25 patients treated with omalizumab at a dose of 300 mg every 4 weeks for 12 weeks, 10 will experience clinically meaningful improvement. These data imply the effects of omalizumab in properly selected patients with CSU are robust and consistent. Individuals with chronic inducible urticaria (CIndU) were excluded from these clinical trials; however, subsequent studies have shown benefit in patients with cold, cholinergic, delayed pressure, dermatographic, and solar urticaria treated with omalizumab.[15–19] Optimal duration of omalizumab treatment of CSU, and optimal strategies for suspending omalizumab, merit clarification in future studies.[20]

In addition, the psychiatric comorbidities of CSU cannot be understated. A recent systemic review and meta-analysis demonstrated CSU patients receiving omalizumab were more likely to have improved symptoms of depression, anxiety, and sleep disturbances, and resolution of CSU-associated depression. These findings were independent of cutaneous responses of patients with CSU.[21]

Ligelizumab

Ligelizumab is a high-affinity, monoclonal anti-IgE antibody that can provide greater and longer suppression of skin tests and free IgE compared with omalizumab, and it was shown to be efficacious and safe in patients with antihistamine-resistant CSU.[22] In a phase IIb dose-ranging study, compared with omalizumab, ligelizumab was associated with a higher proportion of subjects experiencing complete control of CSU, as gauged by a hives severity score of 0 at week 12 of study participation.[23] Of 382 who were randomized, 30%, 51%, and 42% of subjects receiving 24, 72, and 240 mg of ligelizumab, respectively, every 4 weeks achieved this primary endpoint, compared with 26% who received omalizumab 300 mg every 4 weeks, and none who received placebo every 4 weeks. In this clinical trial, the salutary effect of ligelizumab was observed rapidly and was sustained, and no remarkable untoward effects of ligelizumab were described. However, in 2 multicenter, multinational, double-blind, active-controlled, and placebo-controlled RCTs, in which more than 2000 subjects with antihistamine-resistant CSU were enrolled, both 72 mg q 4 week and 120 mg q 4 week doses of ligelizumab were superior to placebo q 4 weeks ($P < .0001$), but demonstrated no statistically significant difference in change from baseline in weekly UAS7 scores at week 12 compared to omalizumab 300 mg every 4 weeks.[24] Based on findings of this phase III study, further trials of ligelizumab for CSU were halted.

THERAPIES IN MANAGEMENT OF CHRONIC SPONTANEOUS URTICARIA TARGETING TYPE 2 INFLAMMATION
Background

The pathogenesis of CSU involves a complex interplay between a number of effector cells—including mast cells, basophils, eosinophils, epithelial cells, and lymphocytes through innate, adaptive, and autoimmune biologic pathways.[25] Th2 cells are known to stimulate IgE, mast cell-mediated and eosinophil-mediated reactions. Th2 differentiation is dependent on the cytokine interleukin (IL)-4, which activates the transcription factor signal transducer and activator of transcription 6 (STAT6) and GATA-binding protein 3 (GATA3), leading to the expression of Th2 cytokines IL-4, IL-5, and IL-13.

Furthermore, upstream alarmins such as IL-25, IL-33, and thymic stromal lympho-poietin (TSLP), produced by damaged epithelial cells, can induce Th2 inflammation by enhancing this IL-4-mediated pathway and also through the activation of type 2 innate lymphoid cells (**Fig. 2**).[26]

Whereas IL-5 is an activator of eosinophils, IL-4 and IL-13 have more diverse functions, including the ability to stimulate the production of specific IgE antibodies that

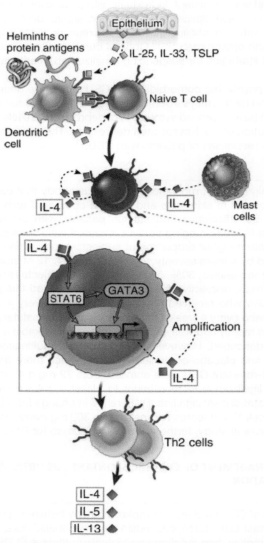

Fig. 2. *Development of Th2 cells.* Dendritic cells are stimulated by epithelial alarmins and/or antigen, leading to the activation of T cells. IL-4 is produced by T cells, as well as mast cells, thereby activated transcription factors STAT6 and GATA3, which stimulates differentiation of naïve CD4[+] T cells to the Th2 subset. (*Figure from* Abul, A., L. Andrew, and P. Shiv, Cellular and Molecular Immunology. Tenth ed. 2022: Elsevier.)

can bind to high-affinity IgE receptors (FcER1α) on mast cells, which can lead to mast cell activation and release of bioactive mediators (**Fig. 3**).[26]

Regarding Th2 inflammation, IL-4 has been an effective regulator of human mast cell phenotype, growth, and differentiation.[27] Additionally, survival of skin mast cells was enhanced by IL-4 treatment, suggesting IL-4 may act as a regulator of the mast cell lineage.[28]

In terms of the interaction between mast cells and eosinophils, there have been studies to suggest these cells adhere to each other during coculture in vitro and that they may be colocalized in urticarial wheals.[29,30] Mast cells have been shown to recruit

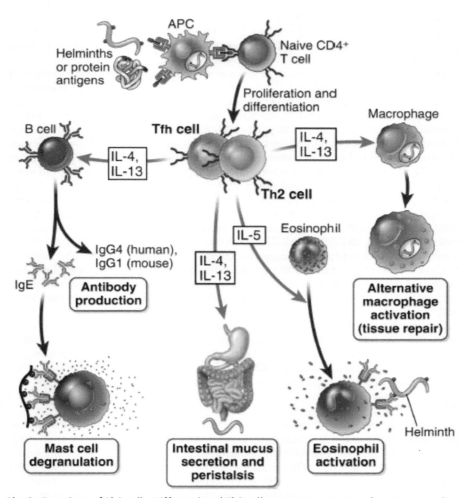

Fig. 3. Functions of Th2 cells. Differentiated Th2 cells secrete IL-4, IL-5, and IL-13. IL-4 and IL-13 act on B cells to stimulate antibody production of IgE, which binds to mast cells and eosinophils. IL-4 and IL-13 are also involved in immunity at mucosal barriers, induction of alternative pathway of macrophage activation, and inhibition of Th1 macrophage activation. IL-5 activates eosinophils. (*Figure from* Abul, A., L. Andrew, and P. Shiv, Cellular and Molecular Immunology. Tenth ed. 2022: Elsevier.)

eosinophils to diseased skin by releasing eotaxin, which binds to C-C Motif Chemokine Receptor 3 (CCR3) on the eosinophil surface, and mast cells themselves are a significant source of IL-5.[31,32] Activated eosinophils also release inflammatory mediators including major basic protein, eosinophil cationic protein, and eosinophil peroxidase, which induce histamine release from mast cells and basophils by binding to the MAS-related G protein-coupled receptor-X2 (MRGPRX2).[25,33,34]

Anti-interleukin-4/Interleukin-13 Therapy

Dupilumab, a fully human monoclonal antibody (mAb) targeting IL-4Rα, leading to the inhibition of IL-4 and IL-13, has shown efficacy across multiple diseases involving Th2 inflammation, and currently has FDA approval for the treatment of steroid-dependent or eosinophilic asthma, atopic dermatitis, prurigo nodularis, eosinophilic esophagitis in both adults and children, and chronic rhinosinusitis with nasal polyposis.[35] Furthermore, the use of dupilumab has been shown to reduce total IgE in these type 2 diseases.[36–38]

Table 2 describes dupilumab and other emerging agents currently being investigated in patients with CSU and CIndU. Dupilumab has been studied in the management of CSU unresponsive to up to 4 times the FDA-approved dose of second-generation H-1 antihistamines in a 2 part, randomized, double-blind, placebo-controlled phase III clinical trial, referred to as the LIBERTY-CSU CUPID studies.[39] Study A enrolled omalizumab-naïve patients aged 6 years or older to receive dupilumab (n = 70) verses placebo (n = 68) to investigate changes in the primary endpoints: UAS7 and ISS7 at week 24. Study B measured the same endpoints at week 24 in patients enrolled aged 12 years or older who were omalizumab-intolerant/incomplete responders to receive dupilumab (n = 54) or placebo (n = 54). In study A, dupilumab was superior to placebo at improving UAS7 and ISS7 (difference 28.5 [95% CI, 213.2–23.9; $P < .0003$] and 24.2 [95% CI, 26.6–21.8; $P < .0005$], respectively). However, the primary endpoint for study B was not achieved, as UAS7 and ISS7 scores did not demonstrate a statistically significant reduction in symptoms compared to placebo.[39] Furthermore, although the interim analysis for futility was met with the first 83 patients analyzed, the final analysis of 108 patients showed that the change in UAS7 at week 24 was statistically significant/nominally significant, ISS7 at week 24 was not significant and HSS7 at week 24 was nominally significant.

Dupilumab has been approved for CSU in Japan as of February 2024. On the other hand, the FDA rejected the application for approval in the United States in October 2023, requesting more efficacy data, although it did not cite any manufacturing or safety issues. The Liberty-CSU CUPID C study, which is similarly designed to CUPID A study, as well as a pediatric study—CUPIDKids, is currently in progress.

Anti-interleukin-5 Therapy

Targeted IL-5 therapies for the management of CSU have been largely ineffective. Benralizumab, an anti-IL5 receptor alpha mAb, was initially investigated in an open label study in 12 patients with CSU and was associated with a statistically significant reduction in UAS7 scores.[40] This prompted further investigation in patients with CSU refractory to second-generation H-1 antihistamines over 24 weeks in a phase IIb, double-blind, placebo-controlled study called the ARROYO trial.[41] Despite near complete depletion of blood eosinophils, there was no statistically significant change from baseline in ISS7 or UAS7 at week 12 between benralizumab and placebo.

These findings provide further support for the assertion that eosinophil-targeted therapies may be too immunologically limited in addressing the diverse pathways of mast cell activation in the pathogenesis of CSU.

Table 2
Emerging treatments for chronic spontaneous urticaria with ongoing clinical trials

Emerging Agent	Mechanism of Action	Clinical Trials Identifiers (clintrials.gov)	Phase	CSU	CIndU	Active Comparator: Omalizumab
Remibrutinib	BTK inhibitor	NCT05030311, NCT05032157, NCT06042478, NCT05513001, NCT05795153, and NCT05976243	3	Yes	Yes	Yes
Rilzabrutinib	BTK inhibitor	NCT05107115	2	Yes	—	—
Dupilumab	IL4Rα inhibitor	NCT04180488 and NCT05526521	3	Yes	—	Yes
Tezepelumab	Anti-TSLP	NCT04833855	2	Yes	—	Yes
AK006	Anti-Siglec-6	NCT06072157	1	Yes	—	—
EP262	MRGPRX2 antagonist	NCT06077773	2	Yes	—	—
Barzolvolimab (CDX-0159)	Anti-KIT	NCT05405660, NCT05368285	2	Yes	Yes	—
Briquilimab	Anti-KIT	NCT06162728	1,2	Yes	—	—

Abbreviations: BTK, Bruton's tyrosine kinase; CIndU, chronic inducible urticaria; CSU, chronic spontaneous urticaria; MRGPRX2, mas-related G protein-coupled receptor-X2; Siglec, sialic acid-binding immunoglobulin-like lectin; TSLP, thymic stromal lymphopoietin.

Alarmins: Background and Emerging Clinical Trials

Alarmins, most notably IL-25, IL-33, and TSLP, are upstream cytokines that have been shown to be increased in the dermis of lesional skin in patients with CSU.[42] Recently, increased levels of the alarmins, IL-33 more than TSLP, were found to correlate more closely with increases in the UAS7 and decreases in the Dermatology Life Quality Index in patients with CSU compared to controls.[43]

With the recent FDA approval of the anti-TSLP mAb, tezepelumab, as adjuvant therapy in severe, uncontrolled asthma, alarmins have emerged as promising therapeutic targets for other type 2 diseases, including CSU.[44]

A phase IIb INCEPTION study, evaluating tezepelumab in second-generation antihistamine refractory, anti-IgE naïve patients with CSU, as noted in **Table 2**, was recently completed. The primary endpoint was the change in UAS7 from baseline to week 16. Results demonstrated numeric improvement in UAS7 with tezepelumab at week 16, although the primary endpoint was not met (least square mean, LSM [SE]: tezepelumab 210 mg, -17.0 [2.0]; tezepelumab 420 mg, -16.9 [1.9]; placebo, -14.7 [1.9]; $P > .05$ tezepelumab versus placebo; omalizumab 300 mg, -19.5 [2.0]).[45]

Interestingly, there was a sustained effect of tezepelumab in UAS7 from baseline to week 32, 18 to 20 weeks after the last dose for tezepelumab 210 mg (-18.0 [2.1], $P = .037$) and tezepelumab 420 mg (-17.2 [2.1], $P = .062$) verses placebo (-11.7 [2.1]), which was independent of baseline IgE and was not observed with omalizumab (-12.6 [2.1]).[45]

Sialic Acid-Binding Immunoglobulin-Like Lectins: Background

Sialic acid-binding immunoglobulin-like lectins (Siglecs) are a family of immune regulatory receptors found primarily on immune cells containing immunoreceptor tyrosine-based inhibitory motifs that function to counteract activating signals via recruitment of tyrosine phosphatases such as src homology region 2 domain-containing phosphatase-1 (SHP-1) and SHP-2.[46] Mast cells and eosinophils express several inhibitory Siglecs including Siglec-2, Siglec-3, Siglec-6, Siglec-7, and Siglec-8.[47]

Siglec-8 is an inhibitory receptor selectively expressed on mast cells and eosinophils, and to a lesser extent, on basophils. Siglec-8 engagement by antibodies showed in vitro inhibition of mast cell activation and induction of eosinophil apoptosis.[48]

Siglec-6 (CD327) has also been identified using multicolor flow cytometry as a differentially regulated surface antigen on human mast cells and basophils.[49] It was shown to be induced by IL-3 on basophils of healthy individuals and in patients with chronic myeloid leukemia, as well as by stem cell factor on tissue mast cells. Interestingly, IgE-dependent activation resulted in upregulation of Siglec-6 in mast cells but resulted in downregulation in basophils, suggesting unique, cell-specific responses to IgE-receptor cross-linking.[49]

A recent study evaluated Siglec-6 mAb clones to demonstrate epitope-dependent receptor internalization and inhibitory activity.[50] One specific Siglec-6 mAb clone, AK04, required Fc-mediated interaction for receptor internalization and induced inhibition and antibody-dependent cellular phagocytosis against mast cells. Furthermore, treatment of humanized mice with AK04 inhibited systemic anaphylaxis with a single dose and reduced mast cells with chronic dosing.[50]

Siglec-6 expressing transgenic mice were generated to evaluate Siglec-6 mAb activity after intragastric ovalbumin (OVA) challenge and IL-33/LL37 intradermal injections. Siglec-6 mAb treatment reduced OVA-mediated inflammation, including mast cell and eosinophil numbers. Siglec-6 mAb treatments also led to reduction in LL37-induced skin lesions, as well as inhibition of IL-33.[51]

Given these promising findings, anti-Siglec monoclonal antibodies have been investigated as a way to silence mast cells in a variety of diseases, especially in CSU (**Fig. 4**).[52,53]

Clinical Trials Evaluating Anti-Siglec-8 Monoclonal Antibody

A phase 2a proof of concept clinical trial evaluating lirentelimab, an anti-Siglec-8 mAb., was investigated as an open trial in patients with H-1 antihistamine refractory CSU and patients with CIndU, demonstrating an improvement in the urticaria control test (UCT) over time.[54] However, in January 2024, the company announced its phase 2b clinical trial in patients with CSU (MAVERICK) did not meet its primary endpoint in change of UAS7 at 12 weeks, and investigation of this compound was discontinued.

Clinical Trials Evaluating Anti-Siglec-6 Monoclonal Antibody

Preclinical research on primary mouse mast cells suggested a potentially broader role for Siglec-6 than Siglec-8 since treatment with an anti-Siglec-6 antibody significantly inhibited SCF-mediated mast cell (MC) activation more so than targeting Siglec-8.[55]

As shown in **Table 2**, a phase 1 double-blind, sequential, single-ascending and multiple-ascending dose RCT to evaluate safety, tolerability, pharmacokinetics, and immunogenicity of AK006, a selective anti-Siglec-6 mAb, is currently underway in the evaluation of H-1 antihistamine refractory CSU in adults aged 18 years or older.

Novel Therapies in Management of Chronic Spontaneous Urticaria Targeting the Mast Cell

Despite the success of targeted anti-IgE monoclonal antibodies in the treatment of CSU, at least 50% of patients will remain symptomatic after treatment with licensed

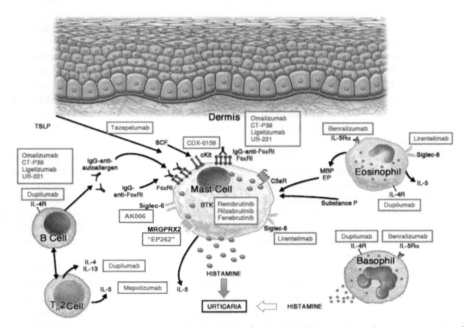

Fig. 4. Biologics and novel targets for CSU. This figure describes various therapeutic sites of interest including inhibition of IgE, IL-4/IL-13, IL-5, TSLP, Siglec 6, Siglec 8, BTK, c-kit, and MRGPRX2. (*Figure adapted from* Casale, T.B., Novel biologics for treatment of chronic spontaneous urticaria. J Allergy Clin Immunol, 2022. 150(6): p. 1256-1259.)

doses of omalizumab for at least 6 months.[56] This suggests a potentially important role for agents that impact alternative routes of mast cell stimulation independent of cross-linking at FcεR1 via IgE or IgG antibodies. Novel areas of active clinical investigation include inhibitors of the protein kinase Bruton's tyrosine kinase (BTK), as well as antagonists of the MRGPRX2 and the c-kit tyrosine kinase receptor, both of which are expressed on the mast cell surface (see **Fig. 4**).[52,53,57]

BTK Inhibitors

BTK is a protein tyrosine kinase of the hepatocellular carcinoma (TEC) kinase family, expressed in selected cells of the adaptive and innate immune system, including B cells, mast cells, basophils, natural killer cells, macrophages, neutrophils, dendritic cells, monocytes, and osteoclasts.[57] BTK has been shown to play a role in immune-mediated pathogenesis of CSU, both through IgE-mediated and IgG-mediated signaling in mast cells and basophils, as well as in the development of autoreactive B cells. Although they are technically small molecule drugs rather than biologics, BTK inhibitors with improved selectivity (fenebrutinib, remibrutinib, and rilzabrutinib) are being explored as a novel pharmacologic approach to treatment of CSU.[57]

Fenebrutinib was randomly administered in a phase II double-blind, placebo-controlled RCT in a dose-ranging protocol (50 mg/d, 150 mg/d, 200 mg bid) to 93 adults with antihistamine-resistant CSU for 8 weeks.[58] Fenebrutinib demonstrated statistically significantly greater efficacy that was quite similar when assessed at 4 weeks and 8 weeks. Equivalent efficacy was observed in subjects with and without type IIb autoimmunity; interestingly, subjects with markers of type IIb autoimmunity exhibited greater reduction in disease activity compared with placebo than subjects without these markers, at lower doses of fenebrutinib. Transient asymptomatic liver enzyme elevations were observed in subjects randomized to fenebrutinib 150 mg daily and 200 mg twice daily. Further development of fenebrutinib is uncertain at the time of this publication.

In a double-blind dose ranging RCT, remibrutinib was administered at doses of 10 mg/d, 35 mg/d, 100 mg/d, 10 mg bid, 25 mg bid, and 100 mg bid for 12 weeks in 311 adults with antihistamine-resistant CSU.[59] Statistically significantly greater reductions in UAS scores were observed from week 1 to week 12 in subjects randomized to all doses of remibrutinib compared with placebo-treated subjects. No difference was observed in outcomes of treatment in prior omalizumab-treated compared with omalizumab-naïve subjects.

Efficacy and safety of rilzalbrutinib was also assessed in a double-blind RCT in a dose-ranging study (400 mg/d, 400 mg bid, and 400 mg tid) in 160 adults whose CSU was not controlled with H-1 antihistamine alone.[60] In subjects randomized to rilzalbrutinib 400 mg tid compared with placebo, statistically significant reduction in UAS7 was observed at week 12. Statistically significant benefit in itch severity scores was also observed at week 12 in subjects randomized to rilzalbrutinib 400 mg tid. Rilzalbrutinib was associated with prompt benefit: significant changes in itch severity scores were observed at week 1.

Safety was assessed in a 52 week extension study in which subjects received 100 mg remibrutinib twice daily; treatment-emergent adverse effects were mild–moderate in nature and considered unrelated to remibrutinib by investigators.[61] Concern has been raised that BTK inhibitors may be associated with immunomodulatory effects including an increased risk for infection; however, no remarkable changes in total serum immunoglobulin levels or elevation in rates of infection have been observed in clinical trials of BTK inhibitors.[58,61] Further data on safety parameters will be important to document in future clinical trials. Evidence has also demonstrated reduction of wheal size with remibrutinib, supporting the assertion that the drug can achieve potent effects in patients with basophil and mast cell-driven CSU.[62]

BTK inhibitors have been shown to be efficacious for both type I and type IIb CSU endotypes. Rapid benefit in urticaria disease activity was observed in RCTs with fenebrutinib, remibrutinib, and rilzabrutinib.[58,61] BTK inhibitors have exhibited efficacy in CSU subjects with or without prior omalizumab treatment and show promise as effective and well-tolerated oral agents for the treatment of antihistamine-resistant CSU.

MRGPRX2: Background

Mast cell G protein-coupled receptors are a family of 7 transmembrane domain receptors that couple via heterotrimeric G-proteins to regulate cell proliferation, development, metabolism, survival, and neuronal signal transmission.[34] MRGPRX2, also known as MRGX2, has been shown to mediate IgE-independent activation of mast cells, basophils, and eosinophils.[63]

Human skin mast cells are activated by neuropeptides, such as substance P, vasoactive intestinal peptide, pituitary adenylate cyclase-activating polypeptide, and somatostatin.[64] MRGPRX2 has since been identified to be a receptor for these basic peptides.[65]

Further studies have also shown granules of human eosinophils, including major basic protein 1 and 2 eosinophil peroxidase, and eosinophil cationic protein have been able to induce histamine release from mast cells by binding to MRGPRX2.[66] Additionally, MRGRPX2 has been shown to be activated by a variety of other neuropeptides, antimicrobial peptides, such as LL-37 and human β-defensins, proteases such as cathepsin, and a variety of drugs—including opiates, fluoroquinolones, vancomycin, bradykinin receptor antagonists, and neuromuscular blocking agents.[67]

Fujisawa and colleagues[29] compared MRGPRX2 expression using immunofluorescence in skin tissues from normal controls, patients with severe chronic urticaria (UAS7 >30), and on skin-derived cultured mast cells. The number of MRGPRX2 skin mast cells and the percentage of MRGPRX2-positive mast cells in all mast cells in patients with CSU were statistically significantly greater than in normal control subjects.[29] This study provided further support for MRGPRX2 as a potential therapeutic target.

Serum MRGPRX2 levels have been evaluated as a potential marker for severe CSU. Serum MRGPRX2 levels were significantly higher in patients with severe CSU (median [interquartile range], 16.5 [10.8–24.8]) than in healthy controls (11.7 [6.5–21.2], $P = .036$) and in nonsevere patients with CSU (8.7 [4.5–18.8], $P = .002$), although they did not differ significantly between healthy subjects and nonsevere patients with CSU.[68]

MRGPRX2: Clinical Trials

An oral, highly selective once-daily small molecule antagonist of MRGPRX2, called "EP262," is currently being studied in a phase II double-blind RCT in patients with antihistamine refractory CSU. The current estimated primary completion date is October 2024.

C-kit: Background

Mast cells are derived from pluripotent, c-kit+ (CD117+), CD34+ stem cells in the bone marrow. KIT is the receptor for the cytokine SCF, which is the critical growth factor of mast cells. The gene that encodes the receptor kit is the proto-oncogene c-kit.[69]

The KIT receptor is expressed on the surface of uncommitted stem cells, MC progenitor cells, mature MCs, as well as other cell types, including melanocytes, Cajal cells of the gastrointestinal tract, and germ cells.[70]

The binding of SCF to c-kit receptor triggers several membrane and intracellular signaling events in mast cells, leading to differentiation, proliferation, and maturation of cells in the mast cell lineage; promotion of mast cell migration, chemotaxis, and adhesion; and mast cell piecemeal degranulation and the release of bioactive mediators.[71]

Murine mast cells and in vivo mouse models have been helpful in exploring pathogenic roles within mast cells, particularly in IgE-mediated reactions; however, there is a lack of suitable murine models for CSU.[72,73] In vitro stimulation of human mast cells and in vivo human mast cell studies investigating mast cell disorders, represent current gaps in knowledge that have impeded our better understanding of the pathogenesis of CSU.[73]

However, since the dysregulation of SCF/KIT can influence multiple aspects of the mast cell cellular response, blocking the KIT/SCF pathway has become a popular therapeutic target for a variety of disease processes including systemic mastocytosis, CSU, and malignancies.[71,74,75]

Unlike multitargeted tyrosine kinase KIT inhibitors, which can carry risks of off-target toxicities, tissue depleting mast cell therapies such as anti-KIT monoclonal antibodies have shown early therapeutic promise in CSU and CIndU, with greater safety profiles.[73,76,77]

C-kit: Clinical Trials

Barzolvolimab (CDX-0159), a humanized antibody that inhibits KIT activation by SCF, was recently evaluated in phase 1b clinical study in patients with antihistamine-refractory cold-induced urticaria or symptomatic dermatographia.[75] Barzolvolimab was well tolerated and resulted in durable depletion of skin mast cells, circulating tryptase and improvement in UCT.

CDX-0159 is currently being investigated in phase 2 trials in patients with CIndU and in patients with CSU.

Early results from a phase 2 RCT for barzolvolimab in CSU showed that barzolvolimab at doses of 150 mg Q4W and 300 mg Q8W demonstrated clinically meaningful and statistically significant improvement. Specifically, at week 12, LSM change in UAS7 from baseline for the 150 and 300 mg arms versus placebo were −23.02/−10.47 (difference −12.55, $P < .0001$) and −23.87/−10.47 (difference −13.41, $P < .0001$), respectively. Barzolvolimab was well tolerated. Most drug-related toxicities were low grade (hair color changes and neutropenia) and improved with longer term use and/or after discontinuation. There were no drug-related serious adverse events.[78]

Briquilimab, an unconjugated, aglycosylated, anti-c-Kit antibody, is also currently under investigation in a 3 part escalating phase 1 B/2A clinical trial, with part I open label and part II/III randomized, double-blinded, and placebo-controlled trials.

SUMMARY

Biologic agents play an important therapeutic role in the management of patients with allergic/immunologic disorders, particularly involving type 2 inflammation. Although omalizumab has enabled many patients with antihistamine-resistant CSU to achieve the goals of management, including patients with type I and type IIb endotypes, unmet needs persist. A number of emerging agents, including those affecting IL-4/IL-13, mast cell activating and inhibitory receptors, mast cell survival, and alarmins, have shown promise in clinical trials. In the near future, the landscape of biologic agents for the treatment of antihistamine-resistant CSU will be expanding, and this will lead to a greater proportion of patients achieving the goals of management for CSU and CIndU.

CLINICS CARE POINTS

- Despite recent and substantial advances in our understanding of chronic urticaria and the availability of efficacious therapies, many patients with chronic urticaria continue to experience poor control and impaired quality of life.

- Many patients with chronic urticaria do not achieve disease control with H-1 antihistamines, with/without H-2 antihistamine and/or antileukotriene agents; these patients are candidates for treatment with a biologic agent.

- Omalizumab has enabled many patients with antihistamine-resistant chronic urticaria to achieve the goals of management, including patients with type I and type IIb endotypes.

- The landscape of biologic agents for treatment of antihistamine-resistant chronic urticaria will be expanding in the near future; this will lead to a greater proportion of patients achieving the goals of management.

DISCLOSURE

J.S. Bernstein has no conflicts of interest to disclose. *J.A. Bernstein* has served as PI and consultant for Sanofi Regeneron, Novartis, Genentech, Amgen, GSK, Celldex, Jasper, Escient, Astra-Zeneca, Allakos, Blueprint, Cogent, Telios, CSL Behring, Takeda/Shire, Pharming, Biocryst, Kalvista, Ionis, Biomarin, GSK, and Merck. Serves on AAAAI BOD, WAO BOD, Interasma BOD, UCARE COE, and AIM COE as well as on the editorial boards for Journal of Allergy and Clinical Immunology, Journal of Allergy and Clinical Immunology: In Practice, Annals of Allergy, Asthma and Clinical Immunology, Allergy and Asthma Proceedings. *D.M. Lang* has served as a consultant for, received honoraria from, and/or has carried out clinical research with AstraZeneca, Blueprint, Celldex, Genentech, Novartis, Sanofi-Regeneron, serves as Guest Editor for *Journal of Allergy and Clinical Immunology in Practice*, and also on the Editorial Boards of *Allergy and Asthma Proceedings* and *DynaMed*, and Delegate to National Quality Forum representing the American Academy of Allergy, Asthma, and Immunology.

REFERENCES

1. Asero R, Ferrer, Kocaturk, et al. Chronic Spontaneous Urticaria: The Role and Relevance of Autoreactivity, Autoimmunity, and Autoallergy. J Allergy Clin Immunol Pract 2023;11(8):2302–8.
2. Lang DM. Chronic Urticaria. N Engl J Med 2022;387(9):824–31.
3. Amin P, Levin, Holmes, et al. Investigation of patient-specific characteristics associated with treatment outcomes for chronic urticaria. J Allergy Clin Immunol Pract 2015;3(3):400–7.
4. Kolkhir P, Muñoz, Asero, et al. Autoimmune chronic spontaneous urticaria. J Allergy Clin Immunol 2022;149(6):1819–31.
5. Available at: https://www.accessdata.fda.gov/drugsatfda_docs/label/2024/103976s5245lbl.pdf. (Accessed May 1 2024).
6. Long A, Rahmaoui, Rothman, et al. Incidence of malignancy in patients with moderate-to-severe asthma treated with or without omalizumab. J Allergy Clin Immunol 2014;134(3):560.e4.
7. Hide M, Igarashi, Yagami, et al. Efficacy and safety of omalizumab for the treatment of refractory chronic spontaneous urticaria in Japanese patients: Subgroup analysis of the phase 3 POLARIS study. Allergol Int 2018;67(2):243–52.

8. Kaplan A, Ledford, Ashby, et al. Omalizumab in patients with symptomatic chronic idiopathic/spontaneous urticaria despite standard combination therapy. J Allergy Clin Immunol 2013;132(1):101–9.

9. Maurer M, Rosén, Hsieh, et al. Omalizumab for the treatment of chronic idiopathic or spontaneous urticaria. N Engl J Med 2013;368(10):924–35.

10. Saini SS, Bindslev-Jensen, Maurer, et al. Efficacy and safety of omalizumab in patients with chronic idiopathic/spontaneous urticaria who remain symptomatic on H1 antihistamines: a randomized, placebo-controlled study. J Invest Dermatol 2015;135(1):67–75.

11. Yuan W, Hu, Li, et al. Efficacy and safety of omalizumab in Chinese patients with anti-histamine refractory chronic spontaneous urticaria. Dermatol Ther 2022; 35(4):e15303.

12. Zhao ZT, Ji, Yu, et al. Omalizumab for the treatment of chronic spontaneous urticaria: A meta-analysis of randomized clinical trials. J Allergy Clin Immunol 2016; 137(6):1742.e4.

13. Kendziora B,FJ, Beinholz M, Rueff F, et al. Efficacy and safety of medications for antihistamine-refractory chronic spontaneous urticaria: A systematic review and network meta-analysis. Allergo J Int 2023;32:83–92.

14. Casale TB, Bernstein JA, Maurer M, et al. Similar efficacy with omalizumab in chronic idiopathic/spontaneous urticaria despite different background therapy. J Allergy Clin Immunol Pract 2015;3(5):743-50.e1.

15. Metz M, Schütz, Weller, et al. Omalizumab is effective in cold urticaria-results of a randomized placebo-controlled trial. J Allergy Clin Immunol 2017;140(3):864.e5.

16. Gastaminza G, Azofra, Nunez-Cordoba, et al. Efficacy and Safety of Omalizumab (Xolair) for Cholinergic Urticaria in Patients Unresponsive to a Double Dose of Antihistamines: A Randomized Mixed Double-Blind and Open-Label Placebo-Controlled Clinical Trial. J Allergy Clin Immunol Pract 2019;7(5):1599.e1.

17. Veleiro-Pérez B, Alba-Muñoz, Pérez-Quintero, et al. Delayed Pressure Urticaria: Clinical and Diagnostic Features and Response to Omalizumab. Int Arch Allergy Immunol 2022;183(10):1089–94.

18. Cakmak ME, Yeğit OO, Öztop N. Comparison of Omalizumab Treatment Response in Patients with Chronic Spontaneous Urticaria and Symptomatic Dermographism: A Single-Center Retrospective Study. Int Arch Allergy Immunol 2023;184(3):236–42.

19. Casanova-Esquembre A, Lorca-Spröhnle J, Peñuelas-Leal R, et al. Solar Urticaria and Omalizumab: A Retrospective Case-Control Study and Follow-Up. Actas Dermosifiliogr 2024. https://doi.org/10.1016/j.ad.2023.04.044.

20. Lang DM. A critical appraisal of omalizumab as a therapeutic option for chronic refractory urticaria/angioedema. Ann Allergy Asthma Immunol 2014;112(4):276–9.

21. Tan MG, Bailey, Dorus, et al. Clinical Impacts of Omalizumab on the Psychiatric Comorbidities of Chronic Spontaneous Urticaria: A Systematic Review and Meta-Analysis. J Drugs Dermatol 2024;23(4):e116–7.

22. Arm JP, Bottoli, Skerjanec, et al. Pharmacokinetics, pharmacodynamics and safety of QGE031 (ligelizumab), a novel high-affinity anti-IgE antibody, in atopic subjects. Clin Exp Allergy 2014;44(11):1371–85.

23. Maurer M, Giménez-Arnau, Sussman, et al. Ligelizumab for Chronic Spontaneous Urticaria. N Engl J Med 2019;381(14):1321–32.

24. Maurer M, Ensina, Gimenez-Arnau, et al. Efficacy and safety of ligelizumab in adults and adolescents with chronic spontaneous urticaria: results of two phase 3 randomised controlled trials. Lancet 2024;403(10422):147–59.

25. Zhou B, Li, Liu, et al. The Role of Crosstalk of Immune Cells in Pathogenesis of Chronic Spontaneous Urticaria. Front Immunol 2022;13:879754.

26. Abul A, Andrew L, Shiv P. Cellular and molecular immunology. 10th edition. Philadelphia, PA: Elsevier; 2022.

27. Babina M, Guhl, Artuc, et al. IL-4 and human skin mast cells revisited: reinforcement of a pro-allergic phenotype upon prolonged exposure. Arch Dermatol Res 2016;308(9):665–70.

28. Thienemann F, Henz BM, Babina M. Regulation of mast cell characteristics by cytokines: divergent effects of interleukin-4 on immature mast cell lines versus mature human skin mast cells. Arch Dermatol Res 2004;296(3):134–8.

29. Fujisawa D, Kashiwakura, Kita, et al. Expression of Mas-related gene X2 on mast cells is upregulated in the skin of patients with severe chronic urticaria. J Allergy Clin Immunol 2014;134(3):622.e9.

30. Minai-Fleminger Y, Elishmereni, Vita, et al. Ultrastructural evidence for human mast cell-eosinophil interactions in vitro. Cell Tissue Res 2010;341(3):405–15.

31. Mukai K, Tsai, Saito, et al. Mast cells as sources of cytokines, chemokines, and growth factors. Immunol Rev 2018;282(1):121–50.

32. Tedeschi A, Asero, Lorini, et al. Serum eotaxin levels in patients with chronic spontaneous urticaria. Eur Ann Allergy Clin Immunol 2012;44(5):188–92.

33. Altrichter S, Frischbutter, Fok, et al. The role of eosinophils in chronic spontaneous urticaria. J Allergy Clin Immunol 2020;145(6):1510–6.

34. Subramanian H, Gupta K, Ali H. Roles of Mas-related G protein-coupled receptor X2 on mast cell-mediated host defense, pseudoallergic drug reactions, and chronic inflammatory diseases. J Allergy Clin Immunol 2016;138(3):700–10.

35. Le Floc'h A, Allinne, Nagashima, et al. Dual blockade of IL-4 and IL-13 with dupilumab, an IL-4Rα antibody, is required to broadly inhibit type 2 inflammation. Allergy 2020;75(5):1188–204.

36. Bachert C, Han, Desrosiers, et al. Efficacy and safety of dupilumab in patients with severe chronic rhinosinusitis with nasal polyps (LIBERTY NP SINUS-24 and LIBERTY NP SINUS-52): results from two multicentre, randomised, double-blind, placebo-controlled, parallel-group phase 3 trials. Lancet 2019;394(10209):1638–50.

37. Castro M, Corren, Pavord, et al. Dupilumab Efficacy and Safety in Moderate-to-Severe Uncontrolled Asthma. N Engl J Med 2018;378(26):2486–96.

38. Paller AS, Siegfried, Simpson, et al. A phase 2, open-label study of single-dose dupilumab in children aged 6 months to. J Eur Acad Dermatol Venereol 2021;35(2):464–75.

39. Maurer M, Casale TB, Saini SS, et al. Dupilumab in patients with chronic spontaneous urticaria (LIBERTY-CSU CUPID): Two randomized, double-blind, placebo-controlled, phase 3 trials. J Allergy Clin Immunol 2024;154(1):184–94.

40. Bernstein JA, Singh, Rao, et al. Benralizumab for Chronic Spontaneous Urticaria. N Engl J Med 2020;383(14):1389–91.

41. Altrichter S, Giménez-Arnau AM, Bernstein JA, et al. Benralizumab does not elicit therapeutic effect in patients with chronic spontaneous urticaria: results from the phase 2b multinational, randomised, double-blind, placebo-controlled ARROYO trial. Br J Dermatol 2024. https://doi.org/10.1093/bjd/ljae067.

42. Kay AB, Clark, Maurer, et al. Elevations in T-helper-2-initiating cytokines (interleukin-33, interleukin-25 and thymic stromal lymphopoietin) in lesional skin from chronic spontaneous ('idiopathic') urticaria. Br J Dermatol 2015;172(5):1294–302.

43. Dobrican-Baruta CT, Deleanu DM, Muntean IA, et al. The Alarmin Triad-IL-25, IL-33, and TSLP-Serum Levels and Their Clinical Implications in Chronic Spontaneous Urticaria. Int J Mol Sci 2024;25(4):2026.

44. Menzies-Gow A, Corren, Bourdin, et al. Tezepelumab in Adults and Adolescents with Severe, Uncontrolled Asthma. N Engl J Med 2021;384(19):1800–9.

45. Maurer M. Sustained Improvement in UAS7 After 16-Week Treatment With Tezepelumab in Biologic-Naïve Adults with CSU: Results of the Phase 2b INCEPTION Study. J Allergy Clin Immunol 2024;153(2).

46. Macauley MS, Crocker PR, Paulson JC. Siglec-mediated regulation of immune cell function in disease. Nat Rev Immunol 2014;14(10):653–66.

47. O'Sullivan JA, Chang, Youngblood, et al. Eosinophil and mast cell Siglecs: From biology to drug target. J Leukoc Biol 2020;108(1):73–81.

48. Kiwamoto T, Kawasaki, Paulson, et al. Siglec-8 as a drugable target to treat eosinophil and mast cell-associated conditions. Pharmacol Ther 2012;135(3):327–36.

49. Smiljkovic D, Herrmann, Sadovnik, et al. Expression and regulation of Siglec-6 (CD327) on human mast cells and basophils. J Allergy Clin Immunol 2023;151(1): 202–11.

50. Schanin J, Korver, Brock, et al. Discovery of an agonistic Siglec-6 antibody that inhibits and reduces human mast cells. Commun Biol 2022;5(1):1226.

51. Benet Z. An Agonistic Monoclonal Antibody Against Siglec-6 Broadly Inhibits Mast Cell Activation in Transgenic Mice. Journal of allergy and clinical immunology 2023; 151(2).

52. Casale TB. Novel biologics for treatment of chronic spontaneous urticaria. J Allergy Clin Immunol 2022;150(6):1256–9.

53. Metz M, Kolkhir, Altrichter, et al. Mast cell silencing: A novel therapeutic approach for urticaria and other mast cell-mediated diseases. Allergy 2024;79(1):37–51.

54. Altrichter S, Staubach, Pasha, et al. An open-label, proof-of-concept study of lirentelimab for antihistamine-resistant chronic spontaneous and inducible urticaria. J Allergy Clin Immunol 2022;149(5):1683.e7.

55. Korver W, Benet, Wong, et al. Regulation of mast cells by overlapping but distinct protein interactions of Siglec-6 and Siglec-8. Allergy 2024;79(3):629–42.

56. Agache I, Akdis, Akdis, et al. EAACI Biologicals Guidelines-Omalizumab for the treatment of chronic spontaneous urticaria in adults and in the paediatric population 12-17 years old. Allergy 2022;77(1):17–38.

57. Bernstein JA, Maurer M, Saini SS. BTK signaling-a crucial link in the pathophysiology of chronic spontaneous urticaria. J Allergy Clin Immunol 2023;153(5): 1229–40.

58. Metz M, Sussman, Gagnon, et al. Fenebrutinib in H(1) antihistamine-refractory chronic spontaneous urticaria: a randomized phase 2 trial. Nat Med 2021;27(11): 1961–9.

59. Maurer M, Berger, Giménez-Arnau, et al. Remibrutinib, a novel BTK inhibitor, demonstrates promising efficacy and safety in chronic spontaneous urticaria. J Allergy Clin Immunol 2022;150(6):1498.e2.

60. Maurer M,G-AA, Ferrucci S, Mikol V, et al. Efficacy and Safety of Rilzabrutinib in Patients With Chronic Spontaneous Urticaria: 12-Week Results From the RILECSU Phase 2 Dose-Ranging Study. J Allergy Clin Immunol 2024;153.

61. Jain V, Giménez-Arnau, Hayama, et al. Remibrutinib demonstrates favorable safety profile and sustained efficacy in chronic spontaneous urticaria over 52 weeks. J Allergy Clin Immunol 2024;153(2):479.e4.

62. Kaul M, End, Cabanski, et al. Remibrutinib (LOU064): A selective potent oral BTK inhibitor with promising clinical safety and pharmacodynamics in a randomized phase I trial. Clin Transl Sci 2021;14(5):1756–68.

63. Wedi B, Gehring M, Kapp A. The pseudoallergen receptor MRGPRX2 on peripheral blood basophils and eosinophils: Expression and function. Allergy 2020;75(9): 2229–42.

64. Lowman MA, Rees, Benyon, et al. Human mast cell heterogeneity: histamine release from mast cells dispersed from skin, lung, adenoids, tonsils, and colon in response to IgE-dependent and nonimmunologic stimuli. J Allergy Clin Immunol 1988;81(3):590–7.

65. Tatemoto K, Nozaki, Tsuda, et al. Immunoglobulin E-independent activation of mast cell is mediated by Mrg receptors. Biochem Biophys Res Commun 2006; 349(4):1322–8.

66. Ogasawara H, Furuno, Edamura, et al. Peptides of major basic protein and eosinophil cationic protein activate human mast cells. Biochem Biophys Rep 2020;21: 100719.

67. Kühn H, Kolkhir, Babina, et al. Mas-related G protein-coupled receptor X2 and its activators in dermatologic allergies. J Allergy Clin Immunol 2021;147(2):456–69.

68. Cao TBT, Cha, Yang, et al. Elevated MRGPRX2 Levels Related to Disease Severity in Patients With Chronic Spontaneous Urticaria. Allergy Asthma Immunol Res 2021;13(3):498–506.

69. Valent P, Akin, Hartmann, et al. Mast cells as a unique hematopoietic lineage and cell system: From Paul Ehrlich's visions to precision medicine concepts. Theranostics 2020;10(23):10743–68.

70. Valent P, Akin, Hartmann, et al. Drug-induced mast cell eradication: A novel approach to treat mast cell activation disorders? J Allergy Clin Immunol 2022; 149(6):1866–74.

71. Tsai M, Valent P, Galli SJ. KIT as a master regulator of the mast cell lineage. J Allergy Clin Immunol 2022;149(6):1845–54.

72. Galli SJ, Tsai, Marichal, et al. Approaches for analyzing the roles of mast cells and their proteases in vivo. Adv Immunol 2015;126:45–127.

73. Kolkhir P, Elieh-Ali-Komi, Metz, et al. Understanding human mast cells: lesson from therapies for allergic and non-allergic diseases. Nat Rev Immunol 2022;22(5): 294–308.

74. London CA, Gardner, Rippy, et al. KTN0158, a Humanized Anti-KIT Monoclonal Antibody, Demonstrates Biologic Activity against both Normal and Malignant Canine Mast Cells. Clin Cancer Res 2017;23(10):2565–74.

75. Terhorst-Molawi D, Hawro, Grekowitz, et al. Anti-KIT antibody, barzolvolimab, reduces skin mast cells and disease activity in chronic inducible urticaria. Allergy 2023;78(5):1269–79.

76. Shyam Sunder S, Sharma UC, Pokharel S. Adverse effects of tyrosine kinase inhibitors in cancer therapy: pathophysiology, mechanisms and clinical management. Signal Transduct Target Ther 2023;8(1):262.

77. Wedi B. Inhibition of KIT for chronic urticaria: a status update on drugs in early clinical development. Expert Opin Investig Drugs 2023;32(11):1043–54.

78. Maurer M, Kobielusz-Gembala, Mitha, et al. Barzolvolimab Significantly Decreases Chronic Spontaneous Urticaria Disease Activity and is Well Tolerated: Top Line Results from a Phase 2 Trial. Journal of allergy and clinical immunology 2024;153(2):AB366.

Advancements in Biologic Therapies for Eosinophilic Gastrointestinal Diseases
A Comprehensive Review

Racha Abi Melhem, MD[a], Yasmin Hassoun, MD[b],*

KEYWORDS

- Eosinophilic esophagitis • Eosinophilic gastrointestinal diseases
- Eosinophilic gastritis • Eosinophilic enteritis • Biologics • Review

KEY POINTS

- Eosinophilic gastrointestinal diseases (EGIDs) encompass a group of disorders characterized by an abnormal accumulation of eosinophils in various parts of the gastrointestinal tract. These conditions include eosinophilic esophagitis (EoE), gastritis (EoG), enteritis (EoN), and colitis.
- Current treatment options for EGIDs are lacking and biologics have extended more treatment options in the management of patients with eosinophilic gastrointestinal disorders.
- A variety of biologics have been evaluated in the treatment of EGIDs, dupilumab is the only Food and Drug Administration-approved drug.

BIOLOGICS IN EOSINOPHILIC GASTROINTESTINAL DISEASES
Introduction

Eosinophilic gastrointestinal diseases (EGIDs) encompass a group of disorders characterized by an abnormal accumulation of eosinophils in various parts of the gastrointestinal tract. These conditions, including eosinophilic esophagitis (EoE), gastritis (EoG), enteritis (EoN), and colitis. EGIDs, present with a wide range of symptoms such as abdominal pain, vomiting, diarrhea, difficulty swallowing, and food impaction. The exact cause of EGIDs remains unclear, although allergic and immune-mediated responses are believed to play significant roles. These pathologies share skewed immune response to antigens, specifically a skewed TH2 response, leading to abnormal activation of

[a] Department of Internal Medicine, Staten Island University Hospital, 300 Constitution Avenue, Apartment 109, Bayonne, NJ 07002, USA; [b] Division of Allergy and Immunology, Department of Pediatrics, Cincinnati Children's Hospital Medical Center, University of Cincinnati College of Medicine, 3333 Burnet Avenue, ML7028, Cincinnati, OH 45229, USA
* Corresponding author.
E-mail address: Yasminhassou@gmail.com

Immunol Allergy Clin N Am 44 (2024) 615–627
https://doi.org/10.1016/j.iac.2024.07.002   **immunology.theclinics.com**

eosinophils, basophils, and mast cells.[1] The most well-known of these disorders is EoE. The prevalence and incidence of EoE is highly variable. In 2019, a systematic review conducted by Navarro and colleagues, showed the prevalence of EoE was 34.2/100,000 inhabitants, and the incidence of EoE was 4.4/100,000 inhabitants.[2] EoE was 3 times more common in men than in women; however, there was no difference in the severity of disease between the 2 sexes.[3] Diagnosis of EoE necessitates endoscopy with biopsy. Common endoscopic findings include furrows (showing as mucosal vertical lines), trachealization (showing as concentric rings leading to esophageal narrowing), exudates, edema, and strictures.[4] Based on systematic review and expert opinion, consensus led to the following diagnostic criteria for EoE: (a) esophageal symptoms and (b) presence of >15% eosinophils per high power field (HPF) in the esophageal biopsy after ruling out other conditions associated with comparable clinical, endoscopic, and histologic features.[5] This threshold is 100% sensitive and 96% specific to diagnose EoE. A new scoring system has been formed and validated, named the EoE histologic scoring index (HSS), and it takes into consideration additional inflammatory findings besides the eosinophilic count in the esophageal tissue.[6]

Pathophysiology

The pathogenesis of eosinophilic gastrointestinal disorders remains unknown. It is considered multifactorial and results from the interplay of genetic, environmental, and immunologic factors. Several studies describe food allergens having an important role in the pathophysiology of EoE by stimulating an immune response. Elimination diets have led to disease remission in a subset of patients, with reintroduction of food triggers resulting in recurrence of disease. Immunoglobulin E (IgE) has been postulated to be a part of the pathogenesis of EoE; however, a lack of response to omalizumab suggests that IgE may not be a major player.[7,8] Triggering factors are still not completely understood but the most studied factors are food antigens. The proposed mechanism is that they stimulate dendritic and epithelial cells releasing epithelial cytokines (interleukin [IL]-33, IL-25, thymic stromal lymphopoietin) which activate immune cells, such as innate lymphoid type 2 cells (ILC2), CD4 + effector memory Th-2 cells, and invariant natural killer T (iNKT) cells. As a result, Th-2 immune response occurs by secreting Th-2 related cytokines, such as IL-5, IL-4, IL-13, and eotaxin-3.[9,10] IL-5 activates eosinophils to multiply and circulate from the bone marrow into blood and then to the esophagus. These stimulated eosinophils release vascular endothelial growth factor and vascular cell adhesion molecule 1, managing endothelial activation and angiogenesis, respectively; and as a result, inflammatory cells are recruited toward the layers of the esophagus.[11] Continuous transmural inflammation of the esophageal tissue leads to constant remodeling of its wall with smooth muscle hypertrophy, lamina propria fibrosis, and basal cell hyperplasia and thus esophageal dysfunction.[12]

Treatment

The main purpose of treatment of EoE is to decrease inflammation with end goals of eosinophils less than 15 per HPF and a normal appearance of the esophagus during endoscopy. Management of eosinophilic esophagitis can be divided into non-pharmacological and pharmacologic therapies. The former consists of endoscopic interventions for treating disease complications and of diet modification.[13] In children, treatment therapies include empiric elimination diet, proton pump inhibitor (PPI), or swallowed steroids. In adults, PPIs or swallowed corticosteroids represent the mainstay therapy; however, systemic corticosteroids are used in patients with persistent eosinophilia.[14]

Monoclonal antibodies, targeting inflammatory cytokines or eosinophils, are the next emerging therapy for EGIDs. The only FDA- approved monoclonal antibody is dupilumab and it has been approved for the treatment of EoE. Monoclonal antibodies that have been studied for the treatment of EGIDs are listed in **Table 1**. In this article, the authors will discuss biologics that have been used and investigated in the treatment of eosinophilic gastrointestinal diseases.

Biologic in Eosinophilic Gastrointestinal Diseases

Anti-IL5 and anti-IL5-Rα− mepolizumab, reslizumab, benralizumab

Mepolizumab and reslizumab are monoclonal antibodies that work by blocking the binding of IL-5 to its corresponding receptor. In a randomized double blind, placebo-controlled trial, 5 adult patients with active EoE received 750 mg intravenous infusion of mepolizumab for a total of 2 doses separated by 1 week; then after 8 weeks (about 2 months), they were given two 1500 mg doses 4 weeks apart. The trial showed a statistically significant decrease in the number of eosinophils ($P = 0.03$) in esophageal tissues of the group treated with mepolizumab compared to placebo. However, subjects showed minimal improvement in symptoms, specifically dysphagia.[15] Reslizumab in clinical trials showed similar outcomes with regards to a statistically significant decrease in eosinophil counts but no improvement in patient-reported outcomes using the CHQ scores and symptoms.[16] Benralizumab is another IL-5 blocking agent, which is a monoclonal antibody against the IL-5 receptor α subunit, with strong antibody-dependent cellular cytotoxicity against eosinophils and basophils.[17] Benralizumab has been evaluated in the treatment of both EoE and EoG. In EoE, benralizumab was not shown to be efficacious as demonstrated by the Phase 3, MESSINA trial. The trial had to be terminated as the study drug did not meet the primary endpoint.[18] Benralizumab has also been evaluated as a treatment option in EoG in a phase 2 trial on 26 patients age 12 to 60 years of age with EoG, equally randomized to benaralizumab and Placebo.[19] Patients were treated with 30 mg of benralizumab versus placebo.[19] Benralizumab showed a higher histologic remission in patients on the drug compared to placebo (difference of 69% points [95% CI 32–85]; $P = 0.0010$).[19] Patients in the

Table 1
Biologics investigated in the treatment of eosinophilic gastrointestinal diseases

Drug/ Disease	Eosinophilic Esophagitis	Eosinophilic Gastritis	Eosinophilic Enteritis	Eosinophilic Colitis
Mepolizumab	+	-	-	-
Reslizumab	+	-	-	-
Benralizumab	+	+	+	-
Omalizumab	+	+	+	-
Dupilumab	+	*	*	-
QAX576	+	-	-	-
Canakinumab	+	-	-	-
Lirentelimab	+	+	+	-
Vedolizumab	-	+	+	-

+: Has been used in clinical trials in the treatment of the indicated eosinophilic gastrointestinal diseases.

-: Has not been used in clinical trials in the treatment of the indicated eosinophilic gastrointestinal diseases.

*: Studies currently underway.

treatment arm also showed statistically significant lower peak gastric eosinophil count and improvement in histology inflammation score compared to placebo. Benralizumab, however, did not show a statistically significant improvement in eosinophilic gastritis histology structural score or improvement in patient symptom-reported outcomes.[19] The histology inflammation scores refer to the degree of inflammation in the tissue based on the extent of presence of inflammatory cells. Patients did not show improvement in that aspect. Patients however did show an improvement in the EOG histology structural score which reflects distortion of tissue architecture secondary to the disease state. Currently, the Hudson GI study is underway (pending results) evaluating efficacy of benralizumab in patients with EoG or EoN.[20]

Anti-IgE: omalizumab

The initial studies of anti-IgE therapy in GI disease were done in patients with EGIDs. Foroughi and colleagues evaluated the role of omalizumab in 9 patients with EoG and/ or EoN, shown to have ≥ 25 eosinophils per HPF in stomach or duodenal biopsies.[8] Patients were on biweekly omalizumab, and at the end of the 16 -week trial, omalizumab was shown to have a statistically significant decrease in absolute eosinophil count in the peripheral blood compared to baseline (34%, $P=.004$).[8] Omalizumab also led to a reduction in duodenal and antral eosinophil levels, but this drop was not statistically significant.[8] Following this study, Foster and colleagues studied food-allergen-specific T-cell responses to omalizumab over a 16 -week period in 9 patients with EGIDs.[21] The study showed that omalizumab did not inhibit food-allergen-specific T-cell responses and concluded that IgE does not play a role in T-cell antigen presentation.[21] In EoE, there were 2 studies that evaluated the treatment outcomes of anti-IgE antibodies.[7,22] The first study conducted by Clayton and colleagues was a randomized, double-blind, placebo-controlled trial that was 16 weeks in duration. The study recruited 30 patients, 16 of whom were on omalizumab (every 2–4 weeks) and 14 of whom were on placebo.[7] The primary endpoint of the study was a decrease in esophageal eosinophils. The study did not show a statistically significant difference in the esophageal eosinophil count after treatment, nor did it show a statistically significant improvement in dysphagia scores on omalizumab compared to placebo ($P = .95$).[7] Following this study, Loizou et al conducted a single-arm, open label, unblinded study in patients with EoE treated with omalizumab.[22] The study showed a significant reduction of tissue IgE levels, but only 33% of the patients were able to achieve histologic and clinical remission.[22] Patients who were able to achieve remission had low peripheral blood absolute eosinophil counts.[22]

Anti-IL4Rα: dupilumab

Dupilumab is a human monoclonal antibody that targets IL4 receptor-α, thereby blocking signaling of IL4 and IL13.[23] Dupilumab was approved by the FDA for treatment of EoE in May 2022.[24] The efficacy of Dupilumab in EoE was first demonstrated in a phase 2 study in adults with active disease where patients were randomized to weekly injections of 300 mg of dupilumab or to placebo.[23] Patients showed symptomatic improvement as assessed by the Straumann Dysphagia Instrument patient-reported outcome score, with scores improving from 6.4 to 3 ($P = .0304$).[23] Dupilumab also showed histologic and endoscopic feature reduction; at week 12, patients on dupilumab showed a 68.3% drop in their HSS severity score ($P<.0001$) and a mean peak esophageal intraepithelial eosinophil count decrease by 86.8 eosinophils per HPF ($P<.0001$).[23] The most common side effects were erythema at injection site and nasopharyngitis.[23] A phase 3 study- LIBERTY EoE TREET followed, evaluating patients 12 years or older with active EoE and was conducted in 3 parts.[25] Part A patients were randomized in a 1:1 ratio and received either a weekly dose of 300 mg of dupilumab or placebo for 24 weeks.[25] Part B was a 3-group randomization to 1:1:1 randomization receiving either weekly dosing of 300 mg of dupilumab or biweekly dosing of 300 mg of dupilumab or placebo for 24 weeks.[25] Part C group was the long-term extension (LTE) portion of the study (week 24–52) where all patients from group A and B were converted to study drug. Patients from part A were continued on 300 mg of weekly dupilumab and those from part B were continued on the weekly or biweekly dosing.[25] The primary endpoint at week 24 (part A and B) was histologic remission defined as ≤6 eosinophils per HPF and change from baseline in the Dysphagia Symptom Questionnaire (DSQ) score.[25] In group A, dupilumab induced histologic remission in 60% of the patients compared to 5% on placebo (95% confidence interval [CI], 40–71; $P<.001$).[25] DSQ scores in group A showed a difference of −12.32 (95% CI, −19.11 to −5.54; $P<.001$) compared to placebo.[25] Similar success was seen in patients in group B on weekly dupilumab but not on the biweekly dose.[25] Histologic remission was seen in both the weekly and biweekly group in 59% and 60% of the patients, respectively, when compared to placebo, but the difference was only statistically significant in the weekly dosing group but not in the biweekly dosing group.[25] Drop in DSQ scores were statistically significant in the weekly dosing group −9.92 (95% CI, −14.81 to −5.02; $P<.001$) but not in the biweekly dosing group.[25] The LTE arm of the study, part C, showed maintenance of response in the treatment group; patients on placebo who were switched to dupilumab achieved similar results as the treatment groups (**Table 2**). At week 52, all patients were able to achieve a peak intraepithelial esophageal eosinophil count of <6 eosinophils per HPF.[26] Patients on weekly Dupixent who were continued on their dose showed the highest drop in mean percentage change of peak esophageal eosinophil count −95.9% (95% CI -96.9 to −94.9) followed by patients who were previously on placebo and then switched to biweekly dosing with −91.2% (95% CI -95.9 to −86.5).[26] Significant drops were also seen in the biweekly/biweekly and placebo/weekly group.[26] The mean HSS grade score also showed a statistically significant drop across all groups.[26] Patients also showed improvement in their EoE symptoms with the biggest change in DSQ score recorded in the weekly/weekly dupilumab group.[26] The Endoscopic Reference Score (EREFS) also showed improvements across all groups, with the highest change seen in the placebo/weekly dupilumab group (see **Table 2**).[26] Dupilumab was very recently approved (January 2024) for pediatric patients 1 year and older based on data from parts A (week 16) and B (week 52) of the phase 3 EoE KIDS trial.[27] Patients who were 1 to 11 years of age were randomized to receive a weight-tiered, high-dose or low-dose dupilumab, or placebo.[27] Patients showed statistically significant improvements in regards to HSS grade and stage, EREFS score, and caregiver-reported proportion of days experiencing ≥1 EoE sign.[27] Patients also showed reduced peak intraepithelial eosinophil counts at week 52 with 62.9% of the patients showing ≤6 eosinophils per HPF and 85.7% of the patients showing <15 eosinophils per HPF in patients who were on dupilumab in part A and continued on the drug in part B.[27] Similar responses were seen in patient on placebo in part A who were then switched to dupilumab in part B (52.9% and 64.7% achieved ≤6 and <15 eosinophils per HPF, respectively).[27] There are multiple clinical trials underway evaluating the efficacy of dupilumab in non EoE EGIDs (NCT03678545, NCT05831176).

Anti-IL-13: QAX576, cendakimab

The role of IL-13 has been shown in vitro to be central to the pathophysiology of EoE.[28] Eotaxin 3, an eosinophil chemoattractant, is upregulated by IL-13, leading to eosinophilic esophageal infiltration. IL-13 also promotes its effects through periostin, which promotes both eosinophilic influx and adhesion.[28] IL-13 has also been implicated in

Table 2
Results of the long-term extension arm of the LIBERTY EoE TREET, part C cohort at week 52

Part C Groups	Weekly/Weekly	Biweekly/Biweekly	Placebo/Weekly	Placebo/Biweekly
Mean percentage change of peak esophageal eosinophil count.	−95·9% (95% CI −96·9 to −94·9	−84·8% (95% CI −94·3 to −75·2)	−84·2% (95% CI −98·3 to −70·2)	−91·2% (95% CI −95·9 to −86·5)
Mean change in HSS grade score	−30·3 points (95% CI −34·5 to −26·1)	−20·9% (95% CI −25·4 to −16·3)	−27·3 points (95% CI −32·1 to −22·4)	23·7% (95% CI −29·1 to −18·3)
Mean change in EREFS	−5·4 points (95% CI −6·1 to −4·6)	−5·2% (95% CI −6·0 to −4·4)	−6·1 points (95% CI −7·3 to −4·9)	−4·3% −5·4 to −3·1) (95% CI

Weekly/weekly: Part A and B patients who were on weekly dupilumab and continued on their weekly dosing.
Biweekly/biweekly: Part B patients who were on biweekly dupilumab and continued on their biweekly dosing.
Placebo/weekly: Part A and B patients who were on placebo and switched to weekly dupilumab dosing.
Placebo/biweekly: Part B patients who were on placebo and switched to biweekly dupilumab dosing.

the pathogenesis of non-EoE EGIDs particularly EOG (Eosinophilic Gastritis).[29] QAX576 was the first antibody developed targeting IL-13. Adult patients 18 to 50 years of age with PPI-resistant EoE received 6 mg/kg of QAX576 or placebo (2:1 ratio). The study failed to meet its primary endpoint of a greater than 75% decrease in peak eosinophil counts at week 12.[30] The antibody, however, did show a 60% decrease in the mean eosinophil count with QAX576 compared to 23% with placebo ($P =$ .004), and this response was sustained for 6 months after.[30] Clinically, patients reported improved symptoms, specifically related to dysphagia.[30]

Cendakimab (RPC 4046 and CC-93538) was the next IL-13 antibody to be investigated for the treatment of EGIDs, and it was evaluated in the setting of EoE. Cendakimab is a recombinant humanized monoclonal antibody that binds both the IL-13Rα1 and IL-13Rα2 receptor units, preventing the binding of IL-13 to them.[31] The initial double blind phase 2 trial on cendakimab was a 16 -week trial that studied the drug at 2 doses,180 mg and 360 mg, on a weekly basis in patients 18 to 65 years of age who have failed a trial of PPI.[31] Cendakimab showed a clinically significant reduction in esophageal eosinophil count at both doses. The mean EREFS total score was also statistically reduced at all esophageal locations for both doses at week 16, as well as there was a statistically significant reduction in mean adjusted EoEHSS (Eosinophil Histologic Scoring System) at week 16.[31] Reduction in symptoms was evaluated using the patient's global assessment of disease severity score, clinician's global assessment of disease severity, Dysphagia Symptom Diary (DSD) and Eosinophilic Esophagitis Activity Index (EesAI) PRO.[31] The patient's global assessment of disease severity score showed a statistically significant mean reduction at week 16, at the 360 mg dose 2.01 ± 1.68 and 2.8 ± 2.71.[31] The mean reduction in the clinician's global assessment of disease severity score was statistically significant for both doses at week 16. Neither the EesAI score nor the DSD showed a statistically significant improvement at week 16 when compared to placebo.[31]

The study then proceeded with subgroup analysis of patients with steroid refractory EoE and showed statistically significant mean reductions in esophageal eosinophil count at week 16 at both doses (103.53 ± 89.166, $P=$.0001 for the 180 mg dose [n = 14] and 130.12 ±± 73.993, $P\leq$.0001 for the 360 mg dose doses[n = 17]).[31] The EesAI PRO score showed a statistically significant improvement for the 360 mg dose ($P=$.0393) but not for the 180 mg dose.[31] DSD scores for both doses did not show a statistically significant change.[31] Patients showed statistically significant improvement in the endoscopic score (at all esophageal locations), EREFS, and histologic EoEHSS scores.[31]

Patients of the initial phase 2 trial were then given the option to enroll in a phase 3 open-label LTE over a 52-week period. Eighty six patients continued into the phase 3 trial; 28 patients were on the 180 mg dose, 29 on the 360 mg dose and 29 were on placebo.[32] The phase 3 trial administered the 360 mg to all patients on a weekly basis with outcomes evaluated for the 3 groups. Cendakimab showed a drop in the esophageal eosinophil count by week 12 of the LTE for patients previously on placebo.[32] Eosinophil levels became comparable to patients on Cendakimab at either dose, and this response was maintained until week 52 of the LTE.[32] The number of patients showing a drop in peak esophageal eosinophil count to less than 15 per HPF increased at week 52 compared to week 12 of the LTE. The group previously on placebo showed a 28.5% increase in the number of responders at week 52 compared to week 12, a 20.3% increase was recorded for the group previously on 180 mg, and there was a 14.7% increase in the group previously on 360 mg.[32] The EREFS score over all esophageal locations decreased in both the group previously on placebo and patients receiving the active drug all along. At week 52 of the LTE, the mean change in EREFS score was greatest in the group previously on placebo (−5) followed by the group previously on 360 mg (−2.9), and the smallest change was seen in patient previously receiving the 180 mg (−1.3).[32] Histologically, at the 52 week mark, the EoEHSS grade scores showed a mean change of −21.5 for the group previously on placebo, −2.9 for the group previously on 180 mg, and 2.1 for the 360 mg group.[32] The EoEHSS stage scores similarly showed a drop in the mean EoEHSS stage score for both subjects previously on placebo or 180 mg at the 52 week mark (−20.8 and −1.9), although this was not seen for patients who were previously on the 360 mg dose (3.5).[32] The study did not show differences in outcomes in patients that were identified as steroid refractory versus those who were not.[32] The most common side effects were upper respiratory tract infection (21%) and nasopharyngitis (14%).[32] Currently, a Phase 3, multicenter, multinational, randomized, double-blind, placebo-controlled study is underway evaluating the efficacy and safety of cendakimab in patients 12 to 75 years of age.[33]

Anti-siglec-8: lirentelimab

Siglec-8 is a surface receptor expressed on the surface of mature eosinophils, and crosslinking of the receptor leads to cell death.[34] AK002 (Lirentelimab) is a humanized IgG1 anti siglec-8 monoclonal antibody that has been shown to promote natural killer cell-mediated antibody-dependent apoptosis of eosinophils.[34] The efficacy of AK002 for the treatment of patients with eosinophilic gastritis and eosinophilic duodenitis was evaluated in the ENIGMA trial (phase 2) and ENIGMA 2 trial (phase 3) on 59 adult patients (18–80 years).[34]

The ENIGMA trial was a dose finding study were AK002 was assessed at low (0.3, 1, 1, and 1 mg per kilogram of body weight) and high-dose AK002 (0.3, 1, 3, and 3 mg per kilogram) compared to placebo.[34] Doses were given every month for a total of 4 months.[34] AK002 showed a bigger mean percentage drop in the number of gastrointestinal eosinophils compared to the placebo group.[34] This was seen in both the intention-to-treat analysis (86% reduction in the combined low and high dose compared to 9% in the placebo group) and the prespecified per-protocol analysis (95% reduction in the combined AK002 groups compared to 10% in the placebo group.)[34] In terms of histologic efficacy, AK002 at both doses showed a statistically significant eosinophilic response of lower than 30 eosinophils per HPF in 95% of the patients in the treatment group (95% CI, 83–99) compared to 15% in the placebo group (95% CI 3–38).[34] A total of 95% of the patients in the treatment arm had less than 6 eosinophils per HPF at the end of treatment and 85% had 0 or 1 eosinophils per HPF compared to 0% of the patients on placebo for both these analysis groups.[34] The patients were also analyzed in regard to improvement of associated esophageal eosinophilia; 93% of the patients in the treatment group showed esophageal histologic remission (≤6 eosinophils per high-power field) compared to 0% in the placebo group.[34] Patients also showed similar trends in mean total symptom scores, with patients in the treatment group showing a greater decrease compared to placebo, which was statistically significant in the high-dose protocol but not statistically significant in the low-dose compared to placebo.[34] Infusion-related reactions was the most common adverse event in patients on AK002 (60%). One patient in the high-dose AK002 group had a grade 4 infusion reaction necessitating withdrawal of the participant from the trial.[34] It is important to note that transient lymphopenia after drug infusion was detected in 86% of the patients in the treatment arms and in 47% of those on placebo.[34] Antidrug antibodies were detected in 2 patients (10%) on high-dose AK002, 2 patients (9%) on low-dose AK002, and 2 patients (9%) on placebo.[34] This trial was followed by a 52 -week open label extension study that recruited 58 of the 59 patients from the ENIGMA study.[35] The study showed a 68% reduction of mean total symptoms score in the intervention group, and 94% of the subjects were able to show histologic remission defined as $\leq$ 4 eosinophils in the stomach and/or $\leq$15 eosinophils in the duodenum.[35]

The ENIGMA 2 trial was a 24 -week trial evaluating AK002 in 3 groups; Arm A received 1.0 mg/kg of AK002 for the first month, followed by 5 doses of 3.0 mg/kg given monthly, Arm B received monthly 1.0 mg/kg of AK002, and Arm C was placebo.[36] The trial showed a statistically significant improvement in terms of histologic endpoints as 84.6% of the patients in the combined treatment group showed a decrease to $\leq$4 eosinophils per HPF in the stomach and/or $\leq$15 eosinophils/hpf in the duodenum, compared to 4.5% in the placebo group (P<.0001).[36] The study did not reach statistical significance in regard to symptomatic endpoints, DSQ was the measure used to evaluate symptoms. Absolute mean change in total symptom score (TSS) in the combined dose AK002 groups showed a -10 point change compared to -11.5 in the placebo group ($P = .343$).[36]

Data on EoE from the ENIGMA trial prompted the evaluation of AK002 as a viable option for the treatment of EoE. The KRYPTOS study is a phase 2/3 Multicenter, Randomized, Double-Blind, Placebo-Controlled 24 -week Study on adolescent and adult patients (12–80 years) with EoE.[37] Patients were randomized to receive 6 monthly doses of 1 mg/kg or 3 mg/kg (this group received an initial dose of 1 mg/kg followed by 5 monthly doses of 3 mg/kg of AK002) or placebo.[37] Results were comparable to outcomes from the ENIGMA2 study where patients did not show a statistically significant improvement in DSQ (-11.9 in the 1 mg/kg group $P = .2470$; -17.4 in the 3 mg/kg group $P = .2372$).[37] The study did show a statistically significant decrease (P<.0001) in peak esophageal intraepithelial eosinophil count from baseline in both the 1 mg/kg group (-98.9) and the 3 mg/kg group (-99.6) compared to placebo (-3.1).[37] Patients also showed a statistically significant decrease in peak esophageal intraepithelial eosinophil count at week 24 at different eosinophil targets, namely $\leq$1, $\leq$ 6, and $\leq$15 eosinophils.[37] A total of 88.2% of the patients receiving the 1 mg/kg and 84.6% of the patients receiving the 3 mg/kg showed $\leq$1 esophageal intraepithelial eosinophil compared to placebo (4.3%).[37] A total of 92.5% of the patients receiving the 1 mg/kg and 87.9% of the patients receiving the 3 mg/kg showed <15 esophageal intraepithelial eosinophil compared to placebo (15.2%).[37] Decrease in EREFS score at week 24 compared to baseline was not statistically significant at either drug dose.[37]

Vedolizumab

Vedolizumab has been evaluated in the treatment of eosinophilic gastroenteritis. Vedolizumab is used in the treatment of inflammatory bowel disease (IBD). It targets $\alpha4\beta7$ integrin and has been shown to block migration of T cells to the gastrointestinal tract.[38] It has been hypothesized that $\alpha4\beta7$ integrin may also play a role in eosinophil migration to the gastrointestinal tract in IBD;[38] therefore, blocking it with vedolizumab could be a viable treatment option for eosinophilic gastroenteritis. This was investigated in 2 studies, the first by Kim and colleagues investigated the therapeutic effect of vedolizumab on 5 adult patients with eosinophilic gastritis and/or gastroenteritis who have failed conventional treatments including oral steroids.[38] Two months after treatment, 3 out of 5 of the patients reported symptom improvement and 2 patients had normal gastric and small intestinal biopsies.[38] None of the patients showed improvement in gross endoscopic findings.[38] Grandinetti and colleagues evaluated the efficacy of vedolizumab in 4 patients with eosinophilic gastroenteritis who did not respond to corticosteroids and/or anti-TNF treatment.[39] Vedolizumab was used in a compassionate manner, and the treatment was successful in 3 out of 4 of the patients with patients showing partial improvement in clinical symptoms.[39] The patients were also able to continue vedolizumab over an extended duration of time, up to 35 months in one of the patients.[39]

SUMMARY

The advent of biologic therapies has extended more potential treatment options in the management of patients with eosinophilic gastrointestinal disorders. Dupilumab is the only biologic that has demonstrated improvement in both endoscopic and histologic endpoints as well as improvement in patient reported symptoms. It is also the only biologic that is FDA approved in the treatment of both pediatric and adult patients with EoE. The use of other biologics in EoE seems to have variable outcomes in regard to endoscopic and histologic endpoints but none showed improvement in patient-reported symptoms. Anti Il-5 monoclonal antibodies, mepolizumab and reslizumab, demonstrated decrease in esophageal eosinophil counts that did not translate in improvement in patient symptoms. Benralizumab was not a successful treatment choice for EoE and failed to meet study endpoints. Similarly, omalizumab did not show improvement in eosinophilic esophageal count or improvement in symptoms. The anti-IL13 cendakimab showed significant improvement in both histologic score and endoscopic endpoints, including peak eosinophil counts. As seen with anti-IL-5 antibodies, these improvements did not reflect on patient-reported symptoms, as there was no improvement in questionnaire scores compared to placebo. The phase 2 trial of cendakimab commented on the improvement of clinician's global assessment of disease severity score in the treatment group compared to placebo. The anti Siglec-8 antibody, lirentelimab, did not show improvement in patient-reported outcome or endoscopic reference score, but it did show a significant decrease in peak esophageal eosinophil count.

Several biologics have also been investigated in EoG/EoN, with lirentelimab (AK002) being the one most rigorously studied. Lirentelimab showed improvement in histology, endoscopic findings as well as symptom improvement. The anti-IL-13 agent QAX576 did not show a statistically significant drop in peak eosinophil count but did show a statistically significant decrease in mean eosinophil count and in dysphagia. Omalizumab in EoG and EoN did not show improvement in endoscopic disease features. Vedolizumab has been evaluated in the treatment of EoG and EoN in a compassionate manner in patients who have failed typical therapies. The number of patients in the 2 studies on vedolizumab was too small to make any generalizable conclusions, but it did show some improvement of symptoms, and endoscopic and histologic outcomes in some of the patients.

Moving forward, ongoing research efforts aimed at optimizing treatment strategies, identifying predictive biomarkers, and expanding the therapeutic options will be crucial. Ultimately, the integration of biologics into the treatment paradigm represents a promising frontier in eosinophilic gastrointestinal disorders, offering personalized and targeted approaches to disease management.

CLINICS CARE POINTS

- EGIDs encompass a group of disorders characterized by an abnormal accumulation of eosinophils in various parts of the gastrointestinal tract.
- Biologics are an emerging and promising form of treatment for EGIDs.

Dupilumab is the only FDA-approved biologic drug in both adult and pediatric in the treatment of EoE. It has shown improvement in both histology and patient-reported symptoms for EoE.

- More rigorous studies are needed to determine the role of biologics in EGIDs other the EoE.
- No biologics have been investigated in the treatment of eosinophilic colitis.

DISCLOSURES

The authors have nothing to disclose.

REFERENCES

1. D'Alessandro A, Esposito D, Pesce M, et al. Eosinophilic esophagitis: From pathophysiology to treatment. World J Gastrointest Pathophysiol 2015;6(4):150–8.
2. Navarro P, Arias Á, Arias-González L, et al. Systematic review with meta-analysis: the growing incidence and prevalence of eosinophilic oesophagitis in children and adults in population-based studies. Aliment Pharmacol Ther 2019;49(9):1116–25.
3. Lipowska AM, Kavitt RT. Demographic Features of Eosinophilic Esophagitis. Gastrointest Endosc Clin N Am 2018;28(1):27–33.
4. Hirano I, Moy N, Heckman MG, et al. Endoscopic assessment of the oesophageal features of eosinophilic oesophagitis: validation of a novel classification and grading system. Gut 2013;62(4):489–95.
5. Spergel JM, Dellon ES, Liacouras CA, et al. Summary of the updated international consensus diagnostic criteria for eosinophilic esophagitis: AGREE conference. Ann Allergy Asthma Immunol 2018;121(3):281–4.
6. Collins MH, Martin LJ, Alexander ES, et al. Newly developed and validated eosinophilic esophagitis histology scoring system and evidence that it outperforms peak eosinophil count for disease diagnosis and monitoring. Dis Esophagus 2017;30(3):1–8.
7. Clayton F, Fang JC, Gleich GJ, et al. Eosinophilic esophagitis in adults is associated with IgG4 and not mediated by IgE. Gastroenterology 2014;147(3):602–9.
8. Foroughi S, Foster B, Kim N, et al. Anti-IgE treatment of eosinophil-associated gastrointestinal disorders. J Allergy Clin Immunol 2007;120(3):594–601.
9. Khokhar D, Marella S, Idelman G, et al. Eosinophilic esophagitis: Immune mechanisms and therapeutic targets. Clin Exp Allergy 2022;52(10):1142–56.
10. Ishimura N, Okimoto E, Shibagaki K, et al. Similarity and difference in the characteristics of eosinophilic esophagitis between Western countries and Japan. Dig Endosc 2021;33(5):708–19.
11. Arias Á, Lucendo AJ. Molecular basis and cellular mechanisms of eosinophilic esophagitis for the clinical practice. Expert Rev Gastroenterol Hepatol 2019;13(2):99–117.
12. Visaggi P, Ghisa M, Marabotto E, et al. Esophageal dysmotility in patients with eosinophilic esophagitis: pathogenesis, assessment tools, manometric characteristics, and clinical implications. Esophagus 2023;20(1):29–38.
13. Gómez-Aldana A, Jaramillo-Santos M, Delgado A, et al. Eosinophilic esophagitis: Current concepts in diagnosis and treatment. World J Gastroenterol 2019;25(32):4598–613.
14. Dellon ES, Gonsalves N, Hirano I, et al. ACG clinical guideline: Evidenced based approach to the diagnosis and management of esophageal eosinophilia and eosinophilic esophagitis (EoE). Am J Gastroenterol 2013;108(5):679–92, quiz 693.

15. Straumann A, Conus S, Grzonka P, et al. Anti-interleukin-5 antibody treatment (mepolizumab) in active eosinophilic oesophagitis: a randomised, placebo-controlled, double-blind trial. Gut 2010;59(1):21–30.
16. Spergel JM, Rothenberg ME, Collins MH, et al. Reslizumab in children and adolescents with eosinophilic esophagitis: results of a double-blind, randomized, placebo-controlled trial. J Allergy Clin Immunol 2012;129(2):456–63, 463.e1-3.
17. Ghazi A, Trikha A, Calhoun WJ. Benralizumab–a humanized mAb to IL-5Rα with enhanced antibody-dependent cell-mediated cytotoxicity–a novel approach for the treatment of asthma. Expet Opin Biol Ther 2012;12(1):113–8.
18. A Study of Benralizumab in Patients With Eosinophilic Esophagitis (MESSINA). 2023. Available at: https://clinicaltrials.gov/study/NCT04543409?cond=Eosinophilic%20 Gastroenteritis&intr=Benralizumab&rank=3.
19. Kliewer KL, Murray-Petzold C, Collins MH, et al. Benralizumab for eosinophilic gastritis: a single-site, randomised, double-blind, placebo-controlled, phase 2 trial. Lancet Gastroenterol Hepatol 2023;8(9):803–15.
20. Efficacy and Safety of Benralizumab in Patients With Eosinophilic Gastritis and/or Gastroenteritis (The HUDSON GI Study) (HUDSON GI). NCT05251909.
21. Foster B, Foroughi S, Yin Y, et al. Effect of anti-IgE therapy on food allergen specific T cell responses in eosinophil associated gastrointestinal disorders. Clin Mol Allergy 2011;9(1):7.
22. Loizou D, Enav B, Komlodi-Pasztor E, et al. A pilot study of omalizumab in eosinophilic esophagitis. PLoS One 2015;10(3):e0113483.
23. Hirano I, Dellon ES, Hamilton JD, et al. Efficacy of Dupilumab in a Phase 2 Randomized Trial of Adults With Active Eosinophilic Esophagitis. Gastroenterology 2020;158(1):111–22.e10.
24. Dellon ES, Spergel JM. Biologics in eosinophilic gastrointestinal diseases. Ann Allergy Asthma Immunol 2023;130(1):21–7.
25. Dellon ES, Rothenberg ME, Collins MH, et al. Dupilumab in Adults and Adolescents with Eosinophilic Esophagitis. N Engl J Med 2022;387(25):2317–30.
26. Rothenberg ME, Dellon ES, Collins MH, et al. Efficacy and safety of dupilumab up to 52 weeks in adults and adolescents with eosinophilic oesophagitis (LIBERTY EoE TREET study): a multicentre, double-blind, randomised, placebo-controlled, phase 3 trial. Lancet Gastroenterol Hepatol 2023;8(11):990–1004.
27. Chehade M, Dellon E, Spergel J, et al. Dupilumab Improves Histologic And Endoscopic Outcomes In Children Aged 1 To <12 Years With Eosinophilic Esophagitis (EoE): 52-Week Results From The Phase 3 EoE KIDS Trial. J Allergy Clin Immunol 2024;153(2, Supplement):AB266.
28. O'Shea KM, Aceves SS, Dellon ES, et al. Pathophysiology of Eosinophilic Esophagitis. Gastroenterology 2018;154(2):333–45.
29. Shoda T, Wen T, Caldwell JM, et al. Molecular, endoscopic, histologic, and circulating biomarker-based diagnosis of eosinophilic gastritis: Multi-site study. J Allergy Clin Immunol 2020;145(1):255–69.
30. Rothenberg ME, Wen T, Greenberg A, et al. Intravenous anti-IL-13 mAb QAX576 for the treatment of eosinophilic esophagitis. J Allergy Clin Immunol 2015;135(2): 500–7.
31. Hirano I, Collins MH, Assouline-Dayan Y, et al. RPC4046, a Monoclonal Antibody Against IL13, Reduces Histologic and Endoscopic Activity in Patients With Eosinophilic Esophagitis. Gastroenterology 2019;156(3):592–603.e10.
32. Dellon ES, Collins MH, Rothenberg ME, et al. Long-term Efficacy and Tolerability of RPC4046 in an Open-Label Extension Trial of Patients With Eosinophilic Esophagitis. Clin Gastroenterol Hepatol 2021;19(3):473–83.e17.

33. A Study to Evaluate the Efficacy and Safety of CC-93538 in Adult and Adolescent Participants With Eosinophilic Esophagitis. NCT04753697.
34. Dellon ES, Peterson KA, Murray JA, et al. Anti-Siglec-8 Antibody for Eosinophilic Gastritis and Duodenitis. N Engl J Med 2020;383(17):1624–34.
35. Kathryn A, Peterson JAM, Falk GW, et al. Dellon Interim Results of an Open-label Extension Study of Antolimab, an Anti-Siglec-8 Antibody, for the Treatment of Patients with Eosinophilic Gastritis and/or Eosinophilic Duodenitis (ENIGMA OLE; NCT03664960. Available at: https://www.allakos.com/file.cfm/59/docs/Peterson_et_al_DDW_May_2020.pdf.
36. A Study to Assess AK002 in Eosinophilic Gastritis and/or Eosinophilic Duodenitis (Formerly Referred to as Eosinophilic Gastroenteritis) (ENIGMA 2). NCT04322604. Available at: https://clinicaltrials.gov/study/NCT04322604?tab=results.
37. A Study of Lirentelimab (AK002) in Patients With Active Eosinophilic Esophagitis (KRYPTOS). NCT04322708. Available at: https://classic.clinicaltrials.gov/ct2/show/results/NCT04322708.
38. Kim HP, Reed CC, Herfarth HH, et al. Vedolizumab Treatment May Reduce Steroid Burden and Improve Histology in Patients With Eosinophilic Gastroenteritis. Clin Gastroenterol Hepatol 2018;16(12):1992–4.
39. Grandinetti T, Biedermann L, Bussmann C, et al. Eosinophilic Gastroenteritis: Clinical Manifestation, Natural Course, and Evaluation of Treatment with Corticosteroids and Vedolizumab. Dig Dis Sci 2019;64(8):2231–41.

Biologics in Hypereosinophilic Syndrome and Eosinophilic Granulomatosis with Polyangiitis

Ejiofor Ezekwe, MD, PhD[a], Andrew L. Weskamp, DO[b,1],
Luke M. Pittman, MD[c], Amy D. Klion, MD[a,*]

KEYWORDS

- Eosinophilia • Hypereosinophilic syndrome
- Eosinophilic granulomatosis with polyangiitis • Mepolizumab • Benralizumab
- Dupilumab • Reslizumab • Biologic therapy

KEY POINTS

- Hypereosinophilic syndrome (HES) and eosinophilic granulomatosis with polyangiitis (EGPA) are complex disorders defined by blood and tissue eosinophilia and heterogeneous clinical manifestations.
- Biologics that directly or indirectly target eosinophils have provided new avenues for treatment, improving outcomes, and decreasing toxicity.
- Eosinophil-targeted therapies are the best studied biologics for HES and EGPA, are well-tolerated, and offer significant clinical benefit for many patients.

DEFINITIONS

Although the term "hypereosinophilic syndromes" (HES) was coined by Hardy and Anderson in 1968,[1] the first case definition for "idiopathic" HES was not proposed until 7 years later by Chusid, Dale, West, and Wolff.[2] In agreement with prior authors, they noted a "continuum of hypereosinophilic disease" with varied clinical manifestations that could be indistinguishable from those in patients with hypereosinophilic disorders of known etiology. These considerations together with the availability of eosinophil-

[a] Human Eosinophil Section, Laboratory of Parasitic Diseases, National Institute of Allergy and Infectious Diseases, National Institutes of Health, Building 4, Room B1-28, 4 Memorial Drive, Bethesda, MD 20892, USA; [b] National Capital Consortium Allergy & Immunology ellowship, Department of Medicine, Allergy & Immunology Service, Walter Reed National Military Medical Center, Bethesda, MD, USA; [c] National Capital Consortium Allergy & Immunology ellowship, Department of Medicine, Allergy & Immunology Service, Walter Reed National Military Medical Center, 8300 Wisconsin Avenue, Apartment 632, Bethesda, MD 20814, USA
[1] Present address: 2570 West Canyonwood Court, Nixa, MO 65714.
* Corresponding author.
E-mail address: amy.klion@nih.gov

Immunol Allergy Clin N Am 44 (2024) 629–644
https://doi.org/10.1016/j.iac.2024.07.003
0889-8561/24/Published by Elsevier Inc.
immunology.theclinics.com

targeted therapeutics prompted the development and refinement of a consensus definition and classification system for all patients with marked peripheral eosinophilia and eosinophil-related disease manifestations.[3] Whereas this umbrella definition of HES includes eosinophilic myeloid neoplasms and secondary causes of HES, such as helminth infections and drug hypersensitivity reactions, definitive treatment of these conditions is typically directed at the underlying cause rather than the eosinophilia and data on biologics is sparse. Consequently, this review will exclude myeloid and associated forms of HES, recognizing that there may be a role for eosinophil-lowering biologics in some cases.

Eosinophilic granulomatosis with polyangiitis (EGPA) was first reported in 1951 by Churg and Strauss who described necrotizing granulomatous eosinophilic vasculitis of small to medium arteries in autopsy specimens from 13 patients with polyarteritis nodosa, asthma, sinusitis, and eosinophilia.[4] Over the next several decades, it became apparent that not all patients with what was then called Churg-Strauss syndrome had the classic histopathologic findings. Moreover, definitive documentation of vasculitis was precluded in many patients by the lack of easily accessible tissue and/ or treatment with glucocorticoids at the time of presentation. In 1984, Lanham and colleagues described a characteristic temporal progression of clinical manifestations beginning with a prodromal phase of asthma and/or chronic rhinosinusitis (CRS) followed by an eosinophilic phase indistinguishable from HES and ultimately the onset of systemic vasculitis.[5] These clinical findings became the basis for the first consensus definition of EGPA proposed by the American College of Rheumatology (ACR) in 1990 to distinguish between EGPA and other systemic vasculitides in research studies.[6] In 2022, new criteria were developed and validated by the ACR and the European Alliance of Associations for Rheumatology (EULAR).[7] These criteria include the absence of antibodies suggestive of other vasculitides but not the presence of perinuclear anti-neutrophil cytoplasmic antibodies (pANCA)/anti-myeloperoxidase antibodies identified in 40% to 50% of patients with EGPA. While these criteria are highly sensitive and specific for the identification of patients with EGPA among patients with small and medium vessel vasculitis, as with the prior criteria, characteristic histopathology is neither required nor sufficient for a diagnosis of EGPA and overlap with other HES is highlighted but not addressed.

As eluded to aforementioned context, HES can be clinically difficult to distinguish from EGPA. Biomarkers, other than pANCA/anti-myeloperoxidase antibodies, have also proven unhelpful in this regard.[8,9] Further complicating the picture is the fact that eosinophilia, sometimes marked, is a frequent feature of many common diagnoses, including asthma, CRS, and atopic dermatitis, that may be part of HES (ie, hypereosinophilia is driving the clinical manifestations) or a concomitant condition. This overlap between HES and EGPA is highlighted by the similarities in the criteria used to define these syndromes in recent clinical trials of biologics.[10–12] Although this has generally proven to be a successful strategy, some patients with EGPA (eg, those with detectable pANCA) or HES (eg, those with lymphocytic variant) may benefit from biologics that target non-eosinophil pathways or cells. This review will focus on currently available biologics used to treat HES and/or EGPA, including those that are approved for other indications, and a pragmatic approach to their use in these 2 rare disorders.

EOSINOPHIL-TARGETED BIOLOGICS

Interleukin-5 (IL-5) plays a key role in the survival, differentiation, and activation of eosinophils. Thus, the IL-5/IL-5 receptor alpha (IL-5RA) axis is an attractive target for the treatment of both HES and EGPA. Three monoclonal antibodies that bind IL-5 (mepolizumab and reslizumab) or its receptor (benralizumab) are commercially available, and a third (depemokimab, a long-acting anti-IL-5 monoclonal antibody dosed every 6 months), is in clinical trials for the treatment of HES and EGPA (**Tables 1–3**). Rapid and near complete depletion of blood eosinophils has been reported in response to therapies that bind IL-5 in most patients across clinical indications, but they generally lead to only a moderate (50%–60%) reduction in tissue eosinophilia. In contrast, benralizumab has been shown to deplete eosinophils to undetectable (or nearly undetectable) levels in the blood, tissue, and bone marrow.

Mepolizumab was the first therapy used in a placebo-controlled trial in patients with HES[13] and is currently the only biologic with regulatory approval for the treatment of this syndrome. In a landmark phase 2 study, mepolizumab (750 mg iv monthly) was well-tolerated and effective as a glucocorticoid-sparing agent in patients with *PDFGRA*-negative glucocorticoid-responsive HES,[13] albeit less effective at reducing eosinophilia in patients with lymphocytic variant HES.[14] In the subsequent open-label extension, 62 of 78 patients were prednisone-free for greater than or equal to 12 weeks on mepolizumab monotherapy.[15] High-dose mepolizumab (750 mg iv monthly) has also been used successfully for the treatment of patients with life-threatening, treatment-refractory disease with complete and partial response rates of 57% and 20%, respectively.[16]

The phase III trial that led to the approval of mepolizumab for the treatment of non-myeloid HES in patients greater than or equal to 12 years of age demonstrated a 50% reduction in clinical flares over a 32 week period in patients with steroid-responsive *PDGFRA*-negative HES receiving mepolizumab (300 mg subcutaneously monthly) compared to patients in the placebo arm.[12] This effect was irrespective of the baseline eosinophil count, and most patients had undetectable serum IL-5 levels at baseline.[17] As in prior trials, no safety signals were identified. Six symptom domains (abdominal pain/bloating, breathing problems, chills/sweats, muscle/joint pain, nasal/sinus symptoms, and skin symptoms) were assessed using a HES daily symptom questionnaire. In all domains except for skin, patients reported significant improvement on mepolizumab therapy over 32 weeks.[18]

Mepolizumab is also effective for the treatment of EGPA and was approved for this indication in adults in 2017. After several open-label trials showed a steroid-sparing effect of mepolizumab (750 mg iv monthly) in patients with EGPA,[19,20] a phase 3 randomized, placebo-controlled trial of mepolizumab (300 mg sc monthly) was conducted in patients with relapsing or refractory EGPA. Mepolizumab therapy led to significantly more weeks of accrued remission (28% vs 3%) and a significantly higher proportion of patients in remission at weeks 36 and 48 (32% vs 3%) compared to placebo.[11] Post hoc analyses demonstrated no impact of immunosuppressive therapy, EGPA duration, or clinical evidence of a vasculitis phenotype on response rates,[21,22] and clinical benefit was achieved in 78% to 87% of patients receiving mepolizumab using composite clinical endpoints (compared to 32%–52% in the placebo group; $P<.001$).[23]

Prospective studies of the anti-IL-5 antibody, reslizumab in HES and EGPA have been limited to small open-label case series.[24,25] However, its mechanism of action is identical to that of mepolizumab, and the available data suggest that it is effective in the treatment of patients with these syndromes. Currently approved for the treatment of severe asthma in adult patients with an eosinophilic phenotype,[26] reslizumab is administered intravenously using weight-based dosing, a potential advantage for some patients.

Benralizumab is an afucosylated antibody that depletes IL-5RA-bearing cells, of which eosinophils are the major constituent, through enhanced antibody-dependent cell-mediated cytotoxicity.[27] Approved in 2017 for the treatment of severe eosinophilic asthma, benralizumab has shown efficacy in clinical trials in both HES and EGPA. In a placebo-controlled phase 2 trial of benralizumab (30 mg sc monthly) in 20 patients

Table 1
Research definitions of hypereosinophilic syndrome and eosinophilic granulomatosis with polyangiitis

HES			EGPA		
Year	Criteria	Ref	Year	Criteria	Ref
1975	1. A persistent eosinophilia of 1500 eosinophils/mm³ for longer than 6 mo, or death before 6 mo associated with signs and symptoms of hypereosinophilic disease 2. A lack of evidence for parasitic, allergic, or other known causes of eosinophilia 3. Presumptive signs and symptoms of organ involvement	Chusid Lanham et al,[2] 1975	1984	1. Asthma 2. Peak peripheral blood eosinophil count in excess of 1500/mm3 3. Systemic vasculitis involving 2 or mor extrapulmonary organs	Lanham et al,[5] 1984
2012	1. >1500 eosinophils/mm3 on 2 examinations (interval ≥1 mo or immediately in the case of life-threatening disease) and/or tissue HE defined by the following: a) percentage of eosinophils in BM section exceeds 20% of all nucleated cells and/or b) pathologist is of the opinion that tissue infiltration by eosinophils is extensive and/or c) Marked deposition of eosinophil granule proteins is found (in the absence or presence of major tissue infiltration by eosinophils). 2. Organ damage and/or dysfunction attributable to tissue HES 3. Exclusion of other disorders of conditions as major reason for. organ damage	a	1990	At least 4 of the following criteria in a patient with vasculitis: 1. Asthma 2. Eosinophilia >10% 3. Neuropathy, mono or poly 4. Pulmonary infiltrates, non-fixed 5. Paranasal sinus abnormality 6. Extravascular eosinophils	Masi Lanham et al,[6] 1990

Valent et al.,[3] 2023	Grayson et al.,[7] 2022
2023 1. ≥1500 eosinophils/mm³ on at least two occasions (interval ≥2 wk)[b] 2. Organ damage and/or dysfunction attributable to tissue HE 3. Exclusion of other disorders of conditions as a major reason for organ damage	2022 A score of ≥6 in a patient with small or medium vessel vasculitis: Obstructive airway disease +3 Nasal polyps +3 Mononeuritis multiplex +1 Blood eosinophil ≥1000/mm³ +5 Extravascular eosinophil-predominant inflammation on biopsy +2 Positive test for pANCA or antiproteinase 3 antibodies −3 Hematuria −1

Phase 3 Clinical Trial Definition for HES	Phase 3 Clinical Trial Definition for EGPA
1. >1500 eosinophils/mm3 on 2 examinations (interval ≥1 mo or immediately in the case of life-threatening disease) 2. Organ damage and/or dysfunction attributable to tissue HES 3. Exclusion of other disorders of conditions as major reason for organ damage	1. History or presence of: asthma plus eosinophilia 2. Blood eosinophil ≥1000/mm³ and/or >10% of leukocytes 3. At least 2 of the following additional features of EGPA: a biopsy showing histopathologic evidence of eosinophilic vasculitis, or perivascular eosinophilic infiltration, or eosinophil-rich granulomatous inflammation; neuropathy, mono or poly (motor deficit or nerve conduction abnormality); pulmonary infiltrates, non-fixed; sino-nasal abnormality; cardiomyopathy (established by echocardiography or MRI); glomerulonephritis (haematuria, red cell casts, proteinuria); alveolar haemorrhage (by bronchoalveolar lavage); palpable purpura; anti neutrophil cytoplasmic anti-body (ANCA) positive (Myeloperoxidase or proteinease 3)

a Valent P, Klion, AD, Horny, H et al. Contemporary consensus proposal on criteria and classification of eosinophilic disorders and related syndromes. *J Allergy Clin Immunol.* 2012; 130(3):607–612.e9. https://doi.org/10.1016/j.jaci.2012.02.019.

b Tissue restricted HES can be diagnosed when ≥ 1500 eosinophils/mm³ is not present but one of the following is identified: a) the percentage of eosinophils in bone marrow section exceeds 20% of all nucleated cells, and/or b) a pathologist is of the opinion that tissue infiltration by eosinophils is extensive and/or c) marked deposition of eosinophil granule proteins is found (in the absence or presence of tissue infiltration by eosinophils).

Table 2
Biologics and hypereosinophilic syndrome

Biologic	Target	Dose	Boxed Warnings	Trial	n	Primary Endpoint	Outcome	Reference
Mepolizumab	IL-5	300 mg every 4 wk	None	Multicenter, randomized double-blind, placebo controlled, phase 3 trial	108	Proportion of patients with 1 or more flares of disease during study period of 32 wk	Mepolizumab decreased the number of patients experiencing 1 or more flares by 50% compared to placebo (28% vs 56%)	Roufosse et al,[12] 2020
Benralizumab	IL-5R alpha	30 mg every 4 wk	None	Randomized, double-blind, placebo controlled, phase 2 trial	20	Reduction of at least 50% in absolute eosinophil count	90% of patient in the treatment arm vs 30% of participants in the placebo group achieved suppression of blood eosinophils. In the open extension, all 17 patients that had hematological response reported clinical improvement	Kuang et al,[28] 2019
Reslizumab	IL-5	1 mg/kg every 4 wk	Anaphylaxis	Pilot phase 1/2 single-dose study	4	Reduce of eosinophilia and evidence of clincal improvement	Fall in eosinophil counts to normal range in 50% of patient by 48 h with clinical improvement	Klion et al,[25] 2004

Depemokimab	IL-5, long-acting	N/A	N/A	Multicenter, randomized double-blind, placebo controlled, phase 3 trial	120	Frequency of flares	Ongoing	NCT 05534368
Dupilumab	IL-4Rα	N/A	None	Retrospective; no RCTs	9	N/A	6 subjects with I-HES had clinical response; 2 subjects with L-HES did not have clinical response; 1 subject with overlap HES with clinical response	Chen et al,[59] 2022

Biologics that affect eosinophils without data in treatment of HES: tezepelumab, Tralokinumab, Cendakimab, Dectrekumab, Bertilimumab, Itepekimab, Tozorakimab.

Table 3
Biologics and eosinophilic granulomatosis with polyangiitis

Biologic	Target	Dose	Boxed Warnings	Trial	n	Primary Endpoint	Outcome	Reference
Mepolizumab	IL-5	300 mg every 4 wk	None	A multicenter, double blind, parallel group, phase 3 trial	136	1. Total accrued weeks in remission 2. Proportion of participatnts in remission at both weeks 36 and 48	Mepolizumab significantly more accrued week of remission and a higher percentage of participants in remission at noth week 36 and 48	Wechsler et al,[11] 2017
Benralizumab	IL-5R alpha	30 mg every 4 wk	None	Multicenter, double-blind, phase 3, randomized, active-controlled noninferiority trial	140	Remission at weeks 36 and 48	Benralizumab was noninferior to mepolizumab at inducing remission in patient with relapsing or refractory EGPA	Wechsler et al,[10] 2024
Reslizumab	IL-5	3 mg/kg	Anaphylaxis	Open-label pilot study	10	Oral corticosteroid dose, adverse events, exacerbations, symptom control, disease activity, blood markers, and lung function	Significant reduction in daily oral corticosteroid use (Mean prednisone dose from 17.5 mg to 8.12 mg)	Manka et al,[24] 2021
Depemokimab	IL-5, long-acting	N/A	N/A	Multicenter, randomized double-blind, placebo controlled, phase 3 trial vs mepolizumab	160	Remission at 36 and 52 wk	Ongoing	NCT 05263934
Dupilumab	IL-4Rα	Variable	None	Multicenter retrospective; no RCTs	51	N/A	65% had positive response; 35% had	Molina et al,[48] 2023

Tezepelumab	TSLP	N/A	N/A	Phase 2b, multicenter, randomized, double-blinded, placebo-controlled study	66	Clinical remission	AE; 67% had increase in AEC	Ongoing	NCT 06230354
Rituximab	CD-20	Variable	Fatal infusion reactions; tumor lysis syndrome; severe mucocutaneous reactions; PML	Single-center retrospective; no RCTs	69	N/A	Improvement in 76.8% of patients at 6 mo, 82.8% at 12 mo and in 93.2% by 24 mo; relapses in 54% by 24 mo	N/A	Teixeira et al,[64] 2019

Biologics that affect eosinophils without data in treatment of EGPA: tralokinumab, Cendakimab, Dectrekumab, Bertilimumab, Itepekimab, Tozorakimab.

with *PDGFRA*-negative treatment-refractory HES, 9/10 patients receiving benralizumab had a greater than 50% reduction in absolute eosinophil count (AEC) at 3 months compared to 3/10 receiving placebo.[28] During the open-label phase of the trial, 17/19 evaluable participants experienced hematologic and clinical improvement that was sustained at 48 weeks in 14 patients[28] and for greater than or equal to 6 years in 10 patients.[29] Of note, both patients with *JAK2* mutations failed to respond, and all 6 patients with lymphocytic variant HES relapsed after an initial response.[28,29] A phase 3 trial of benralizumab in HES is ongoing (NCT04191304).

After an open-label pilot study of benralizumab in EGPA demonstrated efficacy in 10 patients with a greater than 50% reduction of median prednisone dose and reduction in EGPA flares,[30] a phase 3, placebo-controlled trial comparing benralizumab to mepolizumab was initiated in adults with relapsing or refractory EPGA. Benralizumab was found to be non-inferior to mepolizumab with similar percentages of patients achieving remission at weeks 36 and 48 (59% vs 56%).[10] Other parameters, including adverse events, time to first relapse and reduction in glucocorticoid dose were also comparable between the 2 groups. Based on these results, it seems likely that benralizumab will be approved for use in EGPA.

Lirentelimab is a non-fucosylated antibody to siglec-8 (sialic acid-binding immunoglobulin-like lectin 8), a receptor that is expressed on eosinophils, basophils, and mast cells. It has a similar mechanism of action to benralizumab (ie, induction of antibody-dependent cell cytotoxicity) and has been shown in a placebo-controlled phase 2 trial to deplete eosinophils and basophils in the blood and gastrointestinal tissue of patients with eosinophilic gastritis and duodenitis, including those with peripheral hypereosinophilia.[31,32] Unfortunately, lirentelimab did not meet the primary clinical endpoint in a subsequent phase 3 trial in eosinophilic gastroenteritis (NCT04322708) and is not currently in development for the treatment of these or other hypereosinophilic disorders.

BIOLOGICS THAT INDIRECTLY IMPACT EOSINOPHILS
Eosinophil-Trafficking Interference

Eosinophils are primarily tissue-resident cells that migrate from the bone marrow to the blood and finally the tissue, where they may exert pathologic effects in some individuals. Eosinophil migration to the tissue involves IL-5, chemokines (eotaxins), chemokine receptors (CCR3), and adhesion molecules (VCAM).[33] Interference with any of these may reduce tissue eosinophilia with the potential for concurrent increase in peripheral blood eosinophilia.[34] While no biologics that target eosinophil-trafficking are currently approved for the treatment of HES or EGPA, several are approved for other atopic conditions.[35–39] Biologics in this category target IL-4Ra (dupilumab), IL-13 (tralokinumab, cendakimab, dectrekumab), eotaxin (bertilimumab), and CCR3. Biologics that target IL-5 were discussed previously.

Dupilumab is the best studied and most used biologic that interferes with eosinophil trafficking. It is a fully human monoclonal immunoglobulin (Ig) G4 antibody that blocks IL-4Rα and downstream signaling of both IL-4 and IL-13, thus limiting IgE synthesis, Th2 polarization, and mucus production. IL-4 and 13 are also critical for VCAM-1 expression and production of eotaxin, effects that contribute to dupilumab's inhibition of eosinophil migration into inflamed tissues.[33,34,40] This inhibition commonly results in a mild (300–750 cells/μL) and transient (<6 months) increase in peripheral eosinophil count. Eosinophil-related clinical complications of dupilumab therapy due to secondary hypereosinophilia are uncommon,[34,35] but do occur.[41–43]

Conversely, cases of successful dupilumab treatment of patients with HES or EGPA have been reported,[44–46] and a recent retrospective review of 25 patients with HES and/or EGPA treated with dupilumab with or without a second eosinophil-lowering biologic described a positive clinical response in 82%, although 4/16 patients on dupilumab alone had worsening eosinophilia and associated complications.[47] Another recent study evaluated dupilumab treatment of 51 patients with EGPA who had refractory upper and lower respiratory symptoms on standard treatment. Although 65% of subjects achieved a partial or complete clinical response, 67% of patients experienced worsening eosinophilia, which was associated with an EGPA flare in 41%.[48] Dupilumab has not been used in prospective clinical trials in HES or EGPA to date, and there are no published data on the uses of other agents that interfere with eosinophil-trafficking (ie, anti-IL-13, anti-eotaxin, or anti-CCR3 antibodies) in patients with these disorders.

Upstream Alarmin Interference

Upstream alarmins are innate cytokines secreted by epithelial cells in response to tissue injury, and include IL-25, IL-33, and thymic stromal lymphopoietin (TSLP). Alarmins broadly affect allergic inflammation by promoting differentiation of Th2 lymphocytes via effects on dendritic cells and inducing ILC2 cells to release IL-5 and IL-13. They may also promote Th17 lymphocyte differentiation, resulting in neutrophilic inflammation.[49]

Currently, the only approved biologic that targets alarmins is tezepelumab, a fully human IgG2λ monoclonal antibody that binds TSLP and blocks its interaction with the TSLP receptor. Tezepelumab is approved for the treatment of moderate to severe asthma irrespective of endotype.[50] Whereas no biologics that target upstream alarmins are approved for the treatment of HES or EGPA, tezepelumab is actively being investigated for the treatment of EGPA (NCT06230354). Available clinical data also support a role for IL-25 and IL-33 in the pathogenesis of allergic inflammation[51] and vasculitis,[52] key features of HES and EGPA; however, neither of the IL-33 antibodies currently in clinical trials (itepekimab and tozorakimab) has received regulatory approval for any indication, and there are no ongoing trials of these agents in HES or EGPA.

B-cell Depletion

In contrast to the previously discussed biologics that target allergic inflammation, rituximab is an anti-CD-20 chimeric monoclonal antibody with broad anti-inflammatory activity through depletion of B-cells. It is routinely used for treatment in several hematologic malignancies and autoimmune diseases (ie, rheumatoid arthritis, ANCA-associated vasculitis). There are no randomized, controlled trials evaluating anti-CD-20 monoclonal antibodies for use in EGPA or HES; however, rituximab has been shown to induce and sustain remission in EGPA, especially ANCA-positive disease, in multiple retrospective and 1 small prospective study[53] and is included in the ACR treatment guidelines for severe, active EGPA.[54] Data to support the use of rituximab in HES is limited to a single case report.[55] Caution should be used when using B-cell depleting agents given the risk of humoral immunosuppression, which may persist for extended periods after treatment.[56]

APPROACH TO BIOLOGIC THERAPY

Systemic corticosteroids have served as the historic treatment of HES and EGPA. However, recent availability of targeted biologics has provided new avenues to pursue improved outcomes with decreased toxicity. Mepolizumab is the best studied and only biologic agent with regulatory approval for the treatment of non-myeloid HES. Initial treatment depends on the subtype of disease, severity, and consideration of comorbid conditions.[57,58] Dosing for mepolizumab in HES (and EGPA) is 300 mg subcutaneously monthly (in contrast to the 100 mg monthly dosing approved for asthma and CRSwNP); if treatment failure occurs, an increased dose of 750 mg subcutaneously monthly may be effective, as suggested by the early HES and EGPA trials.[13,15] Reslizumab is an intravenous anti-IL5 option if treatment failure occurs in patients with elevated body mass index, although there are limited data in HES.[25,59]

When initial therapy fails to achieve hematologic remission (AEC <1000 cells/μL) and/ or symptom improvement, off-label use of biologic therapy may be considered. In a multicenter, retrospective study evaluating off-label use of biologics in HES, 27 of 39 patients receiving off-label benralizumab, reslizumab, omalizumab, or dupilumab reported improvement in HES symptoms.[59] As with mepolizumab, patients with lymphocytic variant were less likely to respond than patients with idiopathic or overlap forms of HES. Of note, neither dupilumab nor omalizumab treatment led to hematologic remission in this study, although eosinophil suppression was maintained in 56% of patients.

Multiple groups, including ACR and EULAR, have published recent consensus guidelines for the treatment for EGPA.[54,60] The general approach is the same in all of the guidelines. High-dose systemic glucocorticoids and either cyclophosphamide or rituximab are recommended for acute life-threatening disease. Whether to use rituximab preferentially for ANCA-positive patients remains controversial.[53,54,60] Systemic glucocorticoids with mepolizumab are considered first-line for active, non-severe EGPA. Alternate regimens include glucocorticoids alone, glucocorticoids with immunosuppressive agents (ie, mycophenolate or azathioprine), and glucocorticoids with rituximab. Given the results of the recent non-inferiority trial,[10] benralizumab may soon be an additional option for patients with EGPA.

Since asthma and CRS with nasal polyposis are common manifestations of EGPA (and to a lesser degree HES), biologics approved for the treatment of these conditions are often prescribed. Dupilumab is a tempting option in EGPA since patients often experience severe, uncontrolled sinus symptoms, and dupilumab has been shown in one network analysis to have improved efficacy compared to mepolizumab for this indication.[61] However, dupilumab has been associated with cases of hypereosinophilia and eosinophil-related complications,[41–43,62] and dupilumab efficacy for the treatment of EGPA is mixed.[45–48,59] Theoretically, combination biologic therapy with dupilumab and an eosinophil-lowering biologic could maximize treatment benefit for patients with HES and/or EGPA while limiting potential eosinophil-related adverse events,[47] but current safety and efficacy data are inadequate to advocate this approach. A dual biologic strategy may also be cost-prohibitive for many patients.

Biologic agents in development for the treatment of HES and/or EGPA include depemokimab and tezepelumab. Given the success to date with mepolizumab, it is anticipated that depemokimab will be effective in both HES and EGPA and allow more convenient dosing (every 6 months) and the potential for reduced cost over time. Tezepelumab is an intriguing treatment option, particularly for EGPA, given that it limits both T2 and Th17 inflammation, the latter of which may be prominent in EGPA and is not directly inhibited by currently available biologics.[49,63] As the number of commercially available biologics that directly or indirectly target eosinophilic inflammation continues to increase, good quality clinical trial data upon which to base treatment algorithms are a major unmet need.

CLINICS CARE POINTS

- Mepolizumab is approved for the treatment of both HES and non-severe EGPA and is considered the first-line biologic therapy for these disorders.

- The choice of second-line biologic in the case of mepolizumab treatment failure or intolerance should be based on disease features and comorbid conditions.
- Dupilumab has shown efficacy in improving symptoms in patients with EGPA and HES but should be used with caution due to the risk for eosinophil-related complications.

DISCLOSURE

The authors have nothing to disclose. This work was supported in part by the Division of Intramural Research, NIAID, NIH.

REFERENCES

1. Hardy WR, Anderson RE. The hypereosinophilic syndromes. Ann Intern Med 1968;68(6):1220–9.
2. Chusid MJ, Dale DC, West BC, et al. The hypereosinophilic syndrome: analysis of fourteen cases with review of the literature. Medicine (Baltim) 1975;54(1):1–27.
3. Valent P, Klion AD, Roufosse F, et al. Proposed refined diagnostic criteria and classification of eosinophil disorders and related syndromes. Allergy 2023; 78(1):47–59.
4. Churg J, Strauss L. Allergic granulomatosis, allergic angiitis, and periarteritis nodosa. Am J Pathol 1951;27(2):277–301.
5. Lanham JG, Elkon KB, Pusey CD, et al. Systemic vasculitis with asthma and eosinophilia: a clinical approach to the Churg-Strauss syndrome. Medicine (Baltim) 1984;63(2):65–81.
6. Masi AT, Hunder GG, Lie JT, et al. The American College of Rheumatology 1990 criteria for the classification of Churg-Strauss syndrome (allergic granulomatosis and angiitis). Arthritis Rheum 1990;33(8):1094–100.
7. Grayson PC, Ponte C, Suppiah R, et al. 2022 American College of Rheumatology/European Alliance of Associations for Rheumatology Classification Criteria for Eosinophilic Granulomatosis with Polyangiitis. Ann Rheum Dis 2022;81(3):309–14.
8. Khoury P, Zagallo P, Talar-Williams C, et al. Serum biomarkers are similar in Churg-Strauss syndrome and hypereosinophilic syndrome. Allergy 2012;67(9): 1149–56.
9. Pagnoux C, Nair P, Xi Y, et al. Serum cytokine and chemokine levels in patients with eosinophilic granulomatosis with polyangiitis, hypereosinophilic syndrome, or eosinophilic asthma. Clin Exp Rheumatol 2019;37(Suppl 117):40–4.
10. Wechsler ME, Nair P, Terrier B, et al. Benralizumab versus Mepolizumab for Eosinophilic Granulomatosis with Polyangiitis. N Engl J Med 2024;390(10): 911–21.
11. Wechsler ME, Akuthota P, Jayne D, et al. Mepolizumab or Placebo for Eosinophilic Granulomatosis with Polyangiitis. N Engl J Med 2017;376(20):1921–32.
12. Roufosse F, Kahn J-E, Rothenberg ME, et al. Efficacy and safety of mepolizumab in hypereosinophilic syndrome: A phase III, randomized, placebo-controlled trial. J Allergy Clin Immunol 2020;146(6):1397–405.
13. Rothenberg ME, Klion AD, Roufosse FE, et al. Treatment of patients with the hypereosinophilic syndrome with mepolizumab. N Engl J Med 2008;358(12): 1215–28.
14. Roufosse F, de Lavareille A, Schandené L, et al. Mepolizumab as a corticosteroid-sparing agent in lymphocytic variant hypereosinophilic syndrome. J Allergy Clin Immunol 2010;126(4):828–35.e3.

15. Roufosse FE, Kahn J-E, Gleich GJ, et al. Long-term safety of mepolizumab for the treatment of hypereosinophilic syndromes. J Allergy Clin Immunol 2013;131(2): 461–7.e1.

16. Kuang FL, Fay MP, Ware J, et al. Long-Term Clinical Outcomes of High-Dose Mepolizumab Treatment for Hypereosinophilic Syndrome. J Allergy Clin Immunol Pract 2018;6(5):1518–27.e5.

17. Rothenberg ME, Roufosse F, Faguer S, et al. Mepolizumab Reduces Hypereosinophilic Syndrome Flares Irrespective of Blood Eosinophil Count and Interleukin-5. J Allergy Clin Immunol Pract 2022;10(9):2367–74.e3.

18. Roufosse F, Butterfield J, Steinfeld J, et al. Mepolizumab therapy improves the most bothersome symptoms in patients with hypereosinophilic syndrome. Front Med 2023;10:1035250.

19. Kim S, Marigowda G, Oren E, et al. Mepolizumab as a steroid-sparing treatment option in patients with Churg-Strauss syndrome. J Allergy Clin Immunol 2010; 125(6):1336–43.

20. Moosig F, Gross WL, Herrmann K, et al. Targeting interleukin-5 in refractory and relapsing Churg-Strauss syndrome. Ann Intern Med 2011;155(5):341–3.

21. Jayne DRW, Terrier B, Hellmich B, et al. Mepolizumab has clinical benefits including oral corticosteroid sparing irrespective of baseline EGPA characteristics. ERJ Open Research 2024;10(1). https://doi.org/10.1183/23120541.00509-2023.

22. Terrier B, Jayne DRW, Hellmich B, et al. Clinical benefit of mepolizumab in eosinophilic granulomatosis with polyangiitis for patients with and without a vasculitic phenotype. ACR Open Rheumatol 2023;5(7):354–63.

23. Steinfeld J, Bradford ES, Brown J, et al. Evaluation of clinical benefit from treatment with mepolizumab for patients with eosinophilic granulomatosis with polyangiitis. J Allergy Clin Immunol 2019;143(6):2170–7.

24. Manka LA, Guntur VP, Denson JL, et al. Efficacy and safety of reslizumab in the treatment of eosinophilic granulomatosis with polyangiitis. Ann Allergy Asthma Immunol 2021;126(6):696–701.e1.

25. Klion AD, Law MA, Noel P, et al. Safety and efficacy of the monoclonal anti-interleukin-5 antibody SCH55700 in the treatment of patients with hypereosinophilic syndrome. Blood 2004;103(8):2939–41.

26. Castro M, Zangrilli J, Wechsler ME, et al. Reslizumab for inadequately controlled asthma with elevated blood eosinophil counts: results from two multicentre, parallel, double-blind, randomised, placebo-controlled, phase 3 trials. Lancet Respir Med 2015;3(5):355–66.

27. Kolbeck R, Kozhich A, Koike M, et al. MEDI-563, a humanized anti-IL-5 receptor alpha mAb with enhanced antibody-dependent cell-mediated cytotoxicity function. J Allergy Clin Immunol 2010;125(6):1344–53.e2.

28. Kuang FL, Legrand F, Makiya M, et al. Benralizumab for PDGFRA-Negative Hypereosinophilic Syndrome. N Engl J Med 2019;380(14):1336–46.

29. Kuang FL, Makiya M, Ware J, et al. Long-term Efficacy and Safety of Benralizumab Treatment for PDGFRA-negative Hypereosinophilic Syndrome. J Allergy Clin Immunol 2024;153(2):AB64.

30. Guntur VP, Manka LA, Denson JL, et al. Benralizumab as a Steroid-Sparing Treatment Option in Eosinophilic Granulomatosis with Polyangiitis. J Allergy Clin Immunol Pract 2021;9(3):1186–93.e1.

31. Dellon ES, Peterson KA, Murray JA, et al. Anti-Siglec-8 Antibody for Eosinophilic Gastritis and Duodenitis. N Engl J Med 2020;383(17):1624–34.

32. Youngblood BA, Leung J, Falahati R, et al. Discovery, Function, and Therapeutic Targeting of Siglec-8. Cells 2020;10(1):19.

33. Le Floc'h A, Allinne J, Nagashima K, et al. Dual blockade of IL-4 and IL-13 with dupilumab, an IL-4Rα antibody, is required to broadly inhibit type 2 inflammation. Allergy 2020;75(5):1188–204.

34. Wechsler ME, Klion AD, Paggiaro P, et al. Effect of dupilumab on blood eosinophil counts in patients with asthma, chronic rhinosinusitis with nasal polyps, atopic dermatitis, or eosinophilic esophagitis. J Allergy Clin Immunol Pract 2022; 10(10):2695–709.

35. Castro M, Corren J, Pavord ID, et al. Dupilumab Efficacy and Safety in Moderate-to-Severe Uncontrolled Asthma. N Engl J Med 2018;378(26):2486–96.

36. Bachert C, Han JK, Desrosiers M, et al. Efficacy and safety of dupilumab in patients with severe chronic rhinosinusitis with nasal polyps (LIBERTY NP SINUS-24 and LIBERTY NP SINUS-52): results from two multicentre, randomised, double-blind, placebo-controlled, parallel-group phase 3 trials. Lancet 2019; 394(10209):1638–50.

37. Simpson EL, Bieber T, Guttman-Yassky E, et al. Two Phase 3 Trials of Dupilumab versus Placebo in Atopic Dermatitis. N Engl J Med 2016;375(24):2335–48.

38. Dellon ES, Rothenberg ME, Collins MH, et al. Dupilumab in Adults and Adolescents with Eosinophilic Esophagitis. N Engl J Med 2022;387(25):2317–30.

39. Wollenberg A, Blauvelt A, Guttman-Yassky E, et al. Tralokinumab for moderate-to-severe atopic dermatitis: results from two 52-week, randomized, double-blind, multicentre, placebo-controlled phase III trials (ECZTRA 1 and ECZTRA 2). Br J Dermatol 2021;184(3):437–49.

40. Olaguibel JM, Sastre J, Rodríguez JM, et al. Eosinophilia Induced by Blocking the IL-4/IL-13 Pathway: Potential Mechanisms and Clinical Outcomes. J Investig Allergol Clin Immunol 2022;32(3):165–80.

41. Yamazaki K, Nomizo T, Hatanaka K, et al. Eosinophilic granulomatosis with polyangiitis after treatment with dupilumab. J Allergy Clin Immunol Glob 2022;1(3): 180–2.

42. Kai M, Vion P-A, Boussouar S, et al. Eosinophilic granulomatosis polyangiitis (EGPA) complicated with periaortitis, precipitating role of dupilumab? A case report a review of the literature. RMD Open 2023;9(3). https://doi.org/10.1136/rmdopen-2023-003300.

43. Suzaki I, Tanaka A, Yanai R, et al. Eosinophilic granulomatosis with polyangiitis developed after dupilumab administration in patients with eosinophilic chronic rhinosinusitis and asthma: a case report. BMC Pulm Med 2023;23(1):130.

44. Du X, Chen Y, Chang J, et al. Dupilumab as a novel steroid-sparing treatment for hypereosinophilic syndrome. JAAD Case Reports 2022;29:106–9.

45. Matucci A, Bormioli S, Bercich L, et al. Effect of dupilumab treatment in a severe asthma patient with EGPA. J Allergy Clin Immunol Pract 2021;9(10):3824–5.

46. Caminati M, Scarpieri E, Maule M, et al. Successful switching from mepolizumab to dupilumab in a patient with EGPA in remission phase and persistent nasal polyposis. Rheumatology 2024;63(3):e96–8.

47. Ezekwe E, Weskamp A, Khoury P, et al. Dupilumab Use in Patients with Hypereosinophilic Syndrome: A Multi-Center Case Series. J Allergy Clin Immunol 2024; 153(2):AB61.

48. Molina B, Padoan R, Urban ML, et al. Dupilumab for relapsing or refractory sinonasal and/or asthma manifestations in eosinophilic granulomatosis with polyangiitis: a European retrospective study. Ann Rheum Dis 2023;82(12):1587–93.

49. Pelaia C, Pelaia G, Crimi C, et al. Tezepelumab: A potential new biological therapy for severe refractory asthma. Int J Mol Sci 2021;22(9). https://doi.org/10.3390/ijms22094369.

50. Menzies-Gow A, Corren J, Bourdin A, et al. Tezepelumab in Adults and Adolescents with Severe, Uncontrolled Asthma. N Engl J Med 2021;384(19):1800–9.

51. Gauvreau GM, Bergeron C, Boulet L-P, et al. Sounding the alarmins-The role of alarmin cytokines in asthma. Allergy 2023;78(2):402–17.

52. Kotas ME, Dion J, Van Dyken S, et al. A role for IL-33-activated ILC2s in eosinophilic vasculitis. JCI Insight 2021;6(12).

53. Akiyama M, Kaneko Y, Takeuchi T. Rituximab for the treatment of eosinophilic granulomatosis with polyangiitis: A systematic literature review. Autoimmun Rev 2021;20(2):102737.

54. Chung SA, Langford CA, Maz M, et al. 2021 American College of Rheumatology/Vasculitis Foundation Guideline for the Management of Antineutrophil Cytoplasmic Antibody-Associated Vasculitis. Arthritis Rheumatol 2021;73(8):1366–83.

55. Wetzler L, Panch S, Berry A, et al. Remission of cold-agglutinin autoimmune hemolytic anemia and hypereosinophilic syndrome with rituximab therapy. J Allergy Clin Immunol Pract 2021;9(5):2107–8.e4.

56. Casulo C, Maragulia J, Zelenetz AD. Incidence of hypogammaglobulinemia in patients receiving rituximab and the use of intravenous immunoglobulin for recurrent infections. Clin Lymphoma Myeloma Leuk 2013;13(2):106–11.

57. Han JK, Bachert C, Fokkens W, et al. Mepolizumab for chronic rhinosinusitis with nasal polyps (SYNAPSE): a randomised, double-blind, placebo-controlled, phase 3 trial. Lancet Respir Med 2021. https://doi.org/10.1016/S2213-2600(21)00097-7.

58. Pavord ID, Korn S, Howarth P, et al. Mepolizumab for severe eosinophilic asthma (DREAM): a multicentre, double-blind, placebo-controlled trial. Lancet 2012;380(9842):651–9.

59. Chen MM, Roufosse F, Wang SA, et al. An International, Retrospective Study of Off-Label Biologic Use in the Treatment of Hypereosinophilic Syndromes. J Allergy Clin Immunol Pract 2022;10(5):1217–28.e3.

60. Hellmich B, Sanchez-Alamo B, Schirmer JH, et al. EULAR recommendations for the management of ANCA-associated vasculitis: 2022 update. Ann Rheum Dis 2024;83(1):30–47.

61. Cai S, Xu S, Lou H, et al. Comparison of different biologics for treating chronic rhinosinusitis with nasal polyps: A network analysis. J Allergy Clin Immunol Pract 2022;10(7):1876–86.e7.

62. Tanaka S, Tsuji T, Shiotsu S, et al. Exacerbation of eosinophilic granulomatosis with polyangiitis after administering dupilumab for severe asthma and eosinophilic rhinosinusitis with nasal polyposis. Cureus 2022;14(5):e25218.

63. Wilde B, Thewissen M, Damoiseaux J, et al. Th17 expansion in granulomatosis with polyangiitis (Wegener's): the role of disease activity, immune regulation and therapy. Arthritis Res Ther 2012;14(5):R227.

64. Teixeira V, Mohammad AJ, Jones RB, et al. Efficacy and safety of rituximab in the treatment of eosinophilic granulomatosis with polyangiitis. RMD Open 2019;5(1):e000905.

Biologics in Food Allergies
Emerging Therapies

Michele Beaudoin, MD[a], Chloe Citron, MD[a],
Kanwaljit K. Brar, MD[b],*

KEYWORDS

- Food allergy • Biologic • Omalizumab • Peanut • Monoclonal antibody • Dupilumab
- Milk • Egg

KEY POINTS

- Food allergies are pervasive in our current population, have large financial and emotional burdens, and carry serious risks of anaphylaxis.
- Omalizumab was recently approved for the reduction of allergic reactions associated with multiple foods in children and adults greater than 1 year old.
- There are ongoing studies of omalizumab and other biologics as monotherapy and with oral immunotherapy to treat or modify food allergies.

INTRODUCTION

Immunoglobulin E-mediated food allergies (IgE-FA) are a public health concern impacting patients and their families as a potentially life-threatening condition, affecting approximately 8% of children in the United States, and 10% of adults.[1,2] Historically, the management of food allergies necessitates strict avoidance of the allergen and prompt use of rescue medication in the case of accidental ingestion. Avoidance is an imperfect solution, as individuals with IgE-FA may experience an average of 1 reaction per year due to accidental ingestion of allergens, which can cause significant emotional burden.[3] Studies have shown that anxiety-driven coping skills are increased in those with IgE-FA, including heighted vigilance, and separation-induced panic.[4] After serious allergic reactions, individuals can even experience symptoms of Post-Traumatic Stress Disorder (PTSD).[4]

Over 170 foods have been reported to cause allergic reactions, and the 9 major allergens responsible for the majority of reactions in the United States are milk, egg,

[a] Department of Pediatrics, NYU Grossman School of Medicine, Hassenfeld Children's Hospital, 430 East 34th Street, New York, NY 10016, USA; [b] Division of Allergy and Immunology, Department of Pediatrics, NYU Grossman School of Medicine, Hassenfeld Children's Hospital, 150 East 32nd Street, New York, NY 10016, USA
* Corresponding author.
E-mail address: Kanwaljit.brar@nyulangone.org

Immunol Allergy Clin N Am 44 (2024) 645–655
https://doi.org/10.1016/j.iac.2024.07.004   **immunology.theclinics.com**

peanut, tree nut, wheat, soy, fish, crustacean shellfish, and sesame. The majority of anaphylactic reactions occur outside the home. Twenty-five percent of reactions occur while eating at a restaurant, with 54% of restaurant allergic reactions occurring despite restaurant staff being notified of the allergy.[5] Per the Food Allergen Labeling and Consumer Protection Act and Food Allergy Safety, Treatment, Education, and Research Act of 2021, foods containing the 9 major allergens must be labeled with the allergen. However, there is no equivalent requirement for restaurant food that is not pre-packaged.

Food allergies and subsequent efforts to avoid allergens can have a significant impact on quality of life, as 1 in 3 children with food allergies report being bullied for their allergies.[4] Over 25% of parents of children with food allergies report that they do not allow their children to participate in camp or sleepovers due to their allergies, while over 15% do not eat at restaurants, and over 10% do not allow their children to attend playdates at friend's houses.[4] Additionally, costs associated with food allergen avoidance place increased financial burden on families, especially those from marginalized communities.[1]

PATHOGENESIS

The immunologic mechanism of IgE-FA is a complex cascade involving many different cell types and cytokines, providing multiple potential targets for biologic therapy. A simplified mechanism of IgE-FA involves interleukin (IL)-4 and IL-13-dependent class switching recombination of memory B cells to plasma cells, which then produce allergen-specific IgE antibodies.[6] IgE subsequently binds to the high-affinity IgE receptor (FceRI) on mast cells and basophils leading to degranulation and release of histamine, platelet activating factor, prostaglandin, and other cytokines.[6] Sialic-acid-binding immunoglobulin-like lectin 8 is an inhibitory receptor, which is expressed on mast cells, basophils, and eosinophils.[7] In atopic dermatitis (AD), IL-4 via keratinocyte-derived cytokines also induces type II helper T cell proliferation.[7] Janus tyrosine kinase (JAKs) signaling broadly acts downstream of cytokines involved in food allergy, including IL-4, IL-5, and IL-13, IL-31, and thymic stromal lymphopoietin.[7] Bruton's Tyrosine Kinase (BTK) is another important enzyme that helps FceRI signaling in mast cells and basophils, allowing for a robust allergic response. Therapeutics targeting the underlying mechanisms that drive allergic inflammation have the mechanistic opportunity to increase patients' tolerance to multiple allergens that provoke IgE-mediated reactions.

DISCUSSION
Anti-Immunoglobulin E Treatment

Multiple clinical trials have examined the use of anti-IgE antibodies such as omalizumab as both monotherapy and as adjunct to oral immunotherapy (OIT) in increasing tolerance to allergic foods[8–12] The first trial was a 2003 double-blind, placebo-controlled (DBPC) trial of TNX-901, an early humanized IgG1 monoclonal antibody against IgE. TNX-901 demonstrated an increase in thresholds of peanut dose required to elicit a reaction during oral food challenges (OFC) compared to baseline and placebo. This response was dose-dependent with the highest dose group tolerating 2626 mg of peanut protein (~9 peanut kernels) after 16 weeks compared with 178 mg (~1/2 peanut kernel) at entry OFC.[8]

Omalizumab is a recombinant humanized monoclonal antibody specifically targeting immunoglobulin E (IgE) that has been in use for over 20 years for moderate-to-severe asthma; it is also approved for use in chronic spontaneous urticaria (CSU) and chronic rhinosinusitis with nasal polyps. It was FDA approved in February, 2024 for the treatment of adults and children 1 year or older, weighing more than 10 kg, with 1 or more food allergy for the reduction of allergic reactions, including anaphylaxis.[13] Omalizumab binds to the constant region of IgE, preventing the interaction of IgE with high and low affinity receptors on the surface of basophils and mast cells, thus preventing the activation of the allergic cascade and release of mediators such as histamine. The formation of IgE-antibody complexes decreases the presence of free IgE, which in turn downregulates the IgE receptors on mast cells and basophils, limiting degranulation and mediator release.[14]

A small 2011 Phase 2 trial of 14 patients also demonstrated an increase in tolerability to peanut protein in omalizumab-treated versus placebo-treated participants, with 44% (n = 4) of the omalizumab group tolerating 1000 mg of peanut flour after 24 weeks of treatment compared to 20% (n = 1) of the placebo group.[9] A larger 2012 study examined the kinetics of mast cell and basophil responses in omalizumab-treated adults with peanut allergy, demonstrating that basophil hyporesponsiveness to allergen may be a biomarker for increasing thresholds tolerated in OFC. Unlike basophils, mast cell fluctuations were not as closely correlated with increased clinical thresholds, showing less potential for mast cells as a biomarker.[10]

Ligelizumab is another anti-IgE monoclonal antibody, which binds to the high-affinity IgE type I receptor with 88 times more potency than omalizumab.[15–17] Its ability to decrease circulating IgE appeared promising for success in disease states treated with omalizumab, such as CSU. However, in 2 clinical trials of adolescents and adults, ligelizumab was not superior to omalizumab, though it was superior to placebo, in reducing urticaria scores.[18] In 2021, recruitment began for a phase 3 multi-center, randomized DBPC trial (NCT04984876) of ligelizumab in peanut allergic participants aged 6 to 55, which enrolled 211 participants. In January 2024, the pharmaceutical sponsor terminated the study with plans to begin a 3-year long-term extension study (NCT05678959).[19,20]

Omalizumab as Monotherapy and as Adjunct Therapy to Multi-Allergen Oral Immunotherapy in Food Allergic Children and Adults Study

The Omalizumab as Monotherapy and as Adjunct Therapy to Multi-Allergen Oral Immunotherapy in Food Allergic Children and Adults (OUtMATCH) trial is a Phase 3, 3-stage, multicenter, randomized DBPC trial investigating the use of omalizumab in reducing IgE-mediated allergic reactions to multiple foods.[13] The study population included participants aged 1 to 55 with allergies to peanut and at least 2 of the following foods: cow's milk, egg white, wheat, cashew, hazelnut, and walnut.[21] Study inclusion criteria included dose-limiting symptoms at less than a single dose of 100 mg of peanut protein, and less than 300 mg of other food proteins. Thus, the study population included the most severe, highly-reactive patients. Exclusion criteria included dose-limiting symptoms to the screening, double blind, placebo food challenge; poorly controlled AD; severe asthma; or history of severe anaphylaxis resulting in neurologic compromise or requiring intubation.[13]

In Stage 1 (**Fig. 1**) of the OUtMATCH trial, 177 participants were included in the final patient analysis, including 3 adults.[21] Mean age of participants was 7 years, and 57% were male.[20] Participants represented a diverse patient population, with 13.3% of participants identified as Asian, 6.7% Black, 63% White, and 16.4% multi-racial.[21] In addition, 8.5% of the participants identified as Hispanic.[21] All participants had allergy to peanuts, and 34.5%, 39.4%, and 57% had allergy to milk, egg, and cashew, respectively.[21] Median total IgE of participants was 700 IU/mL, and 54.6% participants had comorbid asthma. Omalizumab dosage and frequency was based on

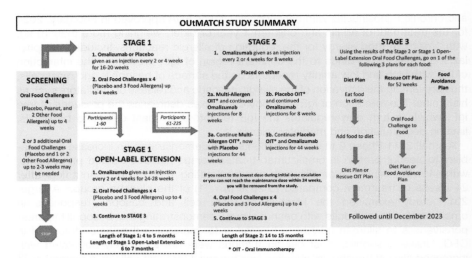

Fig. 1. OUtMATCH study summary. (*From* [Wood RA, Chinthrajah RS, Rudman Spergel AK, et al. Protocol design and synopsis: Omalizumab as Monotherapy and as Adjunct Therapy to Multiallergen OIT in Children and Adults with Food Allergy (OUtMATCH). J Allergy Clin Immunol Glob. 2022;1(4):225-232. Published 2022 Jul 21. doi:10.1016/j.jacig.2022.05.006]; with permission.)

pretreatment serum IgE (IU/mL) and body weight (kg), with 58% of patients dosed every 2 weeks and 42% of patients dosed every 4 weeks (**Table 1**). Patients with IgE levels exceeding the dosing algorithm for their respective weight and with IgE greater than 1850 IU/mL were excluded from the study. Thus, some severely allergic patients were not represented in the study.

Table 1
Omalizumab dosing based on weight and serum immunoglobulin E (IgE) level

Pretreatment Serum IgE (IU/mL)	Body Weight (kg)												
	≥10-12	>12-15	>15-20	>20-25	>25-30	>30-40	>40-50	>50-60	>60-70	>70-80	>80-90	>90-125	>125-150
	Dose (mg)												
≥30 - 100	75	75	75	75	75	75	150	150	150	150	150	300	300
>100 - 200	75	75	75	150	150	150	300	300	300	300	300	450	600
>200 - 300	75	75	150	150	150	225	300	300	450	450	450	600	375
>300 - 400	150	150	150	225	225	300	450	450	450	600	600	450	525
>400 - 500	150	150	225	225	300	450	450	600	600	375	375	525	600
>500 - 600	150	150	225	300	300	450	600	600	375	450	450	600	
>600 - 700	150	150	225	300	225	450	600	375	450	450	525		
>700 - 800	150	150	150	225	225	300	375	450	450	525	600		
>800 - 900	150	150	150	225	225	300	375	450	525	600			
>900 - 1000	150	150	225	225	300	375	450	525	600				
>1000 - 1100	150	150	225	225	300	375	450	600					
>1100 - 1200	150	150	225	300	300	450	525	600					
>1200 - 1300	150	225	225	300	375	450	525						
>1300 - 1500	150	225	300	300	375	525	600						
>1500 - 1850		225	300	375	450	600							

Dosing frequency:
- Dose every 4 weeks
- Dose every 2 weeks
- Do not dose

Participants were assigned to omalizumab monotherapy or placebo for 16 to 20 weeks of treatment, ending in a double-blind placebo-controlled food challenge (DBPCFC). The prespecified threshold dose for peanut was a single dose of at least 600 mg protein (cumulative 1044 mg); for cashew, egg, milk, walnut, hazelnut, and wheat, the prespecified threshold was a single dose of at least 1000 mg protein (cumulative 2044 mg). The study also included a 24-28-week open-label extension to assess the durability of long-term omalizumab therapy in the first 60 patients with an exploratory end point of consumption of 8044 mg cumulative dose of protein for each of 3 foods.

Stage 2, for which results have not yet been published, compares the effect of a short course (8 weeks) of open-label omalizumab monotherapy followed by multi-allergen oral immunotherapy (OIT), with a longer course of omalizumab (52 weeks) without OIT in reducing allergic reactions. Stage 3 is currently underway and consists of long-term safety follow-up of Stage 1 and Stage 2, including patients' ability to consume peanuts and 2 other foods in the diet after omalizumab discontinuation. Participants of stage 3 will be followed for 12 to 24 months.

Sixty-seven percent of peanut-allergic participants receiving omalizumab met the primary endpoint of the study and were able to consume a single dose of ≥600 mg of peanut protein, equivalent to 2 peanut kernels, without dosing-limiting symptoms at post-treatment OFC compared to 7% of those on placebo (P<.00001).[21] The secondary endpoints of the study were similarly met with 65%, 66%, 67%, and 42% of participants allergic to peanut, milk, egg, and cashew, respectively, able to consume a single dose of ≥1000 mg of protein without dosing-limiting symptoms at post-treatment OFC, while only 2%, 10%, 0% and 3%, respectively, in the placebo group could tolerate the above dose (P<.0001).[21] Dose-limiting symptoms included systemic hives, throat tightness, persistent abdominal pain, vomiting, wheezing, hypotension, and change in mental status. Notably, one-third of participants in the omalizumab group did not meet primary endpoint of consuming 600 mg, and 14% in this group could not even consume 30 mg of peanut without dose-limiting symptoms.[21]

There were no significant differences in treatment-related adverse events (AE) between active and placebo groups, with the major side effect being anaphylaxis during OFC. There were no instances of anaphylaxis related to omalizumab. Significant treatment-related AE included injection site reaction and pyrexia.[21] Limited data from 59 participants in the Open Label Extension have been released. The dose tolerated for peanut, egg, and milk at the end of week 24 was comparable to week 16, with no drastic change in AE.[21] Preliminary data suggest those with higher levels of IgE had better success than those with lower IgE levels, suggesting future research should include patients who were excluded from this study due to IgE levels above the dosing threshold for their weight (see **Table 1**).

Advantages of The OUtMATCH trial included high study retention rate (97%). Additionally, treatment was not food-specific, and the study included patients as young as 1 year and with an average age of 7 years. As such, investigators were targeting the most vulnerable of food allergic patients, who require constant vigilance and may unknowingly encounter allergens. Limitations of the study included limited adult participants and exclusion of individuals with the highest IgE levels. The study was least successful in improving reaction thresholds for tree nuts, in particular cashew. However, ultimately, most patients increased the amount of food they could be exposed to, and in OFC settings consumed more protein than what they would encounter in everyday exposures.[21] **Table 2** outlines guidelines for selecting patients that may be good candidates for omalizumab therapy.

Table 2
Proposed criteria for selection of candidates for omalizumab treatment of food allergies

Requirements	Other Supporting Features	Contraindications
• One or more IgE-mediated food allergies	• Food allergens that are difficult to avoid that is, milk, egg, wheat, sesame, peanut	• Non-IgE-mediated food allergies
• Age >1-year-old	• History of life-threatening reactions	• Age <1 y
• Weight > 10 kg	• History of systemic reaction due to cross contamination	• Weight <10 kg
• Patient willing to use in conjunction with allergen avoidance	• Concomitant asthma, chronic urticaria, severe environmental allergies, or atopic dermatitis	• Patients unwilling to comply with subcutaneous injections
• Tolerance of injectable medication	• Significant impact on quality of life from food allergies	• Previous severe reactions to omalizumab
• Willingness to follow anaphylaxis action plan	• Overwhelming anxiety or fears stemming from accidental ingestions or previous reactions	
• Patient and/or caregiver understanding that biologic is not to be used in place of epinephrine for treatment of acute anaphylaxis		

Omalizumab with Oral Immunotherapy

OIT involves daily exposure of allergic individuals to increasing doses of food allergen in order to achieve desensitization, which results in an increased threshold for the amount of food protein that provokes a reaction.[13] The results of OUtMATCH Stage 2, which examines omalizumab with OIT, are not yet reported. However, other clinical trials have shown that omalizumab combined with OIT can increase the tolerated dose of allergens, such as peanut, cow's milk and eggs, and shorten the length of OIT treatment required for successful and safe desensitization.[22] OIT in most studies, including OUtMATCH Stage 2, was started 8 to 16 weeks after initiation of omalizumab treatment.

Pretreatment with omalizumab can increase the starting tolerated dose of OIT. A 2013 study in which peanut-allergic individuals were pre-treated with 12 weeks of omalizumab prior to peanut OIT resulted in 100% of patients tolerating 500 mg (mg) of peanut flour on the initial day of desensitization, equivalent to 2.5 peanuts.[23] In a Phase 1 study of 25 patients on rush, multi-food OIT initially failing DBPCFC of 100 mg of combined allergen protein, pretreatment with omalizumab every 2 to 4 weeks over an 8 -week period allowed 76% of the participants to subsequently tolerate all 6 steps of initial OIT escalation for a maximum of 1250 mg of protein.[24] Pre-treatment also impacts maintenance dose achieved. In a multi-food study, participants were more likely to reach maintenance dose and more likely to pass exit OFC when pre-treated with omalizumab (83% vs 33% of the placebo group).[25]

A 2015 randomized, DBPC trial of omalizumab and milk oral immunotherapy (MOIT) compared 16-month of blinded treatment with omalizumab or placebo. MOIT was initiated 4 months after initiation of omalizumab or placebo treatment, and continued for 12 months. Groups were derandomized after this time, and the treatment group completed an additional 12 months of omalizumab therapy, culminating in an OFC at month 28 with 10 g (g) of milk protein (combined casein and whey). Significantly fewer MOIT doses were required to achieve maintenance in the omalizumab group, resulting in a shorter escalation phase (25.9 vs 30 weeks, $P = .01$).[26] Another study of patients already treated with omalizumab for asthma found that the average tolerated dose for milk increased from 750 mg to 10,000 mg ($P = .04$) after a 4-month period.[27]

In 2020, Palforzia, a peanut powder, was approved for OIT for mitigation of allergic reactions that may occur with accidental exposure.[7] While OIT has demonstrated high rates of desensitization, it is also associated with increased risk of allergic reactions, including anaphylaxis, and large time commitments.[28,29] These studies demonstrate the potential of omalizumab to significantly shorten OIT protocols and increase consumption doses of allergenic foods. This is a clinically meaningful outcome as patient compliance and lack of interest in pursuing prolonged therapies is often cited as a limitation of OIT.

Dupilumab

Dupilumab, a monoclonal antibody against IL-4 receptor alpha, has been studied as monotherapy for food allergy, and as an adjuvant to OIT.[30] A small, open-label phase 2 clinical trial (NCT03793608) evaluated dupilumab as monotherapy for peanut allergy in 25 pediatric patients.[31] Participants (mean age 11.7 years) received either 200 or 300 mg of dupilumab every other week after an initial loading dose. After 24 weeks, all patients underwent a DBPCFC up to 2044 mg of cumulative peanut protein or placebo. Only 8.3% passed the OFC, tolerative of at least 444 mg of peanut protein. This underwhelming result led to the clinical trial being terminated early.[31]

In addition, two phase 2 clinical trials are evaluating dupilumab in combination with OIT for treatment of food allergy in children and adults.[32,33] The first trial[32] focuses on pediatric patients, and recruited 148 individuals to participate. It examined dupilumab combined with peanut OIT versus placebo. Crude results have been released on clinicaltrials.gov, though no official data analysis has been published. Results indicate 55% of patients who received dupilumab in addition to their OIT passed the DBPCFC compared to 35% of patients receiving OIT alone ($P = .04$).[32] A second study included 110 participants, age 4 to 55 year old, all with peanut allergy and 1 or 2 additional food allergies.[33] Results of this study are not yet available.

Other Therapies

Cytokines, such as IL-33, IL-25, and thymic stromal lymphopoietin (TSLP), are alarmins that activate type II cells in response to food allergens, causing subsequent release of other type II cytokines.[34] Etokimab is a monoclonal antibody that targets the alarmin IL-33, and has been studied in a phase 2 trial of food allergy.[35] There were 20 adult participants in this study. Eleven of the 15 patients in the etokimab group passed an OFC to 275 mg of peanut after 45 days compared with 0 of 5 patients in the placebo group. This study was limited by small size and short duration; therefore, further studies are needed.

Although not technically biologic agents, oral agents targeting other immune mediators relevant in food allergy are currently being studied. BTK provides another molecular target with substantial downstream effects that contribute to food allergy pathogenesis. Acalabrutinib, an oral inhibitor of BTK, is approved for malignancy and could potentially be used to prevent anaphylaxis.[36] A Phase 2 study of 10 adult participants with a history of clinical peanut allergy treated with acalabrutinib showed great success. After only 2 days of oral acalabrutinib treatment, 7 out of the 10 patients tolerated the maximum protocol amount (4044 mg) of peanut protein with no clinical reaction, compared with a median threshold dose of 29 mg at study entry OFC.[36] Though the study is small, it highlights the possibility of preventing serious allergic reactions through novel molecular targets in a much shorter time period than conventional, monoclonal antibody treatment. Additionally, acalabrutinib is an oral medication, which may be preferred to injectable options.

Finally, small molecule inhibitors inhibiting JAK are another potential treatment of food allergy.[37] Abrocitinib inhibits JAK1 and is already approved for treatment of refractory moderate-to-severe AD in ages 12 and up as a once-daily oral formulation. It is currently being studied in a phase I clinical trial of peanut, cashew, walnut, hazelnut, sesame, cod, and/or shrimp allergic adults, who also have AD.[37] Results have not yet been published.

SUMMARY

With the FDA approval of omalizumab as the first biologic treatment for IgE-FA, the landscape of food allergy treatment is at an exciting juncture with a promising future for improved patient health, safety, and quality of life. The continued use of omalizumab offers hope that food allergic patients and parents of food allergic children can feel reassurance that they may be protected from unavoidable situations of accidental exposure. It remains unclear what the ultimate duration of omalizumab treatment will be, and at present, continued avoidance of allergens with treatment is recommended. Stage 2 of OUtMATCH will evaluate omalizumab use in combination with OIT, and has the potential to increase the use of OIT as a standard-of-care treatment option.

Dupilumab, an IL-4 receptor alpha antagonist, may be less effective in reducing food allergic reactions. There are a number of new classes of pipeline targets, including IL-33, JAK, and BTK, which are being developed, though studies have been small. Providers seeking to use omalizumab as monotherapy or to combine omalizumab with OIT should use shared decision-making to determine the best options for patients and families.

CLINICS CARE POINTS

- Omalizumab monotherapy may prevent serious allergic reaction in accidental food allergen exposure
- Eligible patients, especially those with multiple food allergies, difficulty to avoid allergens, history of severe reactions, or overwhelming fear/anxiety of accidental exposures, should be strongly considered for omalizumab therapy
- Utility of omalizumab in combination with OIT is currently being studied

DISCLOSURE

K.K. Brar has served as an advisor and received research support from Incyte Pharmaceuticals. She is an investigator for Sanofi, and Siolta Therapeutics.

REFERENCES

1. Gupta RS, Warren CM, Smith BM, et al. The Public Health Impact of Parent-Reported Childhood Food Allergies in the United States. Pediatrics 2018; 142(6):e20181235 [published correction appears in Pediatrics. 2019 Mar; 143(3)].
2. Gupta RS, Warren CM, Smith BM, et al. Prevalence and Severity of Food Allergies Among US Adults. JAMA Netw Open 2019;2(1):e185630.
3. Rotella K, Oriel RC. Accidental Reactions to Foods: Frequency, Causes, and Severity. Curr Treat Options Allergy 2022;9(3):157–68.
4. Feng C, Kim JH. Beyond Avoidance: the Psychosocial Impact of Food Allergies. Clin Rev Allergy Immunol 2019;57(1):74–82.
5. Stankovich GA, Warren CM, Gupta R, et al. Food allergy risks and dining industry - an assessment and a path forward. Front Allergy 2023;4:1060932.
6. Michelet M, Balbino B, Guilleminault L, et al. IgE in the pathophysiology and therapy of food allergy. Eur J Immunol 2021;51(3):531–43.
7. Berin C. Jak out of the box: Targeting Bruton's tyrosine kinase, sialic acid-binding immunoglobulin-like lectin-8, and Janus kinase 1 in food allergy. Ann Allergy Asthma Immunol 2023;131(1):23–8.
8. Leung DY, Sampson HA, Yunginger JW, et al. Effect of anti-IgE therapy in patients with peanut allergy. N Engl J Med 2003;348(11):986–93.
9. Sampson HA, Leung DY, Burks AW, et al. A phase II, randomized, double-blind, parallel-group, placebo-controlled oral food challenge trial of Xolair (omalizumab) in peanut allergy. J Allergy Clin Immunol 2011;127(5):1309–13010.e1.
10. Savage JH, Courneya JP, Sterba PM, et al. Kinetics of mast cell, basophil, and oral food challenge responses in omalizumab-treated adults with peanut allergy. J Allergy Clin Immunol 2012;130(5):1123–9.e2.
11. Brandström J, Vetander M, Lilja G, et al. Individually dosed omalizumab: an effective treatment for severe peanut allergy. Clin Exp Allergy 2017;47(4):540–50.

12. Schneider LC, Rachid R, LeBovidge J, et al. A pilot study of omalizumab to facilitate rapid oral desensitization in high-risk peanut-allergic patients. J Allergy Clin Immunol 2013;132(6):1368–74.

13. Wood RA, Chinthrajah RS, Rudman Spergel AK, et al. Protocol design and synopsis: Omalizumab as Monotherapy and as Adjunct Therapy to Multiallergen OIT in Children and Adults with Food Allergy (OUtMATCH). J Allergy Clin Immunol Glob. 2022;1(4):225–32.

14. Holgate S, Casale T, Wenzel S, et al. The anti-inflammatory effects of omalizumab confirm the central role of IgE in allergic inflammation. J Allergy Clin Immunol 2005;115(3):459–65.

15. Arm JP, Bottoli I, Skerjanec A, et al. Pharmacokinetics, pharmacodynamics and safety of QGE031 (ligelizumab), a novel high-affinity anti-IgE antibody, in atopic subjects. Clin Exp Allergy 2014;44(11):1371–85.

16. Dantzer JA, Wood RA. Anti-immunoglobulin E for food allergy. Ann Allergy Asthma Immunol 2023;131(1):11–22.

17. Wood RA, Chinthrajah RS, Eggel A, et al. The rationale for development of ligelizumab in food allergy. World Allergy Organ J 2022;15(9):100690.

18. Maurer M, Ensina LF, Gimenez-Arnau AM, et al. Efficacy and safety of ligelizumab in adults and adolescents with chronic spontaneous urticaria: results of two phase 3 randomised controlled trials. Lancet 2024;403(10422):147–59.

19. Efficacy and Safety of QGE031 (Ligelizumab) in Patients With Peanut Allergy, Available at: https://www.clinicaltrials.gov/study/NCT04984876. (Accessed March 2 2024). 2023.

20. Long-term Extension Study of Ligelizumab in Food Allergy, Available at: https://classic.clinicaltrials.gov/ct2/show/NCT05678959. (Accessed April 15 2024). 2023.

21. Wood RA, Togias A, Sicherer SH, et al. Omalizumab for the Treatment of Multiple Food Allergies. N Engl J Med 2024;390(10):889–99.

22. Zuberbier T, Wood RA, Bindslev-Jensen C, et al. Omalizumab in IgE-Mediated Food Allergy: A Systematic Review and Meta-Analysis. J Allergy Clin Immunol Pract 2023;11(4):1134–46.

23. Yee CSK, Albuhairi S, Noh E, et al. Long-Term Outcome of Peanut Oral Immunotherapy Facilitated Initially by Omalizumab. J Allergy Clin Immunol Pract 2019;7(2):451–61.e7.

24. Bégin P, Dominguez T, Wilson SP, et al. Phase 1 results of safety and tolerability in a rush oral immunotherapy protocol to multiple foods using Omalizumab. Allergy Asthma Clin Immunol 2014;10(1):7.

25. Andorf S, Purington N, Block WM, et al. Anti-IgE treatment with oral immunotherapy in multifood allergic participants: a double-blind, randomised, controlled trial. Lancet Gastroenterol Hepatol 2018;3(2):85–94.

26. Wood RA, Kim JS, Lindblad R, et al. A randomized, double-blind, placebo-controlled study of omalizumab combined with oral immunotherapy for the treatment of cow's milk allergy. J Allergy Clin Immunol 2016;137(4):1103–10.e11.

27. Fiocchi A, Artesani MC, Riccardi C, et al. Impact of Omalizumab on Food Allergy in Patients Treated for Asthma: A Real-Life Study. J Allergy Clin Immunol Pract 2019;7(6):1901–9.e5.

28. Varshney P, Steele PH, Vickery BP, et al. Adverse reactions during peanut oral immunotherapy home dosing. J Allergy Clin Immunol 2009;124(6):1351–2.

29. Branum AM, Lukacs SL. Food allergy among U.S. children: trends in prevalence and hospitalizations. NCHS Data Brief 2008;(10):1–8.

30. Harb H, Chatila TA. Mechanisms of Dupilumab. Clin Exp Allergy 2020;50(1):5–14.

31. Study to evaluate dupilumab monotherapy in pediatric patients with peanut allergy, Available at: https://clinicaltrials.gov/ct2/show/NCT03793608. (Accessed March 2 2024). 2022.

32. Study in Pediatric Subjects With Peanut Allergy to Evaluate Efficacy and Safety of Dupilumab as Adjunct to AR101 (Peanut Oral Immunotherapy), Available at: https://www.clinicaltrials.gov/study/NCT03682770. (Accessed March 2 2024). 2024.

33. Clinical Study Using Biologics to Improve Multi OIT Outcomes (COMBINE), Available at: https://www.clinicaltrials.gov/study/NCT03679676. (Accessed March 2 2024). 2023.

34. Rizzi A, Lo Presti E, Chini R, et al. Emerging Role of Alarmins in Food Allergy: An Update on Pathophysiological Insights, Potential Use as Disease Biomarkers, and Therapeutic Implications. J Clin Med 2023;12(7):2699.

35. Chinthrajah S, Cao S, Liu C, et al. Phase 2a randomized, placebo-controlled study of anti-IL-33 in peanut allergy. JCI Insight 2019;4(22):e131347.

36. Suresh RV, Dunnam C, Vaidya D, et al. A phase II study of Bruton's tyrosine kinase inhibition for the prevention of anaphylaxis. J Clin Invest 2023;133(16):e172335.

37. JAK Inhibition in Food Allergy, Available at: https://www.clinicaltrials.gov/study/NCT05069831. (Accessed March 2 2024). 2024.

Biologics in Chronic Rhinosinusitis
Current and Emerging

Jacob T. Boyd, MD, PhD, Ashoke R. Khanwalkar, MD*

KEYWORDS

- Chronic rhinosinusitis • Sinusitis • Polyposis • Biologics • Endotype • Phenotype
- Chronic rhinosinusitis with nasal polyps • Chronic rhinosinusitis without nasal polyps

KEY POINTS

- Chronic rhinosinusitis (CRS) is traditionally characterized by phenotype as CRS with nasal polyps (CRSwNP) and CRS without nasal polyps (CRSsNP).
- CRS endotypes are broadly categorized into Type 1, Type 2, and Type 3 (also called Type 17) based on distinct gene signatures and immune cell activity.
- The Type 2 endotype is the most extensively researched and is associated with asthma, atopic disease, and more severe CRS and nasal polyposis presentation.
- There are currently 3 biologics approved as add-on treatment of poorly/inadequately controlled CRSwNP: omalizumab, dupilumab, and mepolizumab.
- There are many active clinical trials in CRSwNP and CRSsNP targeting various cytokines and receptors in the inflammatory cascade.

INTRODUCTION

Chronic rhinosinusitis (CRS) represents an inflammatory state of the sinonasal passageways with persistent associated symptoms. Clinically, CRS in adults is defined as 12 or more weeks of 2 or more cardinal subjective sinonasal symptoms – nasal obstruction, discolored nasal discharge, hyposmia, and facial pressure/pain.[1] Confirmation of the diagnosis requires objective evidence of inflammation (eg, edema or nasal polyps) or purulence on nasal endoscopy, or findings of inflammation on radiographic imaging, most commonly utilizing sinus computed tomography. Prevalence of CRS ranges from 2.1% to 12.0% in the United States and Europe based on epidemiologic surveys and billing codes,[2–4] but with the additional requirement of radiographic

Department of Otolaryngology – Head and Neck Surgery, University of Colorado Anschutz School of Medicine, 12631 East 17th Avenue, MSB 205 Room 3001, Aurora, CO 80045, USA
* Corresponding author.
E-mail address: ashoke.khanwalkar@cuanschutz.edu

Immunol Allergy Clin N Am 44 (2024) 657–671
https://doi.org/10.1016/j.iac.2024.07.005   immunology.theclinics.com

evidence, prevalence narrows to 3.0% to 6.4%.[5] In Asian countries, CRS prevalence ranges from 2.0% to 28.4%.[6]

CRS is a heterogeneous condition that can be subdivided based on clinical phenotypes and pathophysiologic inflammatory endotypes.[7] Phenotypically, CRS is traditionally categorized as CRS with nasal polyps (CRSwNP) and CRS without nasal polyps (CRSsNP).[8] The CRSwNP phenotype may present as various clinical subphenotypes such as allergic fungal rhinosinusitis (AFRS), aspirin-exacerbated respiratory disease (AERD), central compartment atopic disease (CCAD), and cystic fibrosis, among others.[9] While these presentations can often be distinguished clinically to inform treatment recommendations, they lack detailed information regarding the pathophysiologic inflammatory mechanisms underlying the disease.[10] Endotyping is the characterization of the mechanistic disease process and molecular predominance in an individual patient, and a clear understanding may help avoid refractory interventions, inappropriate surgery, and poor outcomes associated with a purely phenotypic approach.[11]

One of the main motivations to transition from a phenotype-based to an endotype-based approach has been the development of immune-modifying biologic agents targeting the specific underlying pathologic mechanisms driving inflammatory and immune cell changes.[10,12,13] To understand the current and future role of biologic therapies in the treatment of CRSwNP, a review of the relevant endotypes is helpful.

ENDOTYPING IN CHRONIC RHINOSINUSITIS

Endotyping refers to the molecular characterization of the heterogenous immunologic responses to pathologic conditions.[14] In CRS, the initial immune response is generated based on intracellular and/or extracellular exposure to specific pathogens or allergens. When the normal immune response becomes dysregulated, chronic inflammation may persist even when the instigating factor has been eliminated or controlled.[15] CRS endotypes are broadly categorized into Type 1, Type 2, and Type 3 (also called Type 17) based on distinct gene signatures and immune cell activity.

Type 1 Endotype

The Type 1 endotype is initiated by response to viruses and intracellular microbes, bacteria, and protozoa with a Th1 predominance and secretion of interferons (IFN)-γ, tumor necrosis factor (TNF)-α, and interleukin (IL)-12.[11,16,17] Type 1 inflammation has traditionally been associated with CRSsNP, but more recent data have shown variation of endotype based on site of biopsy. Some evidence suggests that when polyps do occur in Type 1 inflammation, they are composed of a fibrin matrix similar to Type 2, despite the unique inflammatory profile.[18]

Type 2 Endotype

The Type 2 endotype is the most studied due to its prevalence in Western countries and association with allergic rhinitis, asthma, and nasal polyposis; as such, often endotypes are broadly categorized as Type 2 and non-Type 2.[19] The Type 2 response represents host defense against parasites, but when dysregulated, it is a driver of allergy, eosinophilia, and mast cell and immunoglobulin (Ig) E production with activation of Th2 cells, ILC2 cells, and many associated cytokines, with IL-4, IL-5, and IL-13 being the most established.[11,16,20–24] Epithelial alarmins, including thymic stromal lymphopoietin (TSLP), IL-33, and IL-25, are secreted after environmental triggers and are thought to play a particularly important role in Type 2 inflammation.[11] The Type 2 inflammatory pathway is generally associated with eosinophilia, although certain clinical presentations such as CCAD are characterized by elevated IgE.[25] Clinically, patients tend to demonstrate hyposmia, allergic mucin, edematous eosinophilic polyps, and atopic comorbidities.[26–28] Recurrent disease is common in aggressive Type 2 presentations, sometimes requiring additional therapeutic approaches beyond routine endoscopic sinus surgery and topical steroids and often requiring revision sinus surgery.[29]

Type 3 Endotype

The Type 3 inflammatory endotype develops in response to fungi and extracellular bacteria with upregulation of Th17 and ILC3 cells and production of IL-17 and IL-22 with downstream neutrophil activation.[15,16,30] Both Type 1 and Type 3 inflammation are associated with neutrophilic polyps and the presence of IFN-γ and IL-17, respectively.[31] In patients with CRSwNP, the Type 3 endotype has been associated with purulent nasal drainage, and intraoperative identification of pus is almost exclusively associated with isolated or mixed Type 3 endotypes.[28] Based on these findings, the Type 3 endotype is most strongly associated with bacterial infections, and theoretically may respond most robustly to antibiotics.

Mixed Endotypes and Variability in Phenotypic Relationships

While the Type 2 endotype is most traditionally associated with the CRSwNP phenotype, this is not universally the case, and is particularly called into question within non-Western geographies.[32,33] This variability has implications for the anticipated efficacy of selected treatment options. Further, there are many examples of mixed endotypes among patients with either CRSwNP or CRSsNP.[16,28] Patients with mixed endotypes may experience symptomatology of the individual component endotypes, but the resulting phenotype is far more complex than simply a combination of the individual endotypes. Moreover, therapeutic response to the treatment of a mixed endotype may differ from treatment of an isolated single endotype. Clinical trials are currently underway to evaluate the role of isolated versus mixed endotypes in the context of targeted biologic treatment failure. Given the possibility of a mixed endotype, evaluation of isolated inflammatory markers in a single inflammatory pathway may be insufficient to guide therapy. This highlights the importance of a comprehensive understanding of all the contributing endotypes in an individual patient rather than focusing only on phenotype.

Chronic Rhinosinusitis and Asthma

The concept of endotyping in CRSwNP originated from research in asthma, which shares significant overlap in presentation and pathogenesis. The similarity in upper and lower airway immune mechanisms supports the concept of a unified airway theory.[34] Both asthma and CRSwNP have been broadly divided into Type 2 and non-Type 2 endotypes with Type 2 being the most common in Western countries, although one recent study showed a mixed Type 1/Type 2 endotype has the highest asthma comorbidity in CRSwNP.[28] Multiple studies have also shown that asthma is associated with Type 2 endotype in CRS regardless of polyp status and that nasal cytokine levels, particularly IL-5, predict severity of asthma.[35,36] Elevated IL-5, IL-6, IL-10, and IgE have been observed in CRSwNP patients with asthma compared to non-asthma patients.[36]

Chronic Rhinosinusitis Without Nasal Polyps

CRSsNP accounts for 75% to 90% of all cases of CRS but has not been the primary focus of endotype research, partly because of its more heterogeneous presentation with no consensus tissue to biopsy.[37] Traditionally, CRSsNP was described as Type 1, but this generalization has since been challenged.[33] A recent study showed significant variability in inflammatory biomarkers when comparing inferior turbinate, uncinate, and ethmoid tissue from the same patients with CRSsNP, with higher concentrations of Type 2 and 3 biomarkers in the more inaccessible ethmoids, demonstrating the challenge of a standardized protocol for endotyping this disease process.[38] This site-specific variance could explain the initial assumed association of CRSsNP with Type 1, and why IFN-γ is not in fact elevated in patients with CRSsNP compared to CRSwNP and controls.[32,39] A recent study evaluating inflammatory markers in CRSsNP showed a dramatic predominance of Type 2 and mixed endotypes, with very few exclusively Type 1.[28] To complicate it further, another study showed that over 30% of CRSsNP patients were untypable using known markers.[28] With further understanding of endotypes in CRSsNP, the therapies discussed as follows could play a role in treatment of these patients, many of whom may in fact exhibit Type 2 inflammation. However, at this stage, all approved biologic indications are tied to the phenotype, CRSwNP.

TREATMENT STRATEGY: ROLE OF MEDICAL AND SURGICAL MANAGEMENT

After confirming the diagnosis with clinical history and objective findings, treatment is initiated with nasal saline irrigations and topical corticosteroids to suppress the chronic inflammation. In aggressive disease, it is often necessary to break the cycle of inflammation and mucostasis with functional endoscopic sinus surgery (FESS) and provide a simple widely opened sinonasal cavity for optimal delivery of topical corticosteroids.[40,41] However, even with optimal postoperative management, controlling chronic disease processes can be challenging, especially in patients with asthma, atopy, aspirin sensitivity, and high serum eosinophilia.[42] Oral corticosteroids are often used with temporary success in Type 2 CRSwNP, but long-term use is not recommended given the known side effects.[43] For these patients, novel biologic therapies provide a potential nonsteroidal treatment option, which may obviate the need for repeated FESS and/or systemic steroids.[44]

Biologics are monoclonal antibodies (mAbs) targeted against specific molecules in the inflammatory pathway, and endotype classification using biomarkers can potentially identify patients most likely to respond.[13] Biomarkers have been used to identify Type 2 inflammation, characterize severity of disease, and predict response to individual biologics, although the clinical role is still evolving. Type 2 biomarkers include tissue and serum eosinophilia, ECP, IL-4, IL-5, IL-13, and the eosinophilic cationic protein (ECP)/myeloperoxidase (MPO) ratio, with many others being evaluated.[19]

In 2023, the European Forum for Research and Education in Allergy and Airway Diseases published an update to the European Position Paper on Rhinosinusitis and Nasal Polyps, delineating indications for biologic therapies in CRSwNP. To consider biologics, patients must have bilateral nasal polyps, have had prior FESS (or be medically unable to undergo FESS), and meet 3 of the following criteria: frequent need for systemic steroids (or contraindicated for system steroid use), evidence of Type 2 inflammation, impaired quality of life, loss of smell, or comorbid asthma diagnosis.[45] These strict requirements are partly driven by the high expense of these novel medications. Further research into therapeutic indications, optimal timing of treatment, and biomarkers for biologic selection and outcome prediction is underway and will shape the future of surgical and medical management of CRS.

APPROVED BIOLOGIC TREATMENTS FOR CHRONIC RHINOSINUSITIS

The inflammatory cascade involved with an endotype plays an important role in identifying patients most likely to respond to specific therapies. Multiple biologics have been introduced to target distinct components of the inflammatory cascade.[46] There are currently 3 biologics approved for CRSwNP: omalizumab, dupilumab, and mepolizumab (**Table 1**). Several other agents are in clinical trials.

Dupilumab

Dupilumab is an IL4-Rα blocker targeting the IL-4 and IL-13 shared receptor subunit, thereby inhibiting Type 2 inflammation.[47,48] In 2 phase 3 clinical trials, the SINUS-24 and SINUS-52 trials with a total of 724 subjects, dupilumab was shown to improve subjective nasal symptoms (nasal congestion, hyposmia, or QOL) and objective findings (endoscopic score and Lund-Mackay score).[47] It has also been shown to improve sinonasal symptoms in patients with AERD.[49] Dupilumab is being tested in multiple additional clinical trials, including evaluation in CRSsNP (NCT04362501, NCT04678856), ethnically diverse populations (NCT05246267, NCT05878093), AFRS (NCT05545072), and eosinophilic CRSsNP resistant to topical corticosteroid treatment (NCT04430179). It is currently approved as add-on therapy for patients 18 years and older with poorly controlled CRSwNP, but given its mechanism of action, it is most likely to assist patients with proven Type 2 inflammation.

Mepolizumab

Mepolizumab is a recombinant humanized mAb that targets IL-5, thereby reducing eosinophil recruitment, activation, and survival. In the phase 3 SYNAPSE trial of 407 patients studied for 52 weeks, mepolizumab has shown efficacy in improving nasal polyp score and subjective nasal obstruction in CRSwNP, as well as decreasing need for revision sinus surgery.[50,51] There are several ongoing clinical trials for mepolizumab, investigating markers to predict drug effectiveness in CRSwNP (NCT05708300), use in combination with in-office polypectomy (NCT05923047), and use in comorbid severe asthma and CRSwNP (NCT06069310). During the phase 3 SYNAPSE trial, a subset of patients experienced long-lasting (>48 months) effectiveness after stopping mepolizumab treatment; a clinical trial is now evaluating endotypes and markers to try and predict this durable response (NCT05902325).[52] There is also a clinical trial evaluating the efficacy of mepolizumab compared to dupilumab in CRSwNP (NCT05942222) and a trial evaluating endoscopic sinus surgery and mepolizumab compared to mepolizumab alone (NCT05598814). Currently, mepolizumab is indicated as an add-on therapy in patients 18 years and older with inadequate response to nasal corticosteroids.

Omalizumab

Omalizumab is a mAb that binds circulating IgE on its constant domain, Cε3, which is the same domain that IgE uses to bind to its high-affinity receptor FcεR1, thus neutralizing free IgE and preventing it from binding its receptor on mast cells, basophils, dendritic cells, and eosinophils.[53] Elevated IgE is associated with eosinophilic asthma, severe nasal polyposis, and comorbid asthma.[54–56] Two phase 3 trials, POLYP1 and POLYP2 with a total of 265 patients studied for 24 weeks, demonstrated clinical benefit of omalizumab in CRSwNP, reducing polyp size, improving sinonasal symptoms, and QOL, while decreasing need for revision sinus surgery.[57,58] It was approved in 2020 for use in adults greater than or equal to 18 years with CRSwNP and an inadequate response to nasal corticosteroids. Given its distinct mechanism, omalizumab is likely most suitable for patients with elevated IgE, CCAD, and/or other symptoms of atopy.[59] CCAD is characterized clinically by middle turbinate edema associated with inhaled allergy.[60,61] There is currently 1 active clinical trial evaluating efficacy of omalizumab compared to dupilumab in reducing polyp size and improving sense of smell

Table 1
Summary of chronic rhinosinusitis-approved biologic therapies and their active clinical trials

Agent	Mechanism	Current FDA Approvals	Active Clinical Trials			
			ID	Name	Phase	Condition/Assessment
Dupilumab	Anti-IL-4Rα mAb inhibiting IL-4/13 signaling	CRSwNP; moderate to severe eosinophilic or OCS-dependent asthma; EoE; PN; AD	NCT04678856	Liberty	2	CRSsNP
			NCT04362501	–	2	CRSsNP
			NCT04430179	–	2	Eosinophilic CRSsNP
			NCT05877093	–	3	CRSwNP in Chinese population
			NCT05942222	TORNADO	4	Dup vs Mep in Danish CRSwNP
			NCT06188871	–	4	Early effects in CRSwNP
			NCT04596189	–	4	Pre/periop FESS use in CRSwNP
			NCT04998604	EVEREST	4	Dup vs Oma in Type-2 CRSwNP
			NCT04869436	–	4	CRSwNP olfactory outcomes
			NCT05964465	–	4	Mechanism of smell improvement
			NCT05246267	–	Obs	CRSwNP in diverse populations
			NCT05529784	DUPIREAL	Obs	Real life effectiveness in CRSwNP
			NCT04959448	AROMA	Obs	Real life effectiveness in CRSwNP and CRSwNP Long-term surveillance
Mepolizumab	Anti-IL-5 mAb	CRSwNP; severe eosinophilic asthma; EGPA; HES	NCT05923047	MELYSA	4	Mep + in-office polypectomy
			NCT05942222	TORNADO	4	Mep vs Dup in Danish CRSwNP
			NCT05542806	–	4	Molecular profiling CRS post-Mep
			NCT05902325	RESMEPO	4	Markers to predict length of effect
			NCT05598814	–	4	
			NCT06069310	MepoRiNaPAs	4	
			NCT04823585	AirGOs-biol	4	Mep vs Mep + FESS
			NCT05708300	CALIOPI	Obs	CRSwNP ± asthma
			NCT06258772	MEPOREAL	Obs	AERD/NERD
			NCT05938972	NASUMAB	Obs	CRSwNP ± asthma biomarkers
			NCT05063981	–	Obs	Real life effectiveness in CRSwNP Long-term CRSwNP outcomes Eosinophilic asthma ± CRSwNP
Omalizumab	Anti-IgE Cε3 receptor mAb	CRSwNP; moderate to severe persistent asthma; CSU; Food allergy	NCT04583501	–	1	Ex vivo biomarkers in CRSwNP
			NCT05390255	–	3	Topicals ± OCS ± Oma in CRS
			NCT04998604	EVEREST	4	Oma vs Dup in Type-2 CRSwNP
			NCT05626257	–	Obs	CRSwNP long-term surveillance

Abbreviations: OCS, oral corticosteroid; EoE, eosinophilic esophagitis; PN, prurigo nodularis; AD, atopic dermatitis; EGPA, eosinophilic granulomatosis with polyangiitis; HES, hypereosinophilic syndrome; CSU, chronic spontaneous urticaria; Obs, observational; Dup, dupilumab; Mep, mepolizumab; Oma, Omalizumab.

(NCT04998604). Other IgE-targeting agents such as ligelizumab and quilizumab are being tested in patients with chronic spontaneous urticaria and food allergies and could ultimately provide benefit for CRS patients with elevated IgE levels.

Selection of Biologic Medication

Although there are not yet any published prospective head-to-head trials comparing these Food and Drug Administration (FDA)-approved biologics to each other or to surgery, retrospective studies have evaluated their comparative efficacy. These analyses have generally identified dupilumab as the most effective currently available biologic for sinonasal symptoms – olfaction in particular.[62,63] While FESS has been shown to offer better objective results than any biologic with regards to nasal polyp score, dupilumab was found to potentially offer better olfactory and non-rhinologic (eg, cough, postnasal drip) results.[64] Although surgical intervention and biologics ultimately offer roughly similar disease control and symptom relief, biologics are significantly more expensive and represent an ongoing, indefinitely recurring cost.[65,66] International consensus has evolved to limit the use of biologics in CRSwNP to surgical failures, or if there are independent indications for biologic management such as asthma, in which case the precise selection of biologic may be driven more by the patient's asthma than their CRS.[45] The cost disadvantage for biologics may evolve over time, both with increased competition and potential decreased dosing schedules administered over longer intervals.[67] However, as it stands, the need for indefinite treatment with biologic therapy is a barrier for higher utilization in surgically naïve patients.

EMERGING THERAPIES FOR TYPE 2 AND NON-TYPE 2 ENDOTYPES

Several targeted biologics are currently being investigated for use in Type 2 and non-Type 2 inflammations in both CRSwNP and CRSsNP (**Table 2**). Below, we expound on these agents categorized by mechanism of action. Further research will ideally identify patients who will respond – or even be "super responders" – to targeted therapies, based on endotype and biomarkers.

IL-5

Benralizumab targets the IL-5Rα on eosinophils and basophils and is approved for patients with severe eosinophilic asthma. The phase 3 OSTRO study demonstrated improvement in nasal polyp score, nasal obstruction, and sense of smell at 40 weeks of treatment for patients with CRSwNP.[68] However, the FDA declined approval in 2022, requesting further data. A second multicenter phase 3 trial, ORCHID, is currently underway for eosinophilic CRSwNP (NCT04157335).

Reslizumab, like mepolizumab, is a mAb targeting free IL-5 and is approved for severe uncontrolled eosinophilic asthma. A recent study in 7 patients with severe asthma and comorbid CRSwNP treated with reslizumab demonstrated significant improvement in nasal symptoms, nasal polyp score, Lund-Mackay score, and asthma symptoms.[69]

Depemokimab is an anti-IL-5 mAb engineered for improved affinity and extended half-life. It was well-tolerated in Phase 1 trials and requires less frequent dosing (once every 6 months) compared to other anti-IL-5 mAbs.[70] There are 2 parallel clinical trials evaluating depemokimab in CRSwNP, ANCHOR-1 (NCT05274750), and ANCHOR-2 (NCT05281523).

Thymic Stromal Lymphopoietin

Tezepelumab is a mAb targeting TSLP, a cytokine that activates Type 2 inflammation through multiple cell lineages. Tezepelumab is approved in severe asthma and has

Table 2
Summary of emerging chronic rhinosinusitis biologic therapies in clinical trials

Target	Agent	MOA	Current FDA Approval	Trial Name	Condition	Phase	Trial ID
IL-5	Benralizumab	Anti-IL-5Rα on eosinophils, Activates NK Cell	Severe eosinophilic asthma	OSTRO	CRSwNP	3	Complete[68]
				ORCHID	CRSwNP	3	NCT04157335
	Depemokimab	Long-acting, high affinity anti-IL-5 mAb	—	ANCHOR-1	CRSwNP	3	NCT05274750
				ANCHOR-2	CRSwNP	3	NCT05281523
TSLP	Tezepelumab	mAb against the epithelial cytokine TSLP	Severe uncontrolled a	WAYPOINT	CRSwNP	3	NCT04851964
				TEZARS	Allergic Rhinitis	2	NCT06189742
	TQC2731	mAb against the epithelial cytokine TSLP	—		CRSwNP	2	NCT06036927
	Verekitug	mAb against TSLP receptor	—	VIBRANT	CRSwNP	2	NCT06164704
IL-4	TQH2722	Anti-IL-4Rα mAb inhibiting IL-4/13 signaling	—	—	CRSwNP, CRSsNP	2	NCT06089278
IL-33	Etokimab	Anti-IL33 mAb	—	—	CRSwNP	2	NCT03614923
	PF-06817024	Anti-IL33 mAb	—	—	CRSwNP	1	Complete[76]

Abbreviations: DPP1, dipeptidyl peptidase 1; mAb, monoclonal antibody; NSFB, non-cystic fibrosis bronchiectasis; NSP, neutrophil serine protease; TSLP, thymic stromal lymphopoietin.

shown benefit in both Type 2 and non-Type 2 asthma.[44] In the NAVIGATOR phase 3 trial, tezepelumab demonstrated meaningful improvements in sinonasal symptoms and asthma outcomes in patients with comorbid asthma and CRSwNP.[71] Tezepelumab is currently being evaluated in a clinical trial for CRSwNP (NCT04851964).

Multiple other mAbs targeting the TSLP pathway are currently under investigation in CRS. TQC273, a mAb with high affinity toward TSLP, is in a phase 2 trial for CRSwNP (NCT06036927). Verekitug, a mAb targeting the TSLP receptor, is in a phase 2 clinical trial for CRSwNP (NCT06164704). Ecleralimab, an inhaled TSLP mAb, has shown benefit in allergic asthma and could potentially be used as a topical agent in CRS.[72] TSLP biologics have significant promise in CRS and could provide benefit in both Type 2 and Non-Type 2 endotypes based on the mechanism of action and results of the asthma studies.

IL-4Rα

There is 1 active Phase 2 clinical trial evaluating TQH2722, a humanized mAb targeting IL-4Rα, which leads to the dual-blockade of IL-4 and IL-13, similar to dupilumab (NCT06089278). Phase 1 trials demonstrated acceptable safety and dosing profiles, supporting further clinical development.[73]

IL-33

Etokimab is a mAb against IL-33, which is an epithelial alarmin implicated in the pathogenesis of atopic diseases. Etokimab has been trialed in atopic dermatitis and eosinophilic asthma and has demonstrated a role in both eosinophilic and neutrophilic inflammation.[74] Initial reports from a completed phase 2 clinical trial evaluating etokimab in CRSwNP indicate no significant difference in symptom or nasal polyp scores compared to placebo (NCT03614923). However, since etokimab has been shown to inhibit neutrophilic inflammation and migration,[75] it could suggest a possible use in Type 1 and 3 endotypes – and/or the CRSsNP phenotype – but further studies are necessary. Another IL-33 antibody, PF-06817024, recently completed a phase 1 clinical trial in CRSwNP and atopic dermatitis with promising results justifying further investigation.[76]

Targets of Non-type 2 Inflammation

While biologics for CRSwNP have largely targeted Type 2 inflammation, evaluation of other endotypes and targets in future research will be critical. Currently, no available biologics for CRS target Type 1 and/or Type 3 inflammation. Nevertheless, many possible targets for treating these endotypes exist. For instance, targeting IL-17 could block the Type 3 inflammatory cascade, and multiple mAbs targeting IL-17 are already approved for psoriasis. One of those drugs, brodalumab, has previously been tested in severe asthma without benefit, but could be a possible target in Type 3 CRS.[77] There is an active clinical trial evaluating brensocatib (NCT06013241), a small molecule inhibitor of neutrophil serine proteases, in CRSsNP.

SUMMARY

Endotype classification in CRS has led to a better understanding of an individual patient's disease process and can facilitate precision medicine. Management of CRS will continue to improve with detailed classification of underlying inflammatory pathways and representative biomarkers, helping to establish prognosis for severe and recalcitrant disease and informing appropriate surgical and medical management. Patients with a particular endotype may benefit from corresponding targeted biologic therapy irrespective of the presence of nasal polyps, and hence these medications may ultimately have a role in CRSsNP. Similarly, patients with CRSwNP may not necessarily respond to a particular biologic agent unless their disease corresponds to the appropriate endotype, indicating the importance of tissue analysis and biomarker research.[18]

Sinus irrigations with topical corticosteroids, with appropriate delivery facilitated by well-performed endoscopic sinus surgery, remain the standard-of-care for most patients. However, the use of targeted biologics offers an option for persistent disease despite appropriate routine management, or for those with inflammatory comorbidities, like asthma and atopic diseases.[44] These novel medications offer an exciting advancement in nonsurgical management of this challenging chronic disease process and will likely play an increasingly integral role in the future.

CLINICS CARE POINTS/PITFALLS

- CRS is defined as 12 or more weeks of 2 or more cardinal subjective sinonasal symptoms – nasal obstruction, discolored nasal discharge, hyposmia, and/or facial pressure/pain
- Confirmation of the diagnosis requires objective evidence of inflammation:
- Edema, nasal polyps, and/or purulence on nasal endoscopy, or
- Findings of inflammation (ie, mucosal thickening or opacification) on radiographic imaging
- CRS is traditionally subcategorized into the following phenotypes and subphenotypes:
- CRSwNP
- AFRS
- AERD
- CCAD
- Other CRS associated with systemic disease
- CRSsNP
- Treatment by phenotype alone may be imprecise and ineffective by failing to capture an individual patient's biology
- CRS is more precisely described by endotypes and associated biomarkers:
- Type 1 – Th1 cell predominance secreting IFN-γ, TNF-α, and IL-12
- Type 2 – Th2 and ILC2 cells secreting IL-4, IL-5, IL-33, and IL-13, associated with eosinophilia and/or elevated IgE
- Type 3 – Th17 and ILC3 cells secreting IL-17 and IL-22 leading to neutrophil activation
- Type 2 endotype is most strongly associated with asthma and atopic disease
- There are 3 FDA approved biologics for the treatment of CRSwNP:
- Dupilumab – Anti-IL-4Rα monoclonal antibody
- Mepolizumab – Anti-IL-5 monoclonal antibody
- Omalizumab – Anti-IgE monoclonal antibody
- Many current and novel biologics are in clinical trials, which may expand utilization to other phenotypes (eg, CRSsNP) and/or endotypes (eg, Type 1/3 inflammation)
- Surgery remains the standard of care for routine CRSwNP but biologics play an increasingly critical role for patients with recalcitrant disease, comorbid asthma requiring therapy, and/or poor candidates for general anesthesia

DISCLOSURE

The authors have no relevant disclosures.

REFERENCES

1. Orlandi RR, Kingdom TT, Hwang PH, et al. International consensus statement on allergy and rhinology: rhinosinusitis. Int Forum Allergy Rhinol 2016;6(September 2015):S22–209.
2. Bhattacharyya N, Gilani S. Prevalence of potential adult chronic rhinosinusitis symptoms in the United States. Otolaryngol Head Neck Surg 2018;159(3):522–5.
3. Hirsch AG, Stewart WF, Sundaresan AS, et al. Nasal and sinus symptoms and chronic rhinosinusitis in a population-based sample. Allergy 2017;72(2):274–81.
4. DeConde AS, Soler ZM. Chronic rhinosinusitis: epidemiology and burden of disease. Am J Rhinol Allergy 2016;30(2):134–9.
5. Dietz de Loos D, Lourijsen ES, Wildeman MAM, et al. Prevalence of chronic rhinosinusitis in the general population based on sinus radiology and symptomatology. J Allergy Clin Immunol 2019;143(3):1207–14.
6. Chee J, Pang KW, Low T, et al. Epidemiology and aetiology of chronic rhinosinusitis in Asia-A narrative review. Clin Otolaryngol 2023;48(2):305–12.
7. Grayson J, Hopkins C, Mori E, et al. Contemporary classification of chronic rhinosinusitis beyond polyps vs no polyps: a review. JAMA Otolaryngol Head Neck Surg 2020. https://doi.org/10.1001/jamaoto.2020.1453.
8. Fokkens WJ, Lund VJ, Mullol J, et al. EPOS 2012: European position paper on rhinosinusitis and nasal polyps 2012. A summary for otorhinolaryngologists. Rhinology 2012;50(1):1–12.
9. Cho SH, Hamilos DL, Han DH, et al. Phenotypes of chronic rhinosinusitis. J Allergy Clin Immunol Pract 2020;8(5):1505.
10. Chen CC, Buchheit KM. Endotyping chronic rhinosinusitis with nasal polyps: understanding inflammation beyond phenotypes 2023;37(2):132–9.
11. Cao PP, Wang ZC, Schleimer RP, et al. Pathophysiologic mechanisms of chronic rhinosinusitis and their roles in emerging disease endotypes. Ann Allergy Asthma Immunol 2019;122(1):33–40.
12. Bachert C, Zhang L, Gevaert P. Current and future treatment options for adult chronic rhinosinusitis: Focus on nasal polyposis. J Allergy Clin Immunol 2015; 136(6):1431–40.
13. Bachert C, Gevaert P, Hellings P. Biotherapeutics in chronic rhinosinusitis with and without nasal polyps. J Allergy Clin Immunol Pract 2017;5(6):1512–6.
14. Anderson GP. Endotyping asthma: new insights into key pathogenic mechanisms in a complex, heterogeneous disease. Lancet 2008;372(9643):1107–19.
15. Annunziato F, Romagnani C, Romagnani S. The 3 major types of innate and adaptive cell-mediated effector immunity. J Allergy Clin Immunol 2015;135(3):626–35.
16. Staudacher AG, Peters AT, Kato A, et al. Use of endotypes, phenotypes, and inflammatory markers to guide treatment decisions in chronic rhinosinusitis. Ann Allergy Asthma Immunol 2020;124(4):318–25.
17. Kaech SM, Cui W. Transcriptional control of effector and memory CD8+ T cell differentiation. Nat Rev Immunol 2012;12(11):749–61.
18. Fokkens WJ, Lund VJ, Hopkins C, et al. European position paper on rhinosinusitis and nasal polyps 2020. Official Journal of the European and International Rhinologic Societies and of the Confederation of European ORL-HNS. 2020;29(Suppl): 1–464.

19. De Greve G, Hellings PW, Fokkens WJ, et al. Endotype-driven treatment in chronic upper airway diseases. Clin Transl Allergy 2017;7(1):1–14.
20. Plager DA, Kahl JC, Asmann YW, et al. Gene transcription changes in asthmatic chronic rhinosinusitis with nasal polyps and comparison to those in atopic dermatitis. PLoS One 2010;5(7):1–9.
21. Miljkovic D, Bassiouni A, Cooksley C, et al. Association between group 2 innate lymphoid cells enrichment, nasal polyps and allergy in chronic rhinosinusitis. Allergy 2014;69(9):1154–61.
22. Mahdavinia M, Carter RG, Ocampo CJ, et al. Basophils are elevated in nasal polyps of patients with chronic rhinosinusitis without aspirin sensitivity. J Allergy Clin Immunol 2014;133(6):1759–63.
23. Hammad H, Lambrecht BN. Barrier epithelial cells and the control of type 2 immunity. Immunity 2015;43(1):29–40.
24. Shaw JL, Fakhri S, Citardi MJ, et al. IL-33-responsive innate lymphoid cells are an important source of IL-13 in chronic rhinosinusitis with nasal polyps. Am J Respir Crit Care Med 2013;188(4):432–9.
25. Grayson JW, Cavada M, Harvey RJ. Clinically relevant phenotypes in chronic rhinosinusitis. J Otolaryngol Head Neck Surg 2019;48(1):1–10.
26. Ho J, Hamizan AW, Alvarado R, et al. Systemic predictors of eosinophilic chronic rhinosinusitis. Am J Rhinol Allergy. 2018;32(4):252–7.
27. Couto LGF, Fernades AM, Brandão DF, et al. Histological aspects of rhinosinusal polyps. Braz J Otorhinolaryngol 2008;74(2):207–12.
28. Stevens WW, Peters AT, Tan BK, et al. Associations between inflammatory endotypes and clinical presentations in chronic rhinosinusitis. J Allergy Clin Immunol 2019;7(8):2812–20.e3.
29. Tokunaga T, Sakashita M, Haruna T, et al. Novel scoring system and algorithm for classifying chronic rhinosinusitis: The JESREC Study. Allergy 2015;70(8):995–1003.
30. Bettelli E, Korn T, Kuchroo VK. Th17: the third member of the effector T cell trilogy. Curr Opin Immunol 2007;19(6):652–7.
31. Zhang N, Van Zele T, Perez-Novo C, et al. Different types of T-effector cells orchestrate mucosal inflammation in chronic sinus disease. J Allergy Clin Immunol 2008;122(5):961–8.
32. Wang X, Zhang N, Bo M, et al. Diversity of TH cytokine profiles in patients with chronic rhinosinusitis: A multicenter study in Europe, Asia, and Oceania. J Allergy Clin Immunol 2016;138(5):1344–53.
33. Derycke L, Eyerich S, Van Crombruggen K, et al. Mixed T helper cell signatures in chronic rhinosinusitis with and without polyps. PLoS One 2014;9(6):1–8.
34. Bachert C, Luong AU, Gevaert P, et al. The unified airway hypothesis: evidence from specific intervention with anti-il-5 biologic therapy. J Allergy Clin Immunol Pract 2023;11(9):2630–41.
35. Lee TJ, Fu CH, Wang CH, et al. Impact of chronic rhinosinusitis on severe asthma patients. PLoS One 2017;12(2):1–16.
36. Lin DC, Chandra RK, Tan BK, et al. Association between severity of asthma and degree of chronic rhinosinusitis. Am J Rhinol Allergy. 2011;25(4):205–8.
37. Seshadri S, Rosati M, Lin DC, et al. Regional differences in the expression of innate host defense molecules in sinonasal mucosa. J Allergy Clin Immunol 2013;132(5).
38. Tan BK, Klingler AI, Poposki JA, et al. Heterogeneous inflammatory patterns in chronic rhinosinusitis without nasal polyps in Chicago, Illinois. J Allergy Clin Immunol 2017;139(2):699–703.e7.

39. Van Bruaene N, Pérez-Novo CA, Basinski TM, et al. T-cell regulation in chronic paranasal sinus disease. J Allergy Clin Immunol 2008;121(6):16–8.
40. Orgain CA, Harvey RJ. The role of frontal sinus drillouts in nasal polyposis. Curr Opin Otolaryngol Head Neck Surg 2018;26(1):34–40.
41. Thomas WW, Harvey RJ, Rudmik L, et al. Distribution of topical agents to the paranasal sinuses: An evidence-based review with recommendations. Int Forum Allergy Rhinol 2013;3(9):691–703.
42. Ho J, Li W, Grayson JW, et al. Systemic medication requirement in post-surgical patients with eosinophilic chronic rhinosinusitis. Rhinology journal 2020;0(0). https://doi.org/10.4193/rhin20.073.
43. Walford HH, Lund SJ, Baum RE, et al. Increased ILC2s in the eosinophilic nasal polyp endotype are associated with corticosteroid responsiveness. Clin Immunol 2014;155(1):126–35.
44. Mandl HK, Miller JE, Beswick DM. Current and novel biologic therapies for patients with asthma and nasal polyps. Otolaryngol Clin North Am 2024;57(2): 225–42.
45. Fokkens WJ, Viskens AS, Backer V, et al. EPOS/EUFOREA update on indication and evaluation of Biologics in Chronic Rhinosinusitis with Nasal Polyps 2023. Rhinology 2023;61(3):194–202.
46. Akdis CA. Therapies for allergic inflammation: Refining strategies to induce tolerance. Nat Med 2012;18(5):736–49.
47. Bachert C, Mannent L, Naclerio RM, et al. Effect of subcutaneous dupilumab on nasal polyp burden in patients with chronic sinusitis and nasal polyposis: A randomized clinical trial. JAMA, J Am Med Assoc 2016;315(5):469–79.
48. Ul-Haq Z, Naz S, Mesaik MA. Interleukin-4 receptor signaling and its binding mechanism: A therapeutic insight from inhibitors tool box. Cytokine Growth Factor Rev 2016;32:3–15.
49. Buchheit KM, Sohail A, Hacker J, et al. Rapid and sustained effect of dupilumab on clinical and mechanistic outcomes in aspirin-exacerbated respiratory disease. J Allergy Clin Immunol 2022;150(2):415–24.
50. Han JK, Bachert C, Fokkens W, et al. Mepolizumab for chronic rhinosinusitis with nasal polyps (SYNAPSE): a randomised, double-blind, placebo-controlled, phase 3 trial. Lancet Respir Med 2021;9(10):1141–53.
51. Gevaert P, Van Bruaene N, Cattaert T, et al. Mepolizumab, a humanized anti-IL-5 mAb, as a treatment option for severe nasal polyposis. J Allergy Clin Immunol 2011;128(5):989–95.e8.
52. Fokkens WJ, Mullol J, Kennedy D, et al. Mepolizumab for chronic rhinosinusitis with nasal polyps (SYNAPSE): In-depth sinus surgery analysis. Allergy 2023; 78(3):812–21.
53. Lin H, Boesel KM, Griffith DT, et al. Omalizumab rapidly decreases nasal allergic response and FcεRI on basophils. J Allergy Clin Immunol 2004;113(2):297–302.
54. Bachert C, Gevaert P, Holtappels G, et al. Total and specific IgE in nasal polyps is related to local eosinophilic inflammation. J Allergy Clin Immunol 2001;107(4): 607–14.
55. Van Zele T, Gevaert P, Watelet JB, et al. Staphylococcus aureus colonization and IgE antibody formation to enterotoxins is increased in nasal polyposis. J Allergy Clin Immunol 2004;114(4):979–81.
56. Tomassen P, Vandeplas G, Van Zele T, et al. Inflammatory endotypes of chronic rhinosinusitis based on cluster analysis of biomarkers. J Allergy Clin Immunol 2016;137(5):1449–56.e4.

57. Gevaert P, Calus L, Van Zele T, et al. Omalizumab is effective in allergic and nonallergic patients with nasal polyps and asthma. J Allergy Clin Immunol 2013;131(1):110–6.e1.

58. Gevaert P, Bachert C, Corren J, et al. Omalizumab efficacy and safety in nasal polyposis: results from two parallel, double-blind, placebo-controlled trials. Ann Allergy Asthma Immunol 2019;123(5):S17.

59. Wenzel SE. Asthma phenotypes: the evolution from clinical to molecular approaches. Nat Med 2012;18:716–25.

60. Hamizan AW, Christensen JM, Ebenzer J, et al. Middle turbinate edema as a diagnostic marker of inhalant allergy. Int Forum Allergy Rhinol 2017;7(1):37–42.

61. Brunner JP, Jawad BA, McCoul ED. Polypoid change of the middle turbinate and paranasal sinus polyposis are distinct entities. Otolaryngol Head Neck Surg 2017;157(3):519–23.

62. Dharmarajan H, Falade O, Lee SE, et al. Outcomes of dupilumab treatment versus endoscopic sinus surgery for chronic rhinosinusitis with nasal polyps. Int Forum Allergy Rhinol 2022;12(8):986–95.

63. Miglani A, Soler ZM, Smith TL, et al. A comparative analysis of endoscopic sinus surgery versus biologics for treatment of chronic rhinosinusitis with nasal polyposis. Int Forum Allergy Rhinol 2023;13(2):116–28.

64. Alshatti A, Webb C. Biologics versus functional endoscopic sinus surgery for the treatment of chronic rhinosinusitis with nasal polyps: a literature review. J Laryngol Otol 2023;1–6.

65. Parasher AK, Gliksman M, Segarra D, et al. Economic evaluation of dupilumab versus endoscopic sinus surgery for the treatment of chronic rhinosinusitis with nasal polyps. Int Forum Allergy Rhinol 2022;12(6):813–20.

66. Scangas GA, Wu AW, Ting JY, et al. Cost utility analysis of dupilumab versus endoscopic sinus surgery for chronic rhinosinusitis with nasal polyps. Laryngoscope 2021;131(1):E26–33.

67. Lans RJL van der, Fokkens WJ, Adriaensen GFJPM, et al. Real-life observational cohort verifies high efficacy of dupilumab for chronic rhinosinusitis with nasal polyps. Allergy 2022;77(2):670.

68. Bachert C, Han JK, Desrosiers MY, et al. Efficacy and safety of benralizumab in chronic rhinosinusitis with nasal polyps: A randomized, placebo-controlled trial. J Allergy Clin Immunol 2022;149(4):1309–17.e12.

69. Boiko NV, Lodochkina OE, Kit MM, et al. [Impact of reslizumab on the course of chronic rhinosinusitis in patients with eosinophilic asthma]. Vestn Otorinolaringol 2021;86(2):43–8.

70. Singh D, Fuhr R, Bird NP, et al. A Phase 1 study of the long-acting anti-IL-5 monoclonal antibody GSK3511294 in patients with asthma. Br J Clin Pharmacol 2022; 88(2):702–12.

71. Laidlaw TM, Menzies-Gow A, Caveney S, et al. Tezepelumab efficacy in patients with severe, uncontrolled asthma with comorbid nasal polyps in NAVIGATOR. J Asthma Allergy 2023;16:915.

72. Gauvreau GM, Hohlfeld JM, Mark FitzGerald J, et al. Inhaled anti-TSLP antibody fragment, ecleralimab, blocks responses to allergen in mild asthma. Eur Respir J 2023;61(3).

73. Lin P, Sun F, Xu Y, et al. 565 – Safety and pharmacokinetic profiles of a humanized monoclonal antibody TQH2722 targeting interleukin 4 receptor alpha (IL-4Rα) in health adult subjects. Br J Dermatol 2024;190(Supplement_2):ii59–60.

74. Drake LY, Kita H. IL-33: biological properties, functions and roles in airway disease. Immunol Rev 2017;278(1):173.

75. Chen YL, Gutowska-Owsiak D, Hardman CS, et al. Proof-of-concept clinical trial of etokimab shows a key role for IL-33 in atopic dermatitis pathogenesis. Sci Transl Med 2019;11(515).
76. Danto SI, Tsamandouras N, Reddy P, et al. Safety, tolerability, pharmacokinetics, and pharmacodynamics of pf-06817024 in healthy participants, participants with chronic rhinosinusitis with nasal polyps, and participants with atopic dermatitis: a phase 1, randomized, double-blind, placebo-controlled study. J Clin Pharmacol 2023. https://doi.org/10.1002/JCPH.2360.
77. Busse WW, Holgate S, Kerwin E, et al. Study of brodalumab , a human anti – il-17 receptor monoclonal antibody , in moderate to severe asthma. Am J Respir Crit Care Med 2013;188(11):1294–302.

Biologics in Aspirin-Exacerbated Respiratory Disease and Allergic Bronchopulmonary Aspergillosis

Jenny Huang, MD[a], Andrew A. White, MD[b],*

KEYWORDS

- Aspirin-exacerbated respiratory disease • AERD
- NSAID-exacerbated respiratory disease • N-ERD
- Allergic bronchopulmonary aspergillosis • ABPA • Biologics

KEY POINTS

- Biologic medications should be considered for patients with aspirin-exacerbated respiratory disease (AERD) or allergic bronchopulmonary aspergillosis (ABPA) refractory to first line therapies.
- For the treatment of AERD, both biologics and aspirin therapy after desensitization should be discussed with patients. Patients with AERD may see the most benefit with dupilumab, but other biologics are beneficial.
- More data exist for omalizumab treatment in ABPA, but some data for other biologics support their use if patients do not respond to IgE blockade.
- Patients not responsive to one biologic may be responsive to another, indicating that there may be endotypes of AERD and ABPA, similar to asthma.
- Biologics are not without risks, there have been reports of hypersensitivity reactions with omalizumab and dupilumab induced hypereosinophilia causing an asthma exacerbation complicating the treatment of ABPA.

INTRODUCTION

Biologic medications target specific components of allergic and inflammatory pathways. They are approved for the treatment of many atopic diseases such as asthma, nasal polyposis, and atopic dermatitis, with rapid expansion into additional allergic and hypersensitivity disorders. In this article, we will discuss and review the use of

[a] Division of Allergy, Asthma, and Immunology, Scripps Clinic, 3811 Valley Centre Drive, S99, San Diego, CA 92130, USA; [b] Aspirin Exacerbated Respiratory Disease Clinic, Division of Allergy, Asthma, and Immunology, Scripps Clinic, 3811 Valley Centre Drive, S99, San Diego, CA 92130, USA
* Corresponding author.
E-mail address: white.andrew@scrippshealth.org

Immunol Allergy Clin N Am 44 (2024) 673–692
https://doi.org/10.1016/j.iac.2024.07.006
immunology.theclinics.com
0889-8561/24/© 2024 Elsevier Inc. All rights reserved, including those for text and data mining, AI training, and similar technologies.

biologics for the treatment of aspirin-exacerbated respiratory disease (AERD) and allergic bronchopulmonary aspergillosis (ABPA).

Aspirin-Exacerbated Respiratory Disease

AERD is a disease entity characterized by chronic rhinosinusitis with nasal polyps (CRSwNP), asthma, and respiratory reactions following exposure to nonsteroidal anti-inflammatory medications (NSAIDs) including aspirin. Previously, the only therapy specific for AERD consisted of aspirin therapy after desensitization (ATAD), which involves desensitizing a patient to NSAIDs through gradual introduction of aspirin during a 1 or 2-day procedure, followed by chronic high-dose aspirin therapy. Otherwise, management included topical therapy for nasal polyposis and management of asthma with inhaler therapy and leukotriene modifiers. Many patients who had disease refractory to these treatments were dependent on systemic corticosteroids and repeated sinus surgery. ATAD is not an option for, or effective in, all patients and requires debulking polypectomy prior to employment for optimal effect. Side effects of aspirin might occur; particularly at the doses needed to observe positive effect (325–650 mg twice daily[1]). With the advent of biologic medications, the landscape for the treatment of AERD has shifted significantly.

The gold standard for diagnosing AERD is an oral challenge with aspirin. These oral challenges can be done in different manners, but generally consist of graded challenges occurring over 1 to 2 days with the intention of identifying objective sinonasal reactions (upper airway), bronchospasm, cough or wheeze (lower airway), or a combination of upper and lower airway reactivity. A minority of patients may experience additional symptoms including abdominal pain, flushing, or urticarial-like skin eruptions in addition to respiratory symptoms. However, in patients with a history of hospitalization after taking an NSAID or patients who have had 2 or more respiratory reactions to different NSAIDs, AERD can be diagnosed with history.[2]

Patients with AERD classically have eosinophilic chronic rhinosinusitis with nasal polyposis, which is frequently difficult to control. Additionally, the vast majority of patients have asthma. Following sinus surgery, most patients with AERD have rapid recurrence of nasal polyposis.[3] Additionally, patients with AERD have higher rates of anosmia and worse quality of life when compared with aspirin tolerant patients with nasal polyposis.[1] Similarly, although not all patients with AERD have severe asthma, in the TENOR study, a study of severe asthmatics, 16% of patients with persistent airflow limitation had AERD, compared with 11% of patients with no persistent airflow limitation having comorbid AERD.[4] These findings support the conclusion that once AERD is identified, it predicts that a patient will more likely have disease that is difficult to control and recalcitrant to standard therapy.

In the 1980s, the first use of ATAD was described after the serendipitous discovery of therapeutic benefit in a single patient after an aspirin challenge protocol.[5] This led to the first randomized double-blinded study of ATAD[6] with subsequent work proving the unique effectiveness of this therapy in AERD and not in aspirin tolerant patients.[7] From the 1980s until the early 2000s, ATAD was widely employed for the treatment of AERD combined with leukotriene modifying medications, inhaled therapies for asthma, and topical therapies, namely corticosteroids, to address the concurrent sinus disease. Most patients required multiple functional endoscopic sinus surgeries over the course of their disease. As it became clear that the main effect of ATAD was to slow the rate of polyp growth, but not cause polyp regression, the standard of care was to add ATAD immediately following sinus surgery.[8]

In 2003, omalizumab was the first respiratory biologic approved for the treatment of allergic asthma. Although many patients with AERD did have sensitization to aeroallergens and attempts with omalizumab were often undertaken, there have unfortunately been very limited systematic studies of omalizumab for treatment of AERD despite its existence on the market for over 20 years.

Prior to the coronavirus disease 2019 (COVID-19) pandemic, several respiratory biologics were introduced, including omalizumab, reslizumab, benralizumab, and dupilumab. In 2020, the COVID-19 pandemic began, and simultaneously, there was an increase in the use of biologics. For patients with AERD specifically, the inability to routinely perform procedures, including spirometry, aspirin challenge and desensitization, and sinus surgery (some of which are aerosol-generating), diminished the accessibility and availability of ATAD. As a result, the use of biologics as either a replacement or a stopgap measure emerged. This sequence of events is an important prologue to the subsequent discussion of the biologics which were shown to have effects not just on allergic asthma, but also on nasal polyposis.

Dupilumab

CRSwNP, one of the hallmarks of AERD, has been shown to be predominantly driven by type 2 inflammation,[9,10] of which both IL-4 and IL-13 play a big role in pathogenesis. Because of the type 2 inflammatory signature in nasal polyposis, it is not surprising that some agents which target these pathways, including dupilumab, have been successful in treating AERD.

Dupilumab is a monoclonal antibody which targets IL-4Rα, thereby inhibiting both IL-4 and IL-13. The LIBERTY NP SINUS-24 and LIBERTY NP SINUS-52 trials studied the efficacy of dupilumab for the treatment of nasal polyps. Among the 724 patients enrolled in the 2 studies, 204 patients (28%) had AERD,[11] representing a large proportion of the study population. A subgroup analysis of SINUS-52 showed improvement in nasal polyp score in patients with AERD at week 24 compared to baseline.[11]

In addition to the studies on nasal polyps, there have also been numerous studies published on the use of dupilumab specifically in AERD. Select studies are summarized in **Table 1**. It must be noted that although dupilumab is approved for the treatment of nasal polyps, AERD is not specifically an approved indication for dupilumab or any of the other respiratory biologics discussed here.

In terms of outcomes, patients treated with dupilumab for AERD have shown improvement in symptoms and symptom scores.[12–15] Patients had improvement in smell and nasal symptoms in additional to improvements seen in Sino-Nasal Outcome Test (SNOT-22) scores. SNOT-22 is a questionnaire commonly used to measure symptom burden and monitor treatment response. As asthma is one approved indication for dupilumab, it is not surprising that patients also had improvement in lung function and asthma control.[12,15] Dupilumab use has been shown to reduce polyp recurrence,[16] a common feature of AERD. Though most studies have been done in adults, the use of dupilumab in pediatric patients with AERD has also been reported with positive outcomes.[13]

In addition to the positive symptom outcomes, dupilumab has shown effectiveness in protecting AERD patients from reacting to NSAIDs. One study showed that patients were able to tolerate a higher dose of aspirin during oral challenges while on dupilumab compared to prior: 325 mg compared to 81 mg, respectively.[17] It has been hypothesized that by blocking IL-4, the receptor for PGE2 (EP2) normalizes its previously down-regulated expression. This allows for the appropriate COX-2 mediated synthesis of PGE2, ultimately resolving the sensitivity to COX-1 inhibition.[18]

Biologics Targeting Interleukin-5 Activity

Another important cytokine involved in type 2 inflammation is IL-5, which has been identified in nasal polyp tissue.[10] There are several biologics available which target

Table 1
Summary of select studies on dupilumab for the treatment of aspirin-exacerbated respiratory disease (AERD)

Study	Study Type	Number of Patients	Outcomes
Buchheit et al,[12] 2022	Prospective cohort	22	Improvement in smell, nasal symptoms, and lung function with dupilumab use
Patel et al,[16] 2022	Retrospective cohort	8	Patients with AERD and history of revision endoscopic sinus surgery were subsequently treated with dupilumab with only one patient having polyp recurrence
Bensko et al,[13] 2022	Case series	6	Pediatric patients treated with dupilumab had improvement in SNOT-22 and nasal polyp scores
Mustafa et al,[14] 2021	Prospective case series with placebo run-in phase	10	Patients with AERD and symptoms on standard medical therapy were treated with dupilumab as an add on therapy and saw improvement in SNOT-22 scores
Mustafa et al,[17] 2021	Case series	5	Patients with challenge confirmed AERD underwent repeat aspirin challenge on dupilumab, 4 of which were able to reach a dose of 325 mg, with the previous symptomatic threshold dose being 81 mg
Laidlaw et al,[15] 2019	Clinical trial	19	Patients with AERD enrolled within a larger proof-of-concept study for dupilumab for the treatment of CRSwNP showed improvement in disease outcomes, asthma control, and lung function

the activity of IL-5, namely benralizumab (anti-IL-5Rα), mepolizumab (anti-IL-5), and reslizumab (anti-IL-5). SYNAPSE was the phase 3 clinical trial examining mepolizumab for the treatment of CRSwNP, of which 27% of the patients in the study had AERD.[19] In this study, patients with AERD favored mepolizumab over placebo but there was no significant improvement in symptoms.[19] In the phase 3 clinical trial of benralizumab for CRSwNP (OSTRO), 30% of participants had AERD. Nasal polyp scores were improved on benralizumab compared to placebo, but time to first sinus surgery was not affected.[20]

In terms of studies specifically examining IL-5 blockade for AERD, the most studies exist for mepolizumab, some of which are summarized in **Table 2**. Studies on the use of mepolizumab have showed mixed results. Some reports indicate that mepolizumab may be a viable option with observable symptom control[21] and treatment of concomitant coronary vasospasm[22] and eosinophilic gastroenteritis.[23] There were also reports of successful treatment with mepolizumab my after failure of omalizumab.[24]

However, mepolizumab may not prevent polyp regrowth in patients with severe disease[25] and may not prevent reactions during aspirin challenges or desensitizations.[26] Additionally, reslizumab was seen to deplete peripheral eosinophils but did not seem to have an effect on sinonasal disease, with repeat sinus surgery needed while on therapy.[27]

Omalizumab

POLYP 1 and POLYP 2 were the phase 3 clinical trials for inhibition of IgE with omalizumab for the treatment of CRSwNP. In the studies, between 17% and 39% of study participants had AERD.[28] After 24 weeks of treatment, there was a decrease in nasal polyp scores in the patients with AERD, but it was not significantly different compared to the patients without AERD in the study.[28]

Table 3 summarizes select studies of omalizumab for the treatment of AERD, in which omalizumab has been shown to decrease urinary leukotriene E4[29] and reduce the extra-respiratory symptoms associated with AERD.[30] Patients on omalizumab were also able to decrease steroid and short-acting beta-agonist use.[31] There is also report of aspirin and alcohol tolerance with omalizumab treatment.[32]

The protection from COX-1 inhibitor reactions might be strongest with omalizumab. In a randomized blinded crossover study of AERD patients treated with omalizumab or placebo, 62.5% of patients had their NSAID sensitivity completely silenced on omalizumab treatment.[29] Other studies show that omalizumab can result in decreased reactions during aspirin desensitizations,[33,34] but reactivity may still occur in patients with more severe reactions.[35]

Tezepelumab

Tezepelumab is a monoclonal antibody targeting thymic stromal lymphopoietin (TSLP). It is approved for the treatment of asthma, but being studied for the treatment of nasal polyps. An analysis of the NAVIGATOR phase 3 trial showed that patients with severe asthma and nasal polyps had improvement in sinonasal symptoms and asthma outcomes on tezepelumab.[36]

So far, there are no specific studies on the use of tezepelumab for AERD, but it may be another agent with benefit in AERD.

Comparison Studies Between Biologic Medications for the Treatment of Aspirin-Exacerbated Respiratory Disease

There have been some studies comparing the different biologic medications for the treatment of AERD. These studies do not compare the use of multiple biologics in a

Table 2
Summary of select studies on mepolizumab for the treatment of AERD

Study	Study Type	Number of Patients	Outcomes
Supron et al,[25] 2023	Retrospective cohort	8	In patients with AERD and history of sinus surgery, continuation of mepolizumab treatment after surgery did not prevent recurrence of nasal polyps
Martin et al,[26] 2021	Case series	3	Patients had observed reactions to aspirin during challenge or desensitization while being treated with mepolizumab
Caruso et al,[23] 2020	Case report	1	Successful use of mepolizumab to treat AERD with concomitant eosinophilic gastroenteritis
Mahdavinia et al,[24] 2019	Case report	1	Patient with history of failed aspirin desensitization and disease refractory to omalizumab was able to tolerate desensitization and aspirin therapy while on mepolizumab
Hagin et al,[22] 2019	Case report	1	Patient with AERD-associated coronary vasospasm intolerant to aspirin was successfully treated with mepolizumab
Tuttle et al,[21] 2018	Retrospective cohort	14	Patients with AERD treated with at least 3 doses of mepolizumab showed symptom improvement and decrease in peripheral eosinophilia

Table 3
Summary of select studies on omalizumab for the treatment of AERD

Study	Study Type	Number of Patients	Outcomes
Hayashi et al,[30] 2023	Retrospective cohort; case series	27; 3	Two studies showing that omalizumab decreased extra-respiratory symptoms associated with AERD including chest pain, gastrointestinal, and cutaneous symptoms
Hayashi et al,[29] 2020	Double-blind, randomized, crossover, placebo controlled trial	16	Omalizumab decreased urinary leukotriene E4. Ten out of 16 patients were able to tolerate aspirin challenge
Jean et al,[31] 2019	Retrospective cohort	29	Patients treated with omalizumab showed a decrease in steroid and short-acting beta-agonist use
Lang et al,[33] 2018	Randomized, double-blind, placebo-controlled study	11	Treatment with 16 weeks of omalizumab resulted in a statistically significant likelihood of having no respiratory reaction during aspirin desensitization
Phillips-Angles et al,[34] 2017	Case series	7	Six out of 7 patients with AERD on omalizumab had asymptomatic aspirin challenges
Waldram et al,[35] 2018	Retrospective cohort	167	Single center study of aspirin desensitization for AERD which showed that omalizumab did not prevent symptoms during desensitization in 8 out of 9 patients in the study on omalizumab
Bergmann et al,[32] 2015	Case report	1	Patient with AERD treated with omalizumab resulting in successful aspirin and alcohol challenge (with history of reactions)

single patient. A single-center retrospective cohort study of 74 patients with AERD treated with biologics (data collected in December 2020), showed that patients treated with dupilumab led to statistically significant improved clinical outcomes compared to omalizumab, mepolizumab, and reslizumab.[37] In a separate study, patients reported variable response to biologics, but the majority of patients on dupilumab reported it to be effective.[38] In patients who report inadequate response to IL-5 blockade, dupilumab may be prove to be a successful alternative treatment.[39] Data have indicated that the use of type 2 biologics reduces amount of steroid exposure in AERD.[40] A systematic review and network meta-analysis comparing biologics and aspirin desensitization for the treatment of CRSwNP showed that dupilumab had the most benefit for the outcomes examined, which included quality of life, symptoms, smell, rescue surgery, rescue systemic steroids, nasal polyp size, radiographic severity, and adverse events.[41] Although cost considerations would favor ATAD, aspirin had the most harm with regard to adverse events.[41]

Summary

The emergence of biologic medications has significantly changed the options for treating AERD. Reports have shown that dupilumab may be the most promising option. There has been variable response to IL-5 inhibition and suggestion that dupilumab may be a viable treatment for those with disease refractory to other biologics. The targets of the biologics are quite different, and the improvements in NSAID reactivity versus sense of smell might depend on different cell types; thus, differences in these outcomes might be expected with different biologics. However, results must be interpreted with caution given the lack of studies enrolling well characterized AERD patients, and importantly the lack of any studies truly comparing effectiveness of the biologics head-to-head. Overall, biologics have been shown to be steroid-sparing agents in the treatment of AERD. The choice between ATAD and treatment with biologics should be discussed with all patients.

Allergic Bronchopulmonary Aspergillosis

ABPA results from immune responses to *Aspergillus fumigatus*. Patients with ABPA have most commonly had underlying asthma or cystic fibrosis. A common presentation of ABPA is asthma that is poorly controlled. First line therapy for the treatment of ABPA has included systemic corticosteroids, anti-fungal medications, or a combination of both. However, patients can have disease refractory to first line treatments, requiring consideration of other treatments, including biologic medications.

Although ABPA is not a new entity, understanding of its pathophysiology is unfortunately limited. Type 2 inflammation has been implicated in the pathogenesis of ABPA. In a study of bronchoalveolar lavage fluid from patients with eosinophilic lung diseases, samples from patients with ABPA had significantly increased levels of IL-4 and IL-5.[42] Interestingly, patients with ABPA also had low but significantly elevated levels of IL-2 and interferon-gamma compared to healthy controls and patients with other eosinophilic lung diseases. This indicates a possible role for type 1 inflammation in the pathogenesis of APBA.[42] In a study performed in peripheral blood mononuclear cells, *Aspergillus* stimulated IL-5 and IL-13 production, levels of which were higher in patients with ABPA compared to healthy controls.[43]

There also seems to be a genetic component to the pathogenesis of ABPA. Individuals with certain genetic alleles such as polymorphisms in mannose-binding lectin-2 (*MBL2*) and surfactant protein-A2 (*SP-A2*) have a susceptibility to developing the disease.[44] A polymorphism of toll-like receptor 9 (TLR9) has also been associated with susceptibility to ABPA.[45] Another genetic association study found that ABPA has been associated with single nucleotide polymorphisms in IL13, IL4, and TLR3.[46] This genetic predisposition could provide an explanation as to why all patients with asthma do not have the same likelihood of developing ABPA.

Diagnosis

There have been several diagnostic criteria for ABPA that have been developed over the years. Among the most recently published criteria are the Revised International Society for Human and Animal Mycology (ISHAM)-ABPA working group consensus criteria for diagnosing ABPA published in 2024[47] and the criteria published by Asano and colleagues in 2021.[48] These criteria are summarized in **Table 4**. According to the Revised ISHAM-ABPA working group consensus criteria,[47] the diagnosis of ABPA should be considered in patients with predisposing conditions (asthma, cystic fibrosis, chronic obstructive lung disease, or bronchiectasis) or compatible clinico-radiological presentation. Patients must have *Aspergillus fumigates*-specific IgE greater than or equal to 0.35 kUA/L or positive skin testing, and total serum IgE greater than or equal to 500 IU/mL. Additionally, patients must have at least 2 out of the following 3 criteria: 1) positive *A fumigatus* IgG, 2) blood eosinophil count greater than or equal to 500 cells/uL (could be historical), or 3) thin section chest computed tomography consistent with ABPA (bronchiectasis, mucus plugging and high-attenuation mucus) or fleeting opacities on chest radiograph consistent with ABPA. For the criteria published by Asano and colleagues in 2021, patients need to have at least 6 of the following 10 criteria: current asthma or history of asthma or asthmatic symptoms; an absolute peripheral eosinophil count greater than 500 cells/uL; a total serum IgE level greater than or equal to 417 IU/mL; positive skin testing or the presence of serum IgE to *Aspergillus*; presence of precipitins or IgG against *Aspergillus*; fungal growth in

Table 4
Current diagnostic criteria for allergic bronchopulmonary aspergillosis (ABPA)

Revised International Society for Human and Animal Mycology (ISHAM)-ABPA Working Group Consensus Criteria[47]	Criteria Published by Asano et al. In 2021[48]
Predisposing conditions (asthma, cystic fibrosis, chronic obstructive lung disease, or bronchiectasis) or compatible clinico-radiological presentation Diagnosis requires all of the following: 1. *Aspergillus fumigates*-specific IgE ≥ 0.35 kUA/L or positive skin testing 2. Total serum IgE ≥ 500 IU/mL. And at least 2 of the following: 1. Positive *Aspergillus fumigatus* IgG 2. Blood eosinophil count ≥ 500 cells/uL (could be historical) 3. Thin section chest computed tomography consistent with ABPA (bronchiectasis, mucus plugging and high-attenuation mucus) or fleeting opacities on chest radiograph consistent with ABPA	At least 6 of the following 10 criteria are needed for diagnosis: 1. Current asthma or history of asthma or asthmatic symptoms 2. Absolute peripheral eosinophil count >500 cells/uL 3. Total serum IgE level greater than or equal to 417 IU/mL 4. Positive skin testing or the presence of serum IgE to *Aspergillus* 5. Presence of precipitins or IgG against *Aspergillus* 6. Fungal growth in sputum cultures or bronchial lavage fluid 7. Presence of fungal hyphae in bronchial mucus plugs 8. Central bronchiectasis on chest imaging 9. Presence of mucus plugs based on chest imaging, bronchoscopy, or expectoration 10. Mucus visible on chest imaging

sputum cultures or bronchial lavage fluid; presence of fungal hyphae in bronchial mucus plugs; central bronchiectasis on chest imaging; presence of mucus plugs based on chest imaging, bronchoscopy, or expectoration; and/or mucus visible on chest imaging.

Use of Biologics for the Treatment of Allergic Bronchopulmonary Aspergillosis

First line treatment for ABPA consists of systemic corticosteroids, anti-fungal medications, or a combination of both. Treatment of ABPA requires long courses of oral corticosteroids which need to be tapered off. Unfortunately, there have been higher rates of disease relapse associated with lower dosing of corticosteroids.[49] Anti-fungal agents such as itraconazole have been shown to decrease oral corticosteroid requirements in ABPA, but they are not without adverse effects.[49] It is not uncommon for patients to have refractory symptoms requiring additional treatment. There are an increasing amount of data reporting on the use of biologic medications for ABPA, though most reports consist of case reports and case series. As is the case with AERD, ABPA is not specifically an approved indication for any of the biologics discussed here.

Omalizumab

Omalizumab is a monoclonal antibody directed against IgE. Omalizumab has been available for over 20 years, and as such, more studies exist for omalizumab than the other biologic medications with regard to use for ABPA. The mechanism of action makes omalizumab an attractive choice in ABPA with numerous case reports, case series, and randomized control studies published. Select studies are summarized in **Table 5**.

There are some inconsistencies among studies[50] but, overall, studies have shown that omalizumab is a steroid-sparing agent for the treatment of ABPA.[51–55] In 1 study, 3 out of 9 patients previously on systemic steroids were able to discontinue, 5 out of 9 patients were able to reduce steroid dose by 50% or more, and only 1 patient remained on the same dose of steroids.[55] In a study of patients with cystic fibrosis, 18 out of 32 patients were on systemic steroids prior to the initiation of omalizumab; 5 of those patients were able to discontinue steroids, and 9 patients were able to reduce their daily dose.[53] In another study of cystic fibrosis, there was a trend toward lower cumulative steroids doses on treatment with omalizumab, but this was not statistically significant; 36% of patients in the study were able to decrease their daily dose by more than 50%.[52] A systematic review and meta-analysis of omalizumab in APBA showed statistically significant reductions in annualized exacerbation rates (2.09%), reduction in daily oral corticosteroid dose (14.63%), overall reduction in steroid use (65% of patients), and discontinuation of oral steroids (53%).[51] There was also a 11.9% improvement in FEV1% predicted and 7.73% improvement in Asthma Control Test (ACT) scores.[51]

Data have showed that omalizumab can also be considered in patients with high IgE levels and has been shown to decrease exacerbation frequency in this subset of patients.[56] IgE levels may be a good tool to monitor treatment response even while on omalizumab.[57] Dose of omalizumab has been reduced in some patients without increased exacerbations or need for increasing the amount of systemic steroids.[58]

Biologics Targeting Interleukin-5 Activity

Benralizumab and mepolizumab are monoclonal antibodies directed against IL-5 activity. Benralizumab targets IL-5Rα, while mepolizumab targets IL-5. There are numerous case reports on the use of mepolizumab for the treatment of ABPA; larger

Table 5
Summary of select studies on omalizumab for the treatment of ABPA

Study	Study Type	Number of Patients	Outcomes
Jin et al,[51] 2023	Systematic review and meta-analysis	267	Decreased exacerbations and systemic steroid use with omalizumab treatment
Korkmaz et al,[58] 2022	Retrospective cohort	13	Patients with ABPA on omalizumab had dose reduction without loss of asthma control and need to increase systemic steroids
Koutsokera et al,[52] 2020	Retrospective cohort	27	Study on the use of omalizumab in patients with cystic fibrosis. Eleven patients with ABPA were examined, 4 were able to decreased systemic steroids by more than 50% but IV antibiotics and hospital days did not decrease significantly
Ashkenazi et al,[50] 2018	Retrospective cohort	9	Patients with cystic fibrosis and ABPA on omalizumab did not show any improvement in forced expiratory volume in 1 s, body mass index, exacerbations or steroid sparing effect
Nove-Josserand et al,[53] 2017	Retrospective cohort	32	Omalizumab may be a steroid sparing therapy for patients with cystic fibrosis and ABPA
Perisson et al,[54] 2017	Retrospective cohort	18	Patients with cystic fibrosis on omalizumab had stabilization of decline in lung function and significant decrease in steroid use
Voskamp et al,[56] 2015	Randomized, placebo-controlled study	13	Omalizumab can be used for ABPA in patients with high serum IgE levels
Tillie-Leblond et al,[55] 2011	Prospective, interventional cohort	16	Treatment with omalizumab in patients with ABPA and no cystic fibrosis was associated with fewer exacerbations and reduction in steroid dose

studies are less numerous, those available are summarized in **Table 6**. In 1 case series of 9 patients, 63% of patients on mepolizumab were able to discontinue steroids; there was also an improvement in exacerbation rate, ACT score, and daily steroid dose.[59] Another prospective observational study of 20 patients showed that mepolizumab use resulted in a decrease in daily corticosteroids dose and rate of exacerbations.[60] The use of mepolizumab has also been successful in reducing peripheral eosinophilia in patients with ABPA.[59]

The data for the use of benralizumab in ABPA consist mostly of case reports, also summarized in **Table 6**. Case reports have showed that benralizumab has been used with success in ABPA with concomitant peripheral eosinophilia.[61,62] Successful benralizumab use has also been reported in cases refractory to omalizumab[63] and mepolizumab.[64]

Dupilumab

Dupilumab blocks the activity of both IL-4 and IL-13 through the inhibition of IL-4Rα. Dupilumab has multiple indications, including asthma. The use of dupilumab specifically for the treatment of ABPA has been reported in the literature, mostly through case reports, summarized in **Table 7**. There have been reports of successful treatment with dupilumab after failure of other biologics including omalizumab,[65,66] mepolizumab,[65,67] and benralizumab.[66,68] Patients have been able to discontinue oral steroids on dupilumab.[66,67,69,70] In terms of adverse outcomes, there has been a report of an asthma exacerbation thought to be secondary to dupilumab-induced hypereosinophilia.[70]

Tezepelumab

Tezepelumab is a monoclonal antibody TSLP. It is currently approved for the treatment of asthma, but there are have been reports on its use for ABPA. One patient was successfully treated with tezepelumab when she had relapse and an exacerbation during an attempt to taper steroids.[71] A case was reported of a patient who had appearance of high attenuation mucus after 15 months of mepolizumab treatment and was switched to tezepelumab without the need for systemic steroids.[72]

Concurrent Use of Multiple Biologics to Treat Allergic Bronchopulmonary Aspergillosis

As ABPA is not well understood, it is possible that multiple pathways of inflammation may be at play in the pathogenesis of disease in certain patients and that the pathways may all need to be addressed to have remission of disease. In 2017, a case report was published on the successful use of combination omalizumab and mepolizumab therapy for ABPA with the ability to discontinue systemic corticosteroids.[73] Another case series reported on 3 patients who were also successfully treated with a combination of omalizumab and anti-IL-5/IL-5Rα therapy after having exacerbations on omalizumab. Two patients were treated with the combination of omalizumab and benralizumab, and one patient was treated with the combination of omalizumab and mepolizumab. All 3 of the patients were able to discontinue oral corticosteroids and reduce their dose of omalizumab after the addition of anti-IL-5/5Rα therapy.[74]

Summary

On the continuum of severe asthma, biologics will likely be considered for the treatment of ABPA in many cases that are refractory to first line therapies. Given its longer duration on the market, some data and studies exist for omalizumab, which can be a

Table 6
Summary of select cases and studies on targeting interleukin-5 for the treatment of ABPA

Biologic	Study	Study Type	Number of Patients	Outcomes
Mepolizumab	Caminati et al,[59] 2022	Observational cohort	9	Nine patients with ABPA on mepolizumab were followed for 12 mo and had decrease in oral steroid use, exacerbations, and peripheral eosinophilia
	Schleich et al,[60] 2020	Prospective observational study	20	Patients with ABPA in the Belgian Severe Asthma Registry treated with mepolizumab showed decreased steroid dose, decreased exacerbation rate, and improvement in asthma control
	Soeda et al,[75] 2019	Case series	2	Successful treatment with mepolizumab without the need for steroids or itraconazole
Benralizumab	Alaga et al,[61] 2023	Case report	1	Patient with severe eosinophilic asthma and ABPA refractory to prednisone and itraconazole. She had an allergic reaction to omalizumab. Benralizumab provided rapid clinical improvement
	Tsubouchi et al,[62] 2021	Case report	1	Successful use of benralizumab in a patient with significantly elevated peripheral eosinophilia and high attenuation mucus on imaging
	Tomomatsu et al,[64] 2020	Case series	2	Two patients initially treated with mepolizumab with reduction in peripheral eosinophilia but persistent mucus plugging. Treatment with benralizumab improved mucus plugging and further decreased eosinophilia
	Bernal-Rubio et al,[63] 2020	Case report	1	Patient with clinical improvement on benralizumab after no response to omalizumab
	Soeda et al,[76] 2019	Case report	1	First case report on the successful use of benralizumab for ABPA

Table 7
Summary of select studies on dupilumab for the treatment of ABPA

Study	Study Type	Number of Patients	Outcomes
Kotetsu et al,[68] 2023	Case report	1	Patient with ABPA unresponsive to benralizumab was successfully treated with dupilumab
Lamothe et al,[65] 2023	Case report	2	Case report of identical twins with ABPA, 1 declined treatment with biologics, the other did not have improvement with omalizumab or mepolizumab but had minimal symptoms on dupilumab
Kai et al,[67] 2022	Case report	1	Patient who initially achieved remission with steroids but relapsed 16 months later. Patient did not have improvement on mepolizumab but improved on dupilumab without the need to restart steroids
Nishimura et al,[69] 2021	Case report	1	Patient treated with dupilumab was able to discontinue oral steroids
Ali and Green.[77] 2021	Case report	1	Patient with steroid induced myopathy unable to achieve remission with steroids and voriconazole. The patient had a hypersensitivity reaction to omalizumab. She dramatically improved with dupilumab with reduction in steroid dose
Mummler et al,[66] 2020	Case report	1	Patient refractory to steroids, benralizumab, itraconazole, and omalizumab who was successfully treated with dupilumab with ability to discontinue steroids
Ramonell et al,[70] 2020	Case series	3	Two out of 3 patients were able to discontinue steroids on dupilumab but one had an asthma exacerbation thought to be related to dupilumab-induced hypereosinophilia

steroid sparing-agent. It can be considered even in the case of high levels of serum IgE beyond the current dosing recommendations for asthma.[56] Mepolizumab has also been seen to be a steroid-sparing medication and could be a consideration in most patients with ABPA as the asthmatic component of ABPA is eosinophilic. Given its mechanism of action, benralizumab is another agent to be considered with eosinophilic disease and has been shown to be successful in some cases refractory to omalizumab and mepolizumab. Case reports demonstrate success with dupilumab in disease recalcitrant to omalizumab, mepolizumab, and benralizumab. Systemic corticosteroid withdrawal has been successful in some patients with ABPA on dupilumab. Specific to dupilumab, the eosinophilia associated with treatment can make monitoring of disease much more challenging, especially in the early phases of treatment. Cases of successful treatment of ABPA with tezepelumab indicate there may be a role for TSLP in the pathogenesis of ABPA. Although uncommonly reported, the need for biologics targeting 2 separate components of T2 pathology suggests that this might be necessary in some cases. This also sheds light on the complex immune mechanisms involved in ABPA. Similar to asthma, it appears that there are endotypes of APBA that make patients more or less responsive to biologics depending on their mechanisms of action. Biologics are tools that should be considered in the treatment of patients with ABPA.

DISCUSSION

With time, the approved indications for biologic medications have expanded to include many allergic disorders. However, the use of biologics in AERD and ABPA are unique in that neither condition is an approved indication for any of the biologics available on the market. AERD and ABPA are interesting disorders in that they have components of disease which qualify patients for treatment with biologics, namely asthma and nasal polyposis in AERD and often asthma in ABPA. This is an interesting and unique situation, from a regulatory perspective, because although patients can receive the treatment under an approved indication, the approved dose may not be at the most effective dose to treat AERD or ABPA. Patients with AERD have been included in trials of biologics, but it is quite likely that having ABPA excluded a number of patients from the clinical trials for the use of biologics in asthma. Thus, the specific pathways involved in the disease, the likelihood of benefit, and even the optimal dosing and frequency of the medications for the diseases are all unknown at this time.

As successes have been seen with the use of biologics to treat AERD and ABPA, more work is needed to understand the mechanisms by which these medications work in these disorders. More studies are also needed to optimize dosing and frequency of biologics in AERD and ABPA, as these are not currently approved indications. Despite all of this, biologics have emerged as options for patients with recalcitrant disease or as alternatives to standard therapies that are not without their own risks.

CLINICS CARE POINTS

- Biologic medications should be considered for patients with AERD or ABPA refractory to first line therapies.
- For the treatment of AERD, both biologics and ATAD should be discussed with patients.
- Patients with AERD may see the most benefit with dupilumab, but other biologics are beneficial and head-to-head trials of biologics in AERD are lacking.

- More data exist for omalizumab treatment in ABPA, but limited data for other biologics support their use, including in cases where patients do not respond to IgE blockade.
- Patients not responsive to 1 biologic may be responsive to another, indicating that there may be endotypes of AERD and ABPA similar to asthma.
- Biologics are not without risks; there have been reports of hypersensitivity reactions with omalizumab and of dupilumab-induced hypereosinophilia causing an asthma exacerbation.

DISCLOSURE

J. Huang: nothing to disclose. A.A. White: Speaker Bureau for Regeneron/Sanofi, Optinose, AstraZeneca, Amgen, GSK, Blueprint; Advisory Board: Blueprint, Cogent, GSK, Regeneron; Research Support: Regeneron, United States, AstraZeneca, United Kingdom.

REFERENCES

1. White AA, Stevenson DD. Aspirin-Exacerbated Respiratory Disease. N Engl J Med 2018;379(11):1060–70.
2. Khan DA, Banerji A, Blumenthal KG, et al. Drug allergy: A 2022 practice parameter update. J Allergy Clin Immunol 2022;150(6):1333–93.
3. Kim JE, Kountakis SE. The prevalence of Samter's triad in patients undergoing functional endoscopic sinus surgery. Ear Nose Throat J 2007;86(7):396–9.
4. Lee JH, Haselkorn T, Borish L, et al. Risk factors associated with persistent airflow limitation in severe or difficult-to-treat asthma: insights from the TENOR study. Chest 2007;132(6):1882–9.
5. Stevenson DD, Simon RA, Mathison DA. Aspirin-sensitive asthma: tolerance to aspirin after positive oral aspirin challenges. J Allergy Clin Immunol 1980; 66(1):82–8.
6. Stevenson DD, Pleskow WW, Simon RA, et al. Aspirin-sensitive rhinosinusitis asthma: a double-blind crossover study of treatment with aspirin. J Allergy Clin Immunol 1984;73(4):500–7.
7. Swierczynska-Krepa M, Sanak M, Bochenek G, et al. Aspirin desensitization in patients with aspirin-induced and aspirin-tolerant asthma: a double-blind study. J Allergy Clin Immunol 2014;134(4):883–90.
8. Levy JM, Rudmik L, Peters AT, et al. Contemporary management of chronic rhinosinusitis with nasal polyposis in aspirin-exacerbated respiratory disease: an evidence-based review with recommendations. Int Forum Allergy Rhinol 2016; 6(12):1273–83.
9. Van Zele T, Claeys S, Gevaert P, et al. Differentiation of chronic sinus diseases by measurement of inflammatory mediators. Allergy 2006;61(11):1280–9.
10. Tomassen P, Vandeplas G, Van Zele T, et al. Inflammatory endotypes of chronic rhinosinusitis based on cluster analysis of biomarkers. J Allergy Clin Immunol 2016;137(5):1449–1456 e4.
11. Bachert C, Han JK, Desrosiers M, et al. Efficacy and safety of dupilumab in patients with severe chronic rhinosinusitis with nasal polyps (LIBERTY NP SINUS-24 and LIBERTY NP SINUS-52): results from two multicentre, randomised, double-blind, placebo-controlled, parallel-group phase 3 trials. Lancet 2019;394(10209):1638–50.
12. Buchheit KM, Sohail A, Hacker J, et al. Rapid and sustained effect of dupilumab on clinical and mechanistic outcomes in aspirin-exacerbated respiratory disease. J Allergy Clin Immunol 2022;150(2):415–24.

13. Bensko JC, McGill A, Palumbo M, et al. Pediatric-onset aspirin-exacerbated respiratory disease: Clinical characteristics, prevalence, and response to dupilumab. J Allergy Clin Immunol Pract 2022;10(9):2466–8.

14. Mustafa SS, Vadamalai K, Scott B, et al. Dupilumab as Add-on Therapy for Chronic Rhinosinusitis With Nasal Polyposis in Aspirin Exacerbated Respiratory Disease. Am J Rhinol Allergy 2021;35(3):399–407.

15. Laidlaw TM, Mullol J, Fan C, et al. Dupilumab improves nasal polyp burden and asthma control in patients with CRSwNP and AERD. J Allergy Clin Immunol Pract 2019;7(7):2462–2465 e1.

16. Patel P, Bensko JC, Bhattacharyya N, et al. Dupilumab as an adjunct to surgery in patients with aspirin-exacerbated respiratory disease. Ann Allergy Asthma Immunol 2022;128(3):326–8.

17. Mustafa SS, Vadamalai K. Dupilumab increases aspirin tolerance in aspirin-exacerbated respiratory disease. Ann Allergy Asthma Immunol 2021;126(6): 738–9.

18. Picado C, Mullol J, Roca-Ferrer J. Mechanisms by which dupilumab normalizes eicosanoid metabolism and restores aspirin-tolerance in AERD: A hypothesis. J Allergy Clin Immunol 2023;151(2):310–3.

19. Han JK, Bachert C, Fokkens W, et al. Mepolizumab for chronic rhinosinusitis with nasal polyps (SYNAPSE): a randomised, double-blind, placebo-controlled, phase 3 trial. Lancet Respir Med 2021;9(10):1141–53.

20. Bachert C, Han JK, Desrosiers MY, et al. Efficacy and safety of benralizumab in chronic rhinosinusitis with nasal polyps: A randomized, placebo-controlled trial. J Allergy Clin Immunol 2022;149(4):1309–1317 e12.

21. Tuttle KL, Buchheit KM, Laidlaw TM, et al. A retrospective analysis of mepolizumab in subjects with aspirin-exacerbated respiratory disease. J Allergy Clin Immunol Pract 2018;6(3):1045–7.

22. Hagin D, Shacham Y, Kivity S, et al. Mepolizumab for the treatment of aspirin-exacerbated respiratory disease associated with coronary spasm. J Allergy Clin Immunol Pract 2019;7(3):1076–7.

23. Caruso C, Colantuono S, Pugliese D, et al. Severe eosinophilic asthma and aspirin-exacerbated respiratory disease associated to eosinophilic gastroenteritis treated with mepolizumab: a case report. Allergy Asthma Clin Immunol 2020;16:27.

24. Mahdavinia M, Batra PS, Codispoti C. Mepolizumab utility in successful aspirin desensitization in aspirin-exacerbated respiratory disease in a refractory case. Ann Allergy Asthma Immunol 2019;123(3):311–2.

25. Supron AD, Bergmark RW, Roditi RE, et al. Perioperative mepolizumab in aspirin-exacerbated respiratory disease does not prevent nasal polyp regrowth. Ann Allergy Asthma Immunol 2023;131(3):384–6.

26. Martin H, Barrett NA, Laidlaw T. Mepolizumab does not prevent all aspirin-induced reactions in patients with aspirin-exacerbated respiratory disease: A case series. J Allergy Clin Immunol Pract 2021;9(3):1384–5.

27. Staudacher AG, Peters AT, Carter RG, et al. Decreased nasal polyp eosinophils but increased mast cells in a patient with aspirin-exacerbated respiratory disease treated with reslizumab. Ann Allergy Asthma Immunol 2020;125(4):490–493 e2.

28. Gevaert P, Omachi TA, Corren J, et al. Efficacy and safety of omalizumab in nasal polyposis: 2 randomized phase 3 trials. J Allergy Clin Immunol 2020;146(3): 595–605.

29. Hayashi H, Fukutomi Y, Mitsui C, et al. Omalizumab for Aspirin Hypersensitivity and Leukotriene Overproduction in Aspirin-exacerbated Respiratory Disease. A Randomized Controlled Trial. Am J Respir Crit Care Med 2020;201(12):1488–98.

30. Hayashi H, Fukutomi Y, Mitsui C, et al. Omalizumab ameliorates extrarespiratory symptoms in patients with aspirin-exacerbated respiratory disease. J Allergy Clin Immunol 2023;151(6):1667–1672 e2.

31. Jean T, Eng V, Sheikh J, et al. Effect of omalizumab on outcomes in patients with aspirin-exacerbated respiratory disease. Allergy Asthma Proc 2019;40(5): 316–20.

32. Bergmann KC, Zuberbier T, Church MK. Omalizumab in the treatment of aspirin-exacerbated respiratory disease. J Allergy Clin Immunol Pract 2015;3(3):459–60.

33. Lang DM, Aronica MA, Maierson ES, et al. Omalizumab can inhibit respiratory reaction during aspirin desensitization. Ann Allergy Asthma Immunol 2018;121(1): 98–104.

34. Phillips-Angles E, Barranco P, Lluch-Bernal M, et al. Aspirin tolerance in patients with nonsteroidal anti-inflammatory drug-exacerbated respiratory disease following treatment with omalizumab. J Allergy Clin Immunol Pract 2017;5(3): 842–5.

35. Waldram J, Walters K, Simon R, et al. Safety and outcomes of aspirin desensitization for aspirin-exacerbated respiratory disease: A single-center study. J Allergy Clin Immunol 2018;141(1):250–6.

36. Laidlaw TM, Menzies-Gow A, Caveney S, et al. Tezepelumab Efficacy in Patients with Severe, Uncontrolled Asthma with Comorbid Nasal Polyps in NAVIGATOR. J Asthma Allergy 2023;16:915–32.

37. Wangberg H, Spierling Bagsic SR, Osuna L, et al. Appraisal of the Real-World Effectiveness of Biologic Therapies in Aspirin-Exacerbated Respiratory Disease. J Allergy Clin Immunol Pract 2022;10(2):478–484 e3.

38. Mullur J, Steger CM, Gakpo D, et al. Aspirin desensitization and biologics in aspirin-exacerbated respiratory disease: Efficacy, tolerability, and patient experience. Ann Allergy Asthma Immunol 2022;128(5):575–82.

39. Bavaro N, Gakpo D, Mittal A, et al. Efficacy of dupilumab in patients with aspirin-exacerbated respiratory disease and previous inadequate response to anti-IL-5 or anti-IL-5Ralpha in a real-world setting. J Allergy Clin Immunol Pract 2021; 9(7):2910–2912 e1.

40. Ghiasi Y, Wangberg H, Bagsic SRS, et al. Type 2 biologics reduce cumulative steroid exposure in aspirin-exacerbated respiratory disease. Ann Allergy Asthma Immunol 2022;129(5):642–3.

41. Oykhman P, Paramo FA, Bousquet J, et al. Comparative efficacy and safety of monoclonal antibodies and aspirin desensitization for chronic rhinosinusitis with nasal polyposis: A systematic review and network meta-analysis. J Allergy Clin Immunol 2022;149(4):1286–95.

42. Walker C, Bauer W, Braun RK, et al. Activated T cells and cytokines in bronchoalveolar lavages from patients with various lung diseases associated with eosinophilia. Am J Respir Crit Care Med 1994;150(4):1038–48.

43. Becker KL, Gresnigt MS, Smeekens SP, et al. Pattern recognition pathways leading to a Th2 cytokine bias in allergic bronchopulmonary aspergillosis patients. Clin Exp Allergy 2015;45(2):423–37.

44. Carvalho A, Cunha C, Pasqualotto AC, et al. Genetic variability of innate immunity impacts human susceptibility to fungal diseases. Int J Infect Dis 2010;14(6): e460–8.

45. Carvalho A, Pasqualotto AC, Pitzurra L, et al. Polymorphisms in toll-like receptor genes and susceptibility to pulmonary aspergillosis. J Infect Dis 2008;197(4): 618–21.

46. Overton NL, Denning DW, Bowyer P, et al. Genetic susceptibility to allergic bronchopulmonary aspergillosis in asthma: a genetic association study. Allergy Asthma Clin Immunol 2016;12:47.

47. Agarwal R, Sehgal IS, Muthu V, et al. Revised ISHAM-ABPA working group clinical practice guidelines for diagnosing, classifying and treating allergic bronchopulmonary aspergillosis/mycoses. Eur Respir J 2024;63(4). https://doi.org/10.1183/13993003.00061-2024.

48. Asano K, Hebisawa A, Ishiguro T, et al. New clinical diagnostic criteria for allergic bronchopulmonary aspergillosis/mycosis and its validation. J Allergy Clin Immunol 2021;147(4):1261–1268 e5.

49. Greenberger PA, Bush RK, Demain JG, et al. Allergic bronchopulmonary aspergillosis. J Allergy Clin Immunol Pract 2014;2(6):703–8.

50. Ashkenazi M, Sity S, Sarouk I, et al. Omalizumab in allergic bronchopulmonary aspergillosis in patients with cystic fibrosis. J Asthma Allergy 2018;11:101–7.

51. Jin M, Douglass JA, Elborn JS, et al. Omalizumab in Allergic Bronchopulmonary Aspergillosis: A Systematic Review and Meta-Analysis. J Allergy Clin Immunol Pract 2023;11(3):896–905.

52. Koutsokera A, Corriveau S, Sykes J, et al. Omalizumab for asthma and allergic bronchopulmonary aspergillosis in adults with cystic fibrosis. J Cyst Fibros 2020;19(1):119–24.

53. Nove-Josserand R, Grard S, Auzou L, et al. Case series of omalizumab for allergic bronchopulmonary aspergillosis in cystic fibrosis patients. Pediatr Pulmonol 2017;52(2):190–7.

54. Perisson C, Destruys L, Grenet D, et al. Omalizumab treatment for allergic bronchopulmonary aspergillosis in young patients with cystic fibrosis. Respir Med 2017;133:12–5.

55. Tillie-Leblond I, Germaud P, Leroyer C, et al. Allergic bronchopulmonary aspergillosis and omalizumab. Allergy 2011;66(9):1254–6.

56. Voskamp AL, Gillman A, Symons K, et al. Clinical efficacy and immunologic effects of omalizumab in allergic bronchopulmonary aspergillosis. J Allergy Clin Immunol Pract 2015;3(2):192–9.

57. Kelso JM. Following total IgE concentration in patients with allergic bronchopulmonary aspergillosis on omalizumab. J Allergy Clin Immunol Pract 2016;4(2): 364–5.

58. Korkmaz ET, Aydin O, Mungan D, et al. Can dose reduction be made in patients with allergic bronchopulmonary aspergillosis receiving high-dose omalizumab treatment? Eur Ann Allergy Clin Immunol 2022. https://doi.org/10.23822/EurAnnACI.1764-1489.261.

59. Caminati M, Batani V, Guidolin L, et al. One-year mepolizumab for Allergic bronchopulmonary aspergillosis: Focus on steroid sparing effect and markers of response. Eur J Intern Med 2022;99:112–5.

60. Schleich F, Vaia ES, Pilette C, et al. Mepolizumab for allergic bronchopulmonary aspergillosis: Report of 20 cases from the Belgian Severe Asthma Registry and review of the literature. J Allergy Clin Immunol Pract 2020;8(7):2412–2413 e2.

61. Alaga A, Ashraff K, Din Khan NH. Rapid onset of effect of benralizumab in a severe eosinophilic and allergic asthma patient with allergic bronchopulmonary aspergillosis. Respirol Case Rep 2023;11(6):e01167.

62. Tsubouchi K, Arimura-Omori M, Inoue S, et al. A case of allergic bronchopulmonary aspergillosis with marked peripheral blood eosinophilia successfully treated with benralizumab. Respir Med Case Rep 2021;32:101339.

63. Bernal-Rubio L, de-la-Hoz Caballer B, Almonacid-Sanchez C, et al. Successful Treatment of Allergic Bronchopulmonary Aspergillosis With Benralizumab in a Patient Who Did Not Respond to Omalizumab. J Investig Allergol Clin Immunol 2020;30(5):378–9.

64. Tomomatsu K, Sugino Y, Okada N, et al. Rapid clearance of mepolizumab-resistant bronchial mucus plugs in allergic bronchopulmonary aspergillosis with benralizumab treatment. Allergol Int 2020;69(4):636–8.

65. Lamothe PA, Runnstrom M, Smirnova N, et al. Allergic bronchopulmonary aspergillosis in identical twins: Effectiveness of dupilumab. J Allergy Clin Immunol Pract 2023;11(5):1556–1558 e2.

66. Mummler C, Kemmerich B, Behr J, et al. Differential response to biologics in a patient with severe asthma and ABPA: a role for dupilumab? Allergy Asthma Clin Immunol 2020;16:55.

67. Kai Y, Yoshikawa M, Matsuda M, et al. Successful management of recurrent allergic bronchopulmonary aspergillosis after changing from mepolizumab to dupilumab: A case report. Respir Med Case Rep 2022;39:101723.

68. Kotetsu Y, Ogata H, Sha K, et al. A Case of Allergic Bronchopulmonary Aspergillosis With Failure of Benralizumab and Response to Dupilumab. Cureus 2023;15(7):e42464.

69. Nishimura T, Okano T, Naito M, et al. Complete withdrawal of glucocorticoids after dupilumab therapy in allergic bronchopulmonary aspergillosis: A case report. World J Clin Cases 2021;9(23):6922–8.

70. Ramonell RP, Lee FE, Swenson C, et al. Dupilumab treatment for allergic bronchopulmonary aspergillosis: A case series. J Allergy Clin Immunol Pract 2020;8(2):742–3.

71. Matsuno O. Allergic bronchopulmonary aspergillosis successfully treated with tezepelumab. J Allergy Clin Immunol Pract 2023;11(8):2589–91.

72. Ogata H, Sha K, Kotetsu Y, et al. Tezepelumab treatment for allergic bronchopulmonary aspergillosis. Respirol Case Rep 2023;11(5):e01147.

73. Altman MC, Lenington J, Bronson S, et al. Combination omalizumab and mepolizumab therapy for refractory allergic bronchopulmonary aspergillosis. J Allergy Clin Immunol Pract 2017;5(4):1137–9.

74. Laorden D, Zamarron E, Dominguez-Ortega J, et al. Successful Long-Term Treatment Combining Omalizumab and Anti-IL-5 Biologics in Allergic Bronchopulmonary Aspergillosis. Arch Bronconeumol 2022;58(8):624–6.

75. Soeda S, To M, Kono Y, et al. Case series of allergic bronchopulmonary aspergillosis treated successfully and safely with long-term mepolizumab. Allergol Int 2019;68(3):377–9.

76. Soeda S, Kono Y, Tsuzuki R, et al. Allergic bronchopulmonary aspergillosis successfully treated with benralizumab. J Allergy Clin Immunol Pract 2019;7(5):1633–5.

77. Ali M, Green O. Dupilumab: a new contestant to corticosteroid in allergic bronchopulmonary aspergillosis. Oxf Med Case Reports 2021;2021(4):omaa029.

Asthma Biologics
Lung Function, Steroid-Dependence, and Exacerbations

Justin D. Salciccioli, MBBS, MA[a],*, Elliot Israel, MD[a,b]

KEYWORDS

- Asthma • Bronchodilators • Glucocorticoids • Exacerbation

KEY POINTS

- Asthma biologics are effective add-on therapies for severe, uncontrolled asthma and should be considered in patients who remain symptomatic despite optimized inhaled therapies.
- There are currently six biologic therapies for asthma that offer diverse mechanisms to enhance lung function, reduce exacerbation risk, and potentially decrease oral corticosteroid dependence.
- All the biologic therapies have been shown to reduce asthma exacerbations and appear to have greater effects in individuals with type-2 inflammation.
- Selecting the most-appropriate biologic agent requires careful consideration of patient characteristics such as clinical features, comorbid conditions, and biomarker status.

INTRODUCTION

The development of multiple targeted biologic therapies over the past two decades has revolutionized the management of asthma. Currently, there are six monoclonal antibodies that target specific inflammatory mediators involved in the pathophysiology of asthma, and together, they provide the opportunity for personalized treatment options beyond bronchodilators and inhaled or systemic glucocorticoids in severe and difficult-to-control asthma. These agents are the anti-IgE antibody omalizumab, the anti-IL-5 antibodies mepolizumab and reslizumab, the IL-5 receptor alpha antagonist benralizumab, the IL-4 receptor alpha antagonist dupilumab, and the anti-thymic stromal lymphopoietin (TSLP) antibody tezepelumab.

[a] Division of Pulmonary and Critical Care Medicine, Brigham and Women's Hospital, Harvard Medical School, 75 Francis Street, Boston, MA 02115, USA; [b] Division of Allergy and Immunology, Brigham and Women's Hospital, Harvard Medical School, 75 Francis Street, Boston, MA 02115, USA
* Corresponding author.
E-mail address: jsalciccioli@bwh.harvard.edu

Immunol Allergy Clin N Am 44 (2024) 693–708
https://doi.org/10.1016/j.iac.2024.08.002   immunology.theclinics.com

These agents have collectively improved outcomes for patients with severe asthma, and each medication has distinct mechanisms of action and risk-benefit profiles. Numerous clinical trials have demonstrated the ability of these biologics to improve airway obstruction, minimize steroid exposure, and reduce exacerbation risk in difficult-to-control disease, and in this chapter, we focus our review on placebo-controlled clinical trial evidence for these biologic agents with respect to these three outcome measures. Our discussion herein on the effects of these treatments on meaningful clinical endpoints is essential for asthma care specialists to make informed, personalized therapeutic decisions that optimize asthma control for a patient population often with complex disease characteristics. A subsequent chapter in this edition discusses the real-world evidence of asthma biologics, and therefore, readers are referred to that chapter to supplement the data from placebo-controlled trials summarized here.

Lung function is essential in assessing asthma for the initial diagnosis and monitoring response to therapies. Simple spirometry, including forced expiratory volume in 1 second (FEV_1), forced vital capacity (FVC), and the ratio of FEV_1:FVC, are all useful and immediately available in most clinical settings; however, in the current chapter, we have restricted our discussion of the effects on lung function to pre-bronchodilator FEV_1 as this is most consistently reported in the literature and serves as a strong predictor of decline in asthma control. The oral corticosteroid (OCS)-sparing effects of the agents are slightly more difficult to report as a single metric as there is substantial variation in the way in which this is reported, and although somewhat limited literature exists, we have attempted to consolidate the results where they are available for each agent with respect to this outcome and have summarized these in the accompanying **Table 1**. We report percentage reduction in OCS dosing where available and odds ratio (OR) and 95% confidence intervals (CIs) for 100% and 50% reduction from baseline in OCS dosing for each intervention with available OCS-sparing data. Asthma exacerbations are perhaps the most valuable outcome parameter to gauge therapeutic response and are reported in this chapter as rate ratios (RRs) compared to placebo in controlled trials.

Omalizumab

The earliest available biologic therapy for asthma was the anti-IgE antibody, omalizumab, which was initially approved for use in moderate or severe cases of allergic asthma in the United States as early as 2003. Omalizumab is a humanized IgG1 antibody that binds circulating IgE and prevents it from binding the $F_{c\epsilon}R1$. It is approved for individuals with asthma with evidence of perennial aeroallergen sensitization and a total IgE level between 30 and 700 IU/mL.

Data from randomized trials show omalizumab improves lung function in uncontrolled allergic asthma, but changes are modest. In a 2001 phase 3 study by Busse and colleagues, patients with baseline FEV_1 2.3-2.4 L with add-on omalizumab had increased the mean FEV_1 from 68% to 73% of predicted value versus 68% to 69% with placebo over 28 weeks, a small but statistically significant difference.[1] Another 2001 study by Solèr and colleagues reported statistically significant improvements in percent predicted FEV_1 with omalizumab therapy, although the exact percentage difference is not provided (Solèr and colleagues, 2001).[2] However, studies of omalizumab targeting FEV_1 as the primary endpoint have failed to show robust improvements in lung function, and meta-analyses indicate omalizumab provides limited spirometric changes, with average increases of 68 mL in FEV_1 compared to placebo.[3]

There are no placebo-controlled trials in adult populations that have demonstrated the OCS-sparing effects of omalizumab. A 2023 open-label study revealed

Table 1
Clinical trial characteristics for biologic therapies in asthma

Therapy	Study, Year	Sample Size (Total N)	Sample Size (Biologic Treated N)	Subject Selection	Baseline Pre-BD FEV_1, L (% Predicted)	FEV_1 Improvement, mL (95% CI)	OCS Reduction (OR, 95% CI)	Exacerbations (RR per Year, 95% CI)
Omalizumab	Busse et al,[1] 2001	525	268	• Med-/high-dose ICS • FEV_1 ≥40% and ≤80% predicted • Positive skin prick testing Total serum IgE ≥30 IU/mL to ≤700 IU/mL	2.3–2.4 (68)	3%[h]	Not tested	48% relative reduction
	Hanania et al,[5] 2011	850	427	• High dose ICS/LABA • 1 AEX • FEV_1 ≥40% and ≤80% predicted • Positive skin prick testing Total serum IgE ≥30 IU/mL to ≤700 IU/mL	Not reported (64–65)	Not assessed	Not tested	25% relative reduction

(continued on next page)

Table 1
(continued)

Therapy	Study, Year	Sample Size (Total N)	Sample Size (Biologic Treated N)	Subject Selection	Baseline Pre-BD FEV$_1$, L (% Predicted)	FEV$_1$ Improvement, mL (95% CI)	OCS Reduction (OR, 95% CI)	Exacerbations (RR per Year, 95% CI)
Mepolizumab	Haldar et al,[7] 2009	61	29	• ≥ 2 AEX on high-dose ICS • Sputum Eos ≥3%	78%[c]	−5 (−260 to 150)[a]	Not tested	0.57 (0.32–0.92)
	Pavord et al,[9] 2012 DREAM (75 mg/ 250 mg/ 750 mg IV)	621	462	• ≥2 AEX • Sputum Eos levels ≥3% or FeNO ≥50 ppb or • Blood Eos ≥300	1.81–1.95 (59–61)	6 (−4 to 161)/81 (−19 to 180)/6 (−4 to 155)	Not tested	0.52 (0.39–0.69)/0.61 (0.46–0.81)/0.48 (0.36–0.64)
	Ortega et al,[10] 2014 MENSA (IV/SC)	576	385	• High-dose ICS with an additional controller • ≥2 AEX FEV$_1$, ≤80% • Blood Eos ≥150	1.73–1.86 (59–62)	100 (13–187)/98 (11–184)	Not tested	0.47 (0.28–0.60)/0.53 (0.36–0.65)
	Bel et al,[12] 2014 SIRIUS	135	69	• Daily OCS • High-dose ICS with an additional controller • Blood Eos ≥150	1.90–2.00 (58–60)	140[a,f,g]	100%: 1.67 (0.49–5.75) 50%: 2.26 (1.10–4.65)	0.68 (0.47–0.99)

Reslizumab	Castro et al,[13] 2015	953	477	• Med-/high-dose ICS • 1 AEX • ACQ-7 ≥1.5 Blood Eos ≥400	1.89–2.13 (64–70)	110 (67–150)	Not tested	0.46 (0.37–0.58)
	Bjermer et al,[14] 2016 (0.3 mg/kg vs 3.0 mg/kg)	315	209	• Med-/high-dose ICS • ACQ-7 ≥1.5 Blood Eos ≥400	2.16–2.22 (69–71)	115 (16–215)/160 (60–259)	Not tested	Not tested
	Corren et al,[15] 2016	492	395	• Med-/high-dose ICS • ACQ-7 ≥1.5 FEV_1 reversibility ≥12%	2.10–2.18 (66)	68 (−30 to 165)[a]	Not tested	Not tested
	Castro et al,[16] 2011	106	53	• High-dose ICS and an additional controller • ACQ-7 ≥1.5 Sputum Eos ≥3%	2.1–2.3 (66–69)	240 (88–392)	Not tested	8% vs 19%[a,b]
Benralizumab	Bleecker et al,[18] 2016 SIROCCO (4-wk/8-wk)	1205	798	• Medium-/high-dose ICS/LABA • ≥2 AEX • ACQ-6 ≥1.5 • FEV_1 ≤80% predicted	1.66–1.68 (56–57)	Eos ≥ 300: 106 (16–196)/159 (68–249) Eos <300: −25 (−134 to 83)/102 (3–208)	Not tested	Eos ≥ 300: 0.55 (0.42–0.71)/0.49 (0.37–0.64) Eos <300: 0.70 (0.50–1.0)/0.83 (0.59–1.16)
	Fitzgerald et al,[19] 2016 CALIMA (4-wk/8-wk)	1306	866	• Medium-/high-dose ICS/LABA • ≥2 AEX • ACQ-6 ≥1.5 • FEV_1 ≤80% predicted	1.76–1.77 (58–59)	Eos ≥ 300: 125 (37–213)/116 (28–204) Eos <300: 64 (−49 to 176)/−15 (−127 to 96)	Not tested	Eos ≥ 300: 0.64 (0.49–0.85); 0.72 (0.54–0.95) Eos <300: 0.64 (0.45–0.92); 0.62 (0.42–0.86)
	Nair et al,[22] 2017 ZONDA (4-wk/8-wk)	369	220	• Daily OCS med-/high-dose ICS/LABA • Blood Eos ≥150	1.75–1.93 (57–62)	105 (−40 to 251)[a]	100%: 5.23 (1.92–14.21) 50%: 3.59 (1.79–7.22) 100%: 4.19 (1.58–11.12) 50%: 3.03 (1.57–5.86)	0.45 (0.27–0.76)/0.30 (0.17–0.53)

(continued on next page)

Table 1
(continued)

Therapy	Study, Year	Sample Size (Total N)	Sample Size (Biologic Treated N)	Subject Selection	Baseline Pre-BD FEV$_1$, L (% Predicted)	FEV$_1$ Improvement, mL (95% CI)	OCS Reduction (OR, 95% CI)	Exacerbations (RR per Year, 95% CI)
Dupilumab	Wenzel et al,[24] 2013	104	52	• Med-/high-dose ICS/LABA ≥1 AEX • FEV$_1$ ≥50% ACQ-5 ≥1.5 and ≤3.0 • Blood Eos ≥300 or sputum Eos levels ≥3%	2.47–2.54 (72)	270 (110–420)	Not tested	0.08 (0.02–0.28)[b]
	Wenzel et al,[25] 2016[d]	776	618	• Med-/high-dose ICS/LABA ≥1 AEX ACQ-5 ≥1.5 • FEV$_1$ ≥40% and ≤80% predicted	1.84 (61)	160 (70–240) Eos ≥ 300: 160 (10–300) Eos < 300: 140 (30–240)	Not tested	0.27 (0.16–0.45) Eos ≥ 300: 0.20 (0.08–0.52) Eos < 300: 0.31 (0.17–0.58)
	Castro et al,[26] 2018 LIBERTY QUEST[d,e]	1902	1264	• Med-/high-dose ICS plus additional controllers FEV$_1$ ≤80% predicted	1.78 (58)	130 (8–180) Eos ≥ 300: 240 (160–320) Eos 150–300: 0 (−100 to 100) Eos <150: 90 (−40 to 100)	Not tested	0.54 (0.43–0.68) Eos ≥ 300: 0.33 (0.23–0.45) Eos 150–300: 0.56 (0.35–0.89) Eos <150: 1.15 (0.75–1.77)
	Rabe et al,[27] 2018 LIBERTY VENTURE	210	103	• Daily OCS • High-dose ICS plus additional controller • FEV$_1$ ≥80% predicted	1.58 (52)	220 (90–340) Eos ≥ 300: 320 (100–540) Eos <300: 130 (−20 to 280)	100%: 2.74 (1.47–5.10) 50%: 3.98 (2.06–7.67) Eos ≥ 300: 100% 4.07 (1.46–11.33)	0.41 (0.26–0.63) Eos ≥ 300: 0.29 (0.14–0.60) Eos <300: 0.55 (0.32–0.94)

Tezepelumab	Corren (low/med/high) PATHWAY, 2016	550	412	• Med-/high-dose ICS/LABA • 2 AEX within 1 y • FEV$_1$ ≥40% and ≤80% predicted	1.82–1.91 (not reported)	120 (20–220)/130 (30–230)/150 (50–250)	50% 6.59 (2.13–20.42) Eos <300: 100%, 2.15 (0.96–4.81) 50%, 2.91 (1.28–6.63)	Not tested	−62%/−71%/−66%
	Menzies-Gow et al,[29] 2021 NAVIGATOR	1061	528	• Med-/high-dose ICS and an additional controller • 2 AEX within 1 y • FEV$_1$ of ≤80% predicted	Not reported (63)	130 (80–180)	Not tested	0.44 (0.37–0.53)	
	SOURCE,[34] 2022	150	74	• Med-/High-dose ICS/LABA • 1 AEX within 1 y • FEV$_1$ of ≤80% predicted	1.58 (54)	260 (130–390)	100%: 1.35 (0.68–2.68) 50%: 1.24 (0.60–2.57)[a,h]	0.69 (0.44–1.09)	

Abbreviations: ACQ, asthma control questionnaire; AEX, asthma exacerbation; BD, bronchodilator; Eos, eosinophil; FEV1, forced expiratory volume in 1 second; ICS, inhaled corticosteroid; LABA, long-acting beta-agonist; OCS, oral corticosteroid; OR, odds radio; RR, rate ratio.

a Not significant.
b Event rate ratio not reported.
c Only post-bronchodilator percent predicted reported.
d Only reporting results from dosing at 300 mg q2 in table.
e Tezepelumab: low dose 70 mg every 4 weeks, medium dose 210 mg every 4 weeks, high dose 280 mg every 2 weeks.
f Reported in a figure and confidence estimates are not provided.
g Reported odds of category percentage change in oral corticosteroid dose.
h Absolute differences not reported, only percentage change from baseline.

significantly lower monthly average prednisone doses with omalizumab add-on therapy versus controls after 48 weeks (35 mg vs 217 mg) along with a higher likelihood of steroid withdrawal (75% vs 8%).[4]

Reducing asthma exacerbation risk is omalizumab's most clinically impactful effect. In a 2011 trial by Hanania and colleagues, add-on omalizumab treatment lowered protocol-defined exacerbation rates by 25% over 48 weeks, from 0.88 to 0.66 per patient annually,[5] and the evidence also suggests that individuals with elevated biomarkers (blood eosinophils and FeNO) may have a marginally greater efficacy than those without elevated biomarkers.[6] Preventing exacerbations, rather than markedly improving day-to-day symptoms or lung function, appears to be omalizumab's primary value.

Mepolizumab

Mepolizumab is a humanized IgG1 antibody that inhibits IL-5 from binding to the alpha-subunit of the IL-5 receptor complex on eosinophils and was approved by the FDA for use in severe cases of asthma in 2015.[8] In the United States, this agent is approved for individuals with severe eosinophilic asthma, and the eligibility criteria may be more restrictive in other health jurisdictions.

The pivotal 2012 DREAM trial enrolled patients with pre-bronchodilator FEV_1 of 1.81 to 1.95 L (59%–61% predicted) and demonstrated a trend toward greater increases in pre-bronchodilator FEV_1 at week 52 with intravenous mepolizumab, but none of the dosing regimens produced a statistically significant improvement compared to placebo.[9] The 2014 MENSA study which enrolled patients with baseline FEV_1 between 1.73 and 1.86 L (59%–62% predicted), showed a statistically significant, albeit relatively small, increase in the pre-bronchodilator FEV_1 (100 mL greater than placebo).[10] Other trials have not reproduced significant improvements in lung function with mepolizumab, and overall, changes in spirometric measures, if present, tend to be modest.

A few small trials provide signals regarding mepolizumab's oral OCS-sparing potential. In a 2009 pilot study of 20 patients with persistent sputum eosinophilia (>3%) despite OCS (baseline prednisone dose 10 mg/day) and ICS therapy, mepolizumab allowed an 84% reduction in OCS dose from baseline versus 48% with placebo over 24 weeks.[11] A 2014 phase 3 study for OCS-dependent asthma (baseline OCS dose 12.5 mg and 10 mg in placebo and mepolizumab arms, respectively) demonstrated a near 3-fold higher likelihood of achieving a clinically important (ie, ≥50% reduction from baseline) OCS dose reduction with mepolizumab versus placebo over 20 to 24 weeks.[12] For mepolizumab, the odds of 100% and 50% reduction in baseline OCS dose was 1.67 (95% CI 0.49–5.75) and 2.26 (95% CI 1.10–4.65), respectively. Analyses of larger populations are still needed, but current evidence indicates mepolizumab may enable lowering of maintenance OCS dose.

Multiple trials firmly establish mepolizumab's efficacy in reducing asthma exacerbations in patients with blood/sputum eosinophilia. The dose used for severe asthma control is 100 mg, and clinical trials have tested the effects on exacerbation rates at multiple different dosages. Specifically, the DREAM study compared mepolizumab to placebo and lowered exacerbation rates with RRs at the different doses between 0.48 (95% CI 0.36–0.64) with 750 mg, 0.61 (95% CI 0.46–0.81) with 250 mg, and 0.52 (95% CI 0.39–0.69) with 75 mg dosing,[9] and the MENSA study also demonstrated a decrease compared to placebo in the exacerbation rate by 53% (95% CI 36–65) with 100 mg subcutaneous administration.[10] These effects appear more pronounced in patients with baseline exacerbation history, as the magnitude of the effect of mepolizumab on exacerbations was greater in clinical trials that required exacerbation history

(DREAM & MENSA) compared to the study by Bel and colleagues that did not have a requirement for prior exacerbation.[12]

Reslizumab

Reslizumab is a humanized IgG4 antibody that blocks IL-5 from binding the alpha-subunit of the IL-5 receptor on eosinophils. Multiple randomized placebo-controlled trials have demonstrated significant improvements in pre-bronchodilator FEV_1 with intravenous reslizumab (3 mg/kg every 4 weeks) compared to placebo. The 2011 clinical trial by Castro and colleagues which enrolled patients with baseline FEV_1 between 2.1 and 2.3 L (66%–69% predicted), demonstrated an improvement in pre-bronchodilator FEV_1 of 240 mL (88, 392; $P = .0023$) at 15 weeks of the therapy. The follow-up phase 3 trial in 2015, which enrolled patients with baseline FEV_1 in the range of 1.89 to 2.13 L (64%–70% predicted) demonstrated more modest improvements in FEV_1 of 110 mL (67, 150) which persisted through 52 weeks of therapy.[13] In the 2016 phase 3 study, patients had a baseline FEV_1 in the range of 2.16 to 2.22 L (69%–71% predicted), and reslizumab led to FEV_1 increases over placebo averaging 120–160 L at 16 weeks across dosing levels.[14]

Data regarding reslizumab's OCS-sparing efficacy are limited. A 2020 phase 3 trial did not show significant OCS dose reductions over 24 weeks with fixed-dose subcutaneous reslizumab 110 mg every 4 weeks versus placebo.[17] Only 20% to 25% of patients achieved complete OCS withdrawal in both arms, and no other major trials have reported OCS-sparing effects for reslizumab.

Data regarding the effects of reslizumab on asthma exacerbations are limited. The 2011 trial by Castro and colleagues reported an asthma exacerbation rate of 8% with reslizumab compared to 19% with placebo (OR 0.33; 95% CI 0.10–1.15; $P = .0833$), although this trial was not powered to detect a difference in this outcome. In the subsequent 2015 phase 3 trial, reslizumab lowered adjudicated exacerbation rates by 41% to 55% over 52 weeks compared to placebo (pooled event rate of 0.84 vs 1.81 events per person-year; RR 0.46; 95% CI 0.37–0.58; $P < .0001$).[13]

Clinical trial evidence supports reslizumab's efficacy in improving lung function and to prevent asthma exacerbations. Additional high-quality data are needed to better understand its effects on OCS dependence. While reslizumab is an important targeted biologic treatment approach for inadequately controlled eosinophilic asthma, its intravenous route of delivery may often be a barrier to its routine use, but certain clinical situations exist such as a known allergy to other anti-IL-5 agents in which there is a need for more controlled administration of this anti-IL-5 therapy.

Benralizumab

The humanized IgG1 antibody, benralizumab, has a direct high affinity for the alpha-subunit of the IL-5 receptor and was approved in the US for use in severe cases of asthma in 2017. Unlike the anti-IL-5 antibodies, which block circulating IL-5 itself, benralizumab's affinity for the IL-5 receptor alpha on the surface of eosinophils produces distinct molecular effects: Not only does the IL-5R Ab block IL-5 signaling, it has an effect to deplete eosinophils directly through antibody-dependent cell-mediated cytotoxicity. This secondary effect of benralizumab can lead to rapid and profound depletion of circulating eosinophils.

Several phase 3 trials have shown that add-on benralizumab significantly improves lung function in uncontrolled, severe eosinophilic asthma. Together, these studies enrolled patients with moderately-severe obstruction with baseline pre-bronchodilator FEV_1 in the range of 1.66 to 1.77 L (56% and 62% of predicted). In the 2016 SIROCCO study, benralizumab increased pre-bronchodilator FEV_1 by 110 to 160 mL over 48 to 56 weeks versus placebo.[18] The 2021 ANDHI trial also demonstrated an improved FEV_1 by 160 mL with benralizumab versus placebo at 24 weeks.[20] Notably, the 2017 BISE study in mild-to-moderate cases of asthma showed an 80-mL greater improvement in FEV_1 at 12 weeks with benralizumab compared to placebo, a modest effect which likely reflects the mild severity of the disease in this cohort.[21] The improvements in lung function with benralizumab appear greater in patients with baseline blood eosinophil counts $\geq$300 cells/μL.

There is robust data to support benralizumab's OCS-sparing potential. The 2017 ZONDA trial for severe asthma with blood eosinophils >150 and who were on chronic daily OCS with a median OCS dose at enrollment of 10 mg/day (IQR 7.5–40), demonstrated a 75% median reduction in OCS dose over 28 weeks with benralizumab versus only 25% with placebo.[22] Fifty-six percent of patients treated with benralizumab were able to withdraw OCS entirely. For every 8-week regimen, which was ultimately approved for use in clinical practice, the OR for 100% and 50% reduction in OCS dose with benralizumab compared to placebo was 4.19 (95% CI 1.58–11.12) and 3.03 (1.57–5.86), respectively. In addition, the open-label 2022 PONENTE study showed even greater steroid elimination, with 63% stopping OCS use and 82% attaining $\geq$50% dose reductions over 28 to 32 weeks.[23]

In the SIROCCO study, benralizumab reduced exacerbation for individuals with elevated blood eosinophils with an annual exacerbation RR of 0.55 (95% CI 0.42–0.71) with dosing every 4 weeks and 0.49 (95% CI 0.37–0.64) every 8-week dosing regimen.[18] Furthermore, the CALIMA study demonstrated annual exacerbation RR between 0.64 (95% CI 0.49–0.85) for patients with blood eosinophils <300 and 0.72 (95% CI 0.54–0.95) for patients with blood eosinophils >300, compared to placebo.

Dupilumab

Clinical trials have demonstrated that dupilumab consistently improves lung function in patients with uncontrolled, severe asthma. A phase 2a study by Wenzel and colleagues in 2013, which enrolled patients with baseline pre-bronchodilator FEV_1 between 2.47 and 2.54 L (72% of predicted), showed significant FEV_1 improvements of 270 mL with dupilumab versus placebo over 12 weeks.[24] These improvements appear within 2 weeks of initiation. The 2016 dose-finding trial by Wenzel and colleagues enrolled patients with lower baseline lung function compared to the 2013 trial (pre-bronchodilator FEV_1 1.84 L; 61% of predicted) and demonstrated improvement in FEV_1 at 24 weeks of therapy between 100 and 200 mL compared to placebo. In the 2018 phase 3 study LIBERTY QUEST, participants had a baseline pre-bronchodilator FEV_1 of 1.78 L (58% predicted) and demonstrated an increase in FEV_1 by 140 to 320 mL over 12 to 24 weeks with dupilumab compared to placebo.[26] Multiple analyses indicate greater spirometric responses in patients with elevated baseline eosinophils with improvements in FEV_1 averaging 210 mL higher with dupilumab versus placebo over 12 weeks in those with $\geq$300 cells/μL.[26] Overall, dupilumab leads to rapid, sustained, and clinically meaningful improvements in airflow obstruction.

Importantly, dupilumab facilitates OCS reduction in severe, steroid-dependent asthma. LIBERTY VENTURE, the 2018 phase 3 trial of dupilumab versus placebo for OCS-dependent asthma (baseline OCS dose 11.26 $\pm$ 6.12), demonstrated a 28% greater reduction in OCS dose over 24 weeks with dupilumab compared to placebo while maintaining asthma control.[27] This trial demonstrated a benefit of steroid-sparing efficacy for dupilumab for both individuals with elevated blood eosinophils, as well as for those with blood eosinophils <150, with 75% of patients achieving at least 50% reduction and 62% of patients achieving a reduction of oral glucocorticoid dose to <5 mg per day. Compared to placebo, the OR for 100% and 50% reduction in OCS dose with dupilumab was 2.74 (95% CI 1.47–5.10) and 3.98 (95% CI 2.06–7.67), respectively. Given risks of chronic steroid exposure, these steroid-sparing effects represent an important clinical benefit in patients with difficult-to-control asthma regardless of baseline eosinophil count. Dupilumab is the only FDA-approved agent to carry an indication for severe OCS-dependent asthma irrespective of biomarker status.

Multiple randomized trials have established dupilumab's efficacy in reducing severe exacerbation rates by 45% to 70% annually compared to placebo, and reductions have been consistent across phase 2 through phase 3 studies. The 2016 trial by Wenzel and colleagues revealed a 70.5% risk reduction versus placebo for dupilumab at the dose of 300 mg every 2 weeks (RR 0.265; 95% CI 0.157–0.445). Furthermore, the 2018 LIBERTY Asthma QUEST study showed a 48% lower yearly rate of severe exacerbations, and the LIBERTY VENTURE study in steroid-dependent asthma demonstrated a nearly 60% reduction (RR 0.407; 95% CI 0.263–0.630).[26,27]

Dupilumab also carries FDA approval in non-asthma conditions such as nasal polyps, atopic dermatitis, lupus pernio, and eosinophilic esophagitis, making this an ideal candidate therapy for dual action in individuals who have asthma with overlapping comorbid disease.

Tezepelumab

The anti-TSLP antibody, tezepelumab, was approved by the FDA for use in severe asthma with no phenotype or biomarker limitations in December 2021. TSLP is produced primarily by epithelial cells in the lung and plays a critical role in the activation of the inflammatory and allergic response. It acts on dendritic cells to signal T-cell differentiation into Th2 cells. Blockade of TSLP with tezepelumab, therefore, has the result of acting upstream to the targets of the other available biologic therapies in asthma and, as a result, has the potential for meaningful effects in a broad range of severe asthma populations.

Together, the two pivotal clinical trials, NAVIGATOR and PATHWAY, have produced evidence for the use of tezepelumab on a range of asthma patients at different levels of blood eosinophilia. Specifically, the phase 2 PATHWAY trial enrolled patients with baseline FEV_1 in the range of 1.82 to 1.91 L and showed improvements of 120 to 150 mL in pre-bronchodilator FEV_1 at week 52 across the dosing range in the tezepelumab groups versus placebo.[28] The NAVIGATOR study was a phase 3 trial of 1061 adults and adolescents with severe, uncontrolled asthma and reported a baseline FEV_1 of 63% predicted in which tezepelumab treatment resulted in a statistically significant 130-mL improvement in pre-bronchodilator FEV_1 at week 52 compared to placebo.[29]

Neither of the above trials directly addressed the effects of tezepelumab on steroid-dependence in asthma, and the SOURCE trial was designed to evaluate tezepelumab's steroid-sparing effect in 150 adults with OCS-dependent asthma over 48 weeks.[30] Participants in the trial had a baseline OCS dose of 13.0 mg (±5.7), and the primary outcome of OCS reduction was not met with numeric improvements, with 54% of tezepelumab patients achieving a 90% to 100% reduction versus 46% on placebo. The corresponding ORs for the effect of tezepelumab versus placebo for 100% and 50% reduction in OCS dose were 1.35 (95% CI 0.68–2.68) and 1.24 (95% CI 0.60–2.57), respectively. The pre-specified secondary outcome of reaching 5 mg or less of daily OCS dose while maintaining asthma control numerically favored tezepelumab but did not achieve statistical significance. The authors speculate that the lack of overall difference could be due in part to a large placebo effect and may be related to a longer OCS-reduction phase used in SOURCE compared to other clinical trials. In the pre-specified analysis of participants with elevated blood eosinophil count, tezepelumab resulted in a greater probability of OCS reduction than with placebo (blood eosinophils $\geq$ 150: OR 2.58; 95% CI 1.16–5.75).

The most consistent and strongest evidence for the use of tezepelumab in cases of severe asthma is its ability to prevent asthma exacerbation. Specifically, in the 2021 NAVIGATOR phase 3 study, tezepelumab reduced overall annualized exacerbation rates by 56% over 52 weeks compared to placebo (0.93 vs 2.10 events/year), and in contrast to the biologic agents in other classes (anti-IgE/anti-IL4/anti-IL5), the anti-TSLP agent demonstrated significant reductions in exacerbation rates regardless of baseline eosinophil counts (blood eosinophil < 300: RR 0.59; 95% CI 0.46–0.75 and blood eosinophil count $\geq$ 300: RR 0.30; 95% CI 0.22–0.40). Similarly, the phase 2 trial by Corren and colleagues (2017) showed reductions in exacerbations of 62% to 71% with tezepelumab versus placebo over 52 weeks.[28] Subsequent analyses found consistent exacerbation rate reductions across subgroups, including patients on different inhaled corticosteroid regimens. In the SOURCE trial population of OCS-dependent patients, tezepelumab lowered annualized exacerbation rates by 31% compared to placebo over 48 weeks. The long-term extension DESTINATION trial provides the best evidence regarding durability, demonstrating sustained reductions in exacerbations of 61% with tezepelumab versus placebo after a total treatment period of up to 156 weeks.[31]

Targeting the upstream TSLP appears to produce beneficial effects on lung function and asthma exacerbations in a broad range of patients with varying levels of T2 inflammation, and while there is a decreasing prevalence of OCS-dependent severe asthma, the data to support the use of tezepelumab in this sub-population are less convincing than some of the other targeted agents in severe asthma. Therefore, although these recent pivotal clinical trials make a compelling case for incorporating tezepelumab as a novel, first-in-class biologic option to improve disease control in severe, refractory asthma irrespective of biomarker status, this should not preclude considered decision-making that takes into account the full clinical picture including clinical features, namely comorbid disease and OCS-dependence, especially in patients who are T2 low.

SUMMARY AND FUTURE DIRECTIONS

The advent of targeted biologic agents has transformed the management of severe, uncontrolled asthma over the past two decades. These monoclonal antibodies target specific inflammatory mediators to provide personalized treatment beyond standard inhaled or systemic asthma therapies. The currently available biologics—omalizumab, mepolizumab, reslizumab, benralizumab, dupilumab, and tezepelumab—have varied mechanisms but share the ability to improve lung function and prevent exacerbations in difficult-to-control disease. The OCS-sparing effects appear to be limited to dupilumab, irrespective of type-2 biomarker status, and to the IL-5 agents mepolizumab, benralizumab, and tezepelumab, in patients with eosinophilia.

The increasing availability of biologic therapies has led to a need for a paradigm shift in the manner in which clinicians evaluate and make initial biologic treatment decisions and biologic transitions, as well as how to monitor response. Each of the available agents has demonstrated efficacy and has been incorporated into clinical practice, and while all agents appear to have a greater effect on lung function for individuals with high T2 inflammation, several key differences emerge in the magnitude and consistency of benefits across outcomes. While the anti-IL-5 therapies and omalizumab produce marginal improvements in lung function, the greatest improvements in lung function appear to arise for individuals with T2 inflammation who are treated with dupilumab or tezepelumab.

While the prevalence of steroid-dependent asthma is likely decreasing over time, there are small trials for a benefit of steroid reduction with mepolizumab as well as benralizumab and dupilumab, and the steroid-sparing effects of tezepelumab appear to be restricted to the sub-set of individuals with elevated blood eosinophils. Another key consideration is identifying responsive patient subgroups, and although this chapter does not focus on biomarkers to predict therapeutic response (covered elsewhere), there appears to be greater benefit with respect to exacerbations and lung function (but not steroid dependence) for each of the available agents for individuals with evidence of T2 inflammation.

Several promising novel therapeutic approaches are in process at the time of writing, which may lead to more targeted therapies in a broad range of individuals with asthma. For instance, multiple clinical trials are in process currently to investigate the potential for genetic differences in response to biologic therapies. The PrecISE clinical trial, which uses precision medicine approach to target treatments to individual patients on the basis of prespecified biomarkers, has completed recruitment, and formal results are in process.[32]

While the current chapter focused on key clinical outcomes of lung function, OCS dependence, and asthma exacerbations, an increasing body of literature is helping to clarify whether additional endpoints, such as full clinical remission from asthma, are possible with targeted biologic therapies. One recent study also highlighted additional unanswered questions regarding the role of maintenance inhaled corticosteroids in patients who have achieved stability on biologic therapy, specifically whether they can be safely withdrawn without compromising asthma control and lung function.[33] Other key uncertainties include the ideal sequencing or combinations of biologics, as well as whether earlier intervention meaningfully impacts long-term disease trajectory. Finally, there is an absence of head-to-head trials comparing different agents for the management of severe asthma. Future research addressing these issues will enable further personalization of care to achieve the best-possible outcomes for individuals with severe asthma.

CLINICS CARE POINTS

Pearls
- Dupilumab and tezepelumab appear to have the greatest improvements in lung function and the greatest reduction in exacerbation risk compared to placebo.
- Dupilumab is the only agent with FDA indication for steroid-dependent asthma, irrespective of biomarker status, while mepolizumab and benralizumab have also shown steroid-sparing effects for asthma with type-2 inflammation.
- Tezepelumab is the only biologic therapy with FDA approval for individuals with and without evidence of elevated type-2 biomarkers, although its steroid-sparing effects were limited to subjects with eosinophils $\geq$ 150.

Pitfalls
- There are currently no data from controlled trials to compare biologic therapies head-to-head in asthma, and the selection of a specific agent should be individualized by clinical features including comorbid conditions, biomarker status, steroid dependence, and side effect profile.
- While exacerbations, lung function, and steroid-dependence are important clinical endpoints, additional studies are required to understand the effect of biologics on other outcomes such as long-term disease trajectory and the potential for achieving clinical remission

ACKNOWLEDGMENTS

The authors would like to thank Hanyi Yang BS for her assistance in portions of the literature review and compiling results for this article.

DISCLOSURES

J.D. Salciccioli has no financial disclosures to declare. E. Israel reports the following: grants and contracts: AstraZeneca, Avillion, Gossamer Bio, National Institutes of Health (NIH), Patient-Centered Outcomes Research Institute (PCORI); royalties or licenses: UpToDate; consulting fees: Amgen, Arrowhead Pharmaceuticals, AstraZeneca, GlaxoSmithKline, Merck, Regeneron, Sanofi, TEVA, Guidepoint, Windrose Consulting Group, Reach Market Research, Apogee Therapeutics, Yuhan, Leerink Partners; honoraria: Clearview Health Partners; support for attending meeting/travel: AstraZeneca; participation on a data safety monitoring board: Novartis; receipt of equipment, materials, drugs, medical writing, or other services: Genentech, Sun Pharma, Laurel Pharmaceuticals, Om Pharma, Nestle, CLS Behring, Sanofi-Regeneron.

REFERENCES

1. Busse W, Corren J, Lanier BQ, et al. Omalizumab, anti-IgE recombinant humanized monoclonal antibody, for the treatment of severe allergic asthma. J Allergy Clin Immunol 2001;108(2):184–90.
2. Solèr M, Matz J, Townley R, et al. The anti-IgE antibody omalizumab reduces exacerbations and steroid requirement in allergic asthmatics. Eur Respir J 2001; 18(2):254–61.
3. Normansell R, Walker S, Milan SJ, et al. Omalizumab for asthma in adults and children. Cochrane Airways Group. Cochrane Database Syst Rev 2014. https://doi.org/10.1002/14651858.CD003559.pub4.
4. Domingo C, Mirapeix RM, González-Barcala FJ, et al. Omalizumab in severe asthma: effect on oral corticosteroid exposure and remodeling. a randomized open-label parallel study. Drugs 2023;83(12):1111–23.
5. Hanania NA, Alpan O, Hamilos DL, et al. Omalizumab in severe allergic asthma inadequately controlled with standard therapy. Ann Intern Med 2011;154(9):573–82.
6. Casale TB, Luskin AT, Busse W, et al. Omalizumab effectiveness by biomarker status in patients with asthma: evidence from prospero, a prospective real-world study. J Allergy Clin Immunol Pract 2019;7(1):156–64.e1.
7. Haldar P, Brightling CE, Hargadon B, et al. Mepolizumab and exacerbations of refractory eosinophilic asthma. N Engl J Med 2009;360(10):973–84.
8. Kips JC, O'Connor BJ, Langley SJ, et al. Effect of SCH55700, a humanized anti-human interleukin-5 antibody, in severe persistent asthma: a pilot study. Am J Respir Crit Care Med 2003;167(12):1655–9.
9. Pavord ID, Korn S, Howarth P, et al. Mepolizumab for severe eosinophilic asthma (DREAM): a multicentre, double-blind, placebo-controlled trial. Lancet 2012; 380(9842):651–9.
10. Ortega HG, Liu MC, Pavord ID, et al. Mepolizumab treatment in patients with severe eosinophilic asthma. N Engl J Med 2014;371(13):1198–207.
11. Nair P, Kjarsgaard M, Efthimiadis A, et al. Mepolizumab for prednisone-dependent asthma with sputum eosinophilia. N Engl J Med 2009;360(10):985–93.
12. Bel EH, Wenzel SE, Thompson PJ, et al. Oral glucocorticoid-sparing effect of mepolizumab in eosinophilic asthma. N Engl J Med 2014;371(13):1189–97.

13. Castro M, Zangrilli J, Wechsler ME, et al. Reslizumab for inadequately controlled asthma with elevated blood eosinophil counts: results from two multicentre, parallel, double-blind, randomised, placebo-controlled, phase 3 trials. Lancet Respir Med 2015;3(5):355–66.

14. Bjermer L, Lemiere C, Maspero J, et al. Reslizumab for inadequately controlled asthma with elevated blood eosinophil levels. Chest 2016;150(4):789–98.

15. Corren J, Weinstein S, Janka L, et al. Phase 3 study of reslizumab in patients with poorly controlled asthma. Chest 2016;150(4):799–810.

16. Castro M, Mathur S, Hargreave F, et al. Reslizumab for poorly controlled, eosinophilic asthma: a randomized, placebo-controlled study. Am J Respir Crit Care Med 2011;184(10):1125–32.

17. Bernstein JA, Virchow JC, Murphy K, et al. Effect of fixed-dose subcutaneous reslizumab on asthma exacerbations in patients with severe uncontrolled asthma and corticosteroid sparing in patients with oral corticosteroid-dependent asthma: results from two phase 3, randomised, double-blind, placebo-controlled trials. Lancet Respir Med 2020;8(5):461–74.

18. Bleecker ER, FitzGerald JM, Chanez P, et al. Efficacy and safety of benralizumab for patients with severe asthma uncontrolled with high-dosage inhaled corticosteroids and long-acting β2-agonists (SIROCCO): a randomised, multicentre, placebo-controlled phase 3 trial. Lancet 2016;388(10056):2115–27.

19. FitzGerald JM, Bleecker ER, Nair P, et al. Benralizumab, an anti-interleukin-5 receptor α monoclonal antibody, as add-on treatment for patients with severe, uncontrolled, eosinophilic asthma (CALIMA): a randomised, double-blind, placebo-controlled phase 3 trial. Lancet 2016;388(10056):2128–41.

20. Harrison TW, Chanez P, Menzella F, et al. Onset of effect and impact on health-related quality of life, exacerbation rate, lung function, and nasal polyposis symptoms for patients with severe eosinophilic asthma treated with benralizumab (ANDHI): a randomised, controlled, phase 3b trial. Lancet Respir Med 2021; 9(3):260–74.

21. Ferguson GT, FitzGerald JM, Bleecker ER, et al. Benralizumab for patients with mild to moderate, persistent asthma (BISE): a randomised, double-blind, placebo-controlled, phase 3 trial. Lancet Respir Med 2017;5(7):568–76.

22. Nair P, Wenzel S, Rabe KF, et al. Oral glucocorticoid–sparing effect of benralizumab in severe asthma. N Engl J Med 2017;376(25):2448–58.

23. Menzies-Gow A, Gurnell M, Heaney LG, et al. Oral corticosteroid elimination via a personalised reduction algorithm in adults with severe, eosinophilic asthma treated with benralizumab (PONENTE): a multicentre, open-label, single-arm study. Lancet Respir Med 2022;10(1):47–58.

24. Wenzel S, Ford L, Pearlman D, et al. Dupilumab in persistent asthma with elevated eosinophil levels. N Engl J Med 2013;368(26):2455–66.

25. Wenzel S, Castro M, Corren J, et al. Dupilumab Efficacy and safety in adults with uncontrolled persistent asthma despite use of medium-to-high-dose inhaled corticosteroids plus a long-acting 2 agonist: a randomised double-blind placebo-controlled pivotal phase 2b dose-ranging trial. Lancet 2016;388(10039):31–44.

26. Castro M, Corren J, Pavord ID, et al. Dupilumab efficacy and safety in moderate-to-severe uncontrolled asthma. N Engl J Med 2018;378(26):2486–96.

27. Rabe KF, Nair P, Brusselle G, et al. Efficacy and safety of dupilumab in glucocorticoid-dependent severe asthma. N Engl J Med 2018;378(26):2475–85.

28. Corren J, Parnes JR, Wang L, et al. Tezepelumab in adults with uncontrolled asthma. N Engl J Med 2017;377(10):936–46.

29. Menzies-Gow A, Corren J, Bourdin A, et al. Tezepelumab in adults and adolescents with severe, uncontrolled asthma. N Engl J Med 2021;384(19):1800–9.
30. Wechsler ME, Menzies-Gow A, Brightling CE, et al. Evaluation of the oral corticosteroid-sparing effect of tezepelumab in adults with oral corticosteroid-dependent asthma (SOURCE): a randomised, placebo-controlled, phase 3 study. Lancet Respir Med 2022;10(7):650–60.
31. Menzies-Gow AN, Price DB. Clinical remission in severe asthma. Chest 2023; 164(2):296–8.
32. Israel E, Denlinger LC, Bacharier LB, et al. PreciSE: precision medicine in severe asthma: an adaptive platform trial with biomarker ascertainment. J Allergy Clin Immunol 2021;147(5):1594–601.
33. Jackson DJ, Heaney LG, Humbert M, et al. Reduction of daily maintenance inhaled corticosteroids in patients with severe eosinophilic asthma treated with benralizumab (SHAMAL): a randomised, multicentre, open-label, phase 4 study. Lancet 2023;403(10423):271–81.
34. Wechsler ME, Menzies-Gow A, Brightling CE, et al. Evaluation of the oral corticosteroid-sparing effect of tezepelumab in adults with oral corticosteroid-dependent asthma (SOURCE): a randomised, placebo-controlled, phase 3 study. Lancet Respir Med 2022;10(7):650–60.

Biologics in Asthma
Role of Biomarkers

Gabriel Lavoie, MD, FRCPC, Ian D. Pavord, DM, FRCP, FMedSci*

KEYWORDS

- Asthma • Management • Inflammation • Severe • Biomarker

KEY POINTS

- Biomarkers define asthma endotype—for clinical use, presence, or absence of type-2 inflammation.
- Type-2 inflammation can be conceptualized as 2 complementary axes, each with a surrogate biomarker—IL-5 with blood eosinophils and interleukin (IL)-4/IL-13 with fraction of exhaled nitric oxide (FeNO).
- FeNO and blood eosinophils independently predict disease activity as assessed by risk of exacerbations. Elevation of both results in a multiplicative risk of exacerbations.
- FeNO and blood eosinophils predict response to steroids and to all targeted biologics.
- Management of type-2 low disease remains a challenge. Macrolides work independently of the presence of type-2 disease.

INTRODUCTION

Targeted monoclonal antibodies have had a massive impact on the management of severe asthma by providing treatments effective at preventing exacerbations, reducing exposure to toxic oral steroids, and significantly improving symptoms. However, these drugs need to be used in the right population. This is best exemplified by mepolizumab; early trials were not successful when used in a general severe asthma population,[1] while later trials targeting a population with a particular pattern of disease, eosinophilic asthma, were successful.[2,3] Eosinophilia and history of exacerbations predicted response to treatment and risk of further events. These are what we refer to as biomarkers. The biomarkers best associated with the risk of adverse outcomes in asthma and response to therapy are eosinophilia and fraction of exhaled nitric oxide (FeNO), with immunoglobulin (Ig)E and other biomarkers currently being of more limited use. In this article, the authors will focus on these biomarkers as they define

Respiratory Medicine Unit and Oxford Respiratory NIHR BRC, Nuffield Department of Clinical Medicine, University of Oxford, John Radcliffe Hospital, Headley Way, Headington, Oxford, OX3 9DU, UK
* Corresponding author.
E-mail address: ian.pavord@ndm.ox.ac.uk

Immunol Allergy Clin N Am 44 (2024) 709–723
https://doi.org/10.1016/j.iac.2024.08.003   **immunology.theclinics.com**
0889-8561/24/© 2024 Elsevier Inc. All rights are reserved, including those for text and data mining, AI training, and similar technologies.

different subtypes of disease that are distinct in progression and response to treatments at every level of disease activity.

WHAT ARE BIOMARKERS?

The FDA provides one of the simplest definition of biomarkers as *"a defined characteristic that is measured as an indicator of normal biological processes, pathogenic processes, or biological responses to an exposure or intervention, including therapeutic interventions"*.[4] Biomarkers are the objective measures with which we diagnose, assess, and treat health care conditions. They include blood tests, imaging and physiologic assessment (lung function, symptom scores, etc.). In asthma, we are mostly interested in 2 types; prognostic and predictive biomarkers. Prognostic biomarkers inform us on the risk of events or of disease progression, for instance elevated blood natriuretic peptide and the risk of admission for heart failure. Predictive biomarkers inform us on which patients should respond to specific therapies, such as elevated expression of programmed death ligand 1 (PDL-1) on biopsy predicting response to anti-PDL-1 agents in lung cancer. A diagnostic biomarker, which demonstrates the presence or absence of a disease such as hemoglobin and hematocrit for anemia, would be of great interest but does not currently exist for asthma.

HISTORICAL BACKGROUND ON THE USE OF BIOMARKERS IN ASTHMA

Although our understanding of asthma as a disease started in the Classical era, our current categorization of asthma is a fairly modern one. Nonetheless, the link between asthma and eosinophils goes back to when Ehrilch first described staining techniques to identify eosinophils in the nineteenth century.[5] Pathologic evidence of eosinophilic infiltration in lung tissue in asthma would follow at the dawn of the twentieth century. These also demonstrated the chronic changes and airway remodeling seen in asthma, including mucus hypersecretion, smooth muscle hypertrophy, and basal membrane thickening.[6] Later studies would go on to illustrate the correlation between eosinophilia and the severity of asthma[7] as well as the risk of exacerbations.[8]

Nitric oxide, naturally produced by the lungs, is increased in some patients with asthma. Already known as a muscle relaxant in the blood, endogenous production of nitric oxide was described in the human lungs in 1991.[9] FeNO is measured through sampling of exhaled air, originally through a chemiluminescent analyzer but now more routinely through point-of-care electroluminescent analyzers. Additional work would demonstrate that FeNO is strongly associated with type-2 airway inflammation and is an independent risk factor for asthma exacerbations[10,11] and airway remodeling with worse lung function and greater lung function decline.[12] Trials confirmed FeNO's response to both inhaled and oral corticosteroid treatment in parallel with clinical improvement.[13,14]

Finally, IgE has been described as the driving factor behind allergic sensitization and type-1 hypersensitivity reactions since the 1960s, with clear associations with asthma.[15] This is evident in patients with asthma and frank sensitization to environmental antigens (the old "extrinsic" phenotype of asthma), where specific IgE to sensitizing agents can be identified and exposure may directly trigger asthmatic symptoms.[16] Even in absence of a history of atopy, we can often observe an increase in IgE in asthma.

In short, although asthma is an old disease, with refinements in our understanding of the underlying immunology and the advent of new therapies, these biomarkers have become crucial in identifying high-risk individuals likely to respond to targeted therapies.

DEFINING ASTHMA ENDOTYPES

Our modern definition of asthma revolves around endotypes and mostly concerns the distinction between subjects demonstrating high type-2 inflammation and subjects with low type-2 inflammation, with biologic therapy essentially targeting the former. Tezepelumab is currently the sole exception, with some effectiveness even in patients with low type-2 biomarkers, although clinical trial findings in this population have not been consistent and its effect is clearly greater in the presence of type-2 disease.[17–19]

Type-2 inflammation in asthma is mediated by T helper 2 (Th2) cells and type-2 innate lymphoid cells (ILC2) and results in increased production of certain inflammatory cytokines (interleukin [IL]4, IL5, and IL13). In allergic asthma, exposure to the sensitizing agent results in antigen presentation by dendritic cells to Th2 cells, driving production of inflammatory cytokines, while in non-atopic asthma airway exposure to irritants such as viruses or air pollutants induces epithelium damage and production of alarmins, including IL-25, IL-33, and thymic stromal lymphopoietin, which in turn activate ILC2 cells and secretion of inflammatory cytokines **Fig. 1**.[20]

Upregulation of IL-5 induces growth and differentiation of eosinophil progenitors in the bone marrow, trafficking of eosinophils to the airway, and increased survival by reducing apoptosis, causing circulating and tissue eosinophilia. It also drives maturation of basophils and mast cells.[21,22] Chronic airway infiltration by eosinophils leads to smooth muscle hypertrophy and remodeling even in mild asthma through direct action and co-activation of mast cells, which secrete pro-fibrotic molecules and tumor necrosis factor-alpha (TNF-α), further stimulating eosinophils.[23] Eosinophilia also

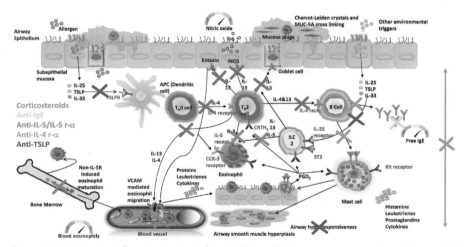

Fig. 1. Type-2 airway inflammation in asthma is driven by immune response to environmental triggers, both allergic and non-allergic, and is mediated by epithelial alarmins (interleukin [IL]-25, IL-33, and thymic stromal lymphopoietin [TSLP]). Activation of these pathways drives further inflammatory cell recruitment and survival in the airways, causing increased and persistent inflammation. Type-2 airway inflammation can be measured with fraction of exhaled nitric oxide (FeNO) (reflecting airway IL-13 activity) and blood eosinophils (reflecting systemic IL-5 activity). Type-2 inflammation causes mucus hypersecretion, airway wall edema and thickening, smooth muscle hyperplasia, and airway hyperresponsiveness. Biologic therapies target different segments of these inflammatory pathways. (Couillard S, Pavord ID, Heaney LG, Petousi N, Hinks TSC. Sub-stratification of type-2 high airway disease for therapeutic decision-making: A 'bomb' (blood eosinophils) meets 'magnet' (FeNO) framework. Respirology. 2022; 27(8): 573–577. https://doi.org/10.1111/resp.14294)

contributes to mucus hypersecretion and plugging, which is associated with physiologic obstruction in acute asthma attacks and chronic disease, and is proportional to the severity of disease.[24] [25] As increased IL-5 leads to both circulating and airway eosinophilia, measures of blood eosinophils are a good surrogate for airway eosinophilia.

The other primary cytokines implicated in type-2 inflammation are IL-4 and IL-13. Their action is conducted through the shared type-2 IL4 receptor α. They facilitate recruitment of eosinophils into the airway through production of eotaxins and upregulation of vascular cell adhesion molecule.[26] They also contribute to airways hyperresponsiveness and goblet cell hyperplasia, causing symptoms and airway obstruction.[26,27] Further, IL-13 also drives a relative preference for MUC5AC over MUC5B, which may also result in qualitative differences in mucus.[28] IL-4 and IL-13 also contribute to B-cell class switch toward IgE production, even outside of allergen stimulation.[27] Finally, IL-13 stimulates inducible nitric oxide synthase, increasing FeNO.[29] FeNO is thus a marker of activity in the IL4/IL13 pathway.

The distinct but complementary actions of the IL-5 and the IL-4/IL-13 pathways in asthma is well illustrated by the conceptual model established by Couillard and colleagues, wherein eosinophils can be thought of as "bombs," effector cells that can cause acute symptoms and long-term damage in the airway, with the IL-4/IL-13 pathway acting as a "magnet" attracting them to the airway.[30] Both high blood eosinophils and high FeNO independently increase the risk of asthma attacks, and both combined results in a multiplicative increase in risk **Fig. 2**.[31,32]

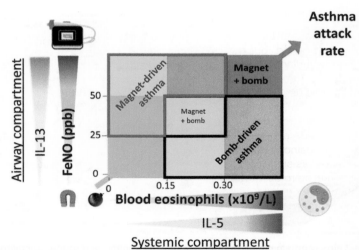

Fig. 2. In severe asthma, FeNO is correlated with increased levels of type-2 cytokines, chemokines, and alarmin in sputum. Blood eosinophils do not correlate with type-2 markers in sputum, but only with serum IL-5. This suggests there are 2 distinct compartments in type-2 inflammation, the interleukin (IL)-4/IL-13 axis driving chemotaxis of inflammatory cells to the airway (the magnet) which correlates with FeNO, and the IL-5 dependent pool of effector cells that can be attracted to the airways (bombs) which are measured with blood eosinophil count. Elevations in either of these result in a higher risk of asthma attacks, but elevation in both results in a further multiplicative increase in risk. (Couillard S, Pavord ID, Heaney LG, Petousi N, Hinks TSC. Sub-stratification of type-2 high airway disease for therapeutic decision-making: A 'bomb' (blood eosinophils) meets 'magnet' (FeNO) framework. Respirology. 2022; 27(8): 573–577. https://doi.org/10.1111/resp.14294)

As we have discussed, B-cell class switch to IgE can occur directly through stimulation of the IL-4/IL-13 pathway. Nonetheless, increased IgE is most associated with allergy and atopic asthma. Indeed, allergen exposure leads to IL-4 and IL-13 secretion, B-cell differentiation, and specific IgE production.[16] These IgE molecules bind to mast cells, priming them to degranulate on allergen re-exposure. This is the key triggering step of the early-phase asthmatic reaction, and also causes secretion of IL-4 and IL-13 driving inflammatory cell recruitment to the airways. This recruitment is associated with the late-phase reaction and sustained inflammation.[33]

In contrast to type-2 high disease, type-2 low disease is not as well understood, with identified clusters including neutrophil-dominant inflammation and paucigranulocytic asthma. Drivers of type 2-low disease are believed to include recurrent or chronic airway insults from infections or environmental irritants.[34] There have been attempts to identify therapeutic targets in this population, but the absence of good biomarkers to identify risk of exacerbation or response to treatment renders this more difficult. What is known is that these individuals show a reduced response to inhaled and systemic steroids.[35,36,37] However, macrolide antibiotics have been shown to reduce exacerbations and improve quality of life in severe asthmatics regardless of presence of type-2 disease.[38,39]

IMPACT OF BIOMARKERS ON ASTHMA TREATMENT
Eosinophils

Eosinophils in blood and the airway are associated with risk of adverse outcomes in asthma. Although there is some correlation between levels of eosinophils in blood, epithelium, and sputum, these associations are moderate at best,[40,41] and likely influenced by factors such as treatment with inhaled corticosteroids.

One may assume that the best assessment of airway eosinophilia may reside in direct epithelial sampling, but this is an invasive procedure that is costly and not without risks, precluding its routine use. Thus, although epithelial eosinophils have been used in phase 1 and 2 trials as markers of drug effect in reducing airway inflammation, their routine use is impractical.

The use of sputum eosinophils provides an evaluation of eosinophilic inflammation within the lungs while remaining accessible and minimally invasive. Sputum eosinophilia is thus considered the optimal marker of eosinophilic airway inflammation, with a cut-off of eosinophils representing $\geq 3\%$ of total non-squamous cells being generally accepted as significant.[42] Older trials have shown that titration of treatment of inhaled[43] or oral steroids[44] to normalize sputum eosinophils leads to reduced risks of exacerbations, although sometimes at the cost of increased steroid doses and side effects.[44] Despite being used to define eosinophilic asthma and qualify subjects for inclusion in some biologic studies,[2,3] sputum eosinophils were not a predictor of response for mepolizumab,[45] and more recent phase 3 trials have not used a cut-off of sputum eosinophils as an inclusion criteria or a predictor of response. This is likely due to limited accessibility outside of specialized centers and the proportion of subjects who are unable to produce sputum despite induction.[46]

Of all the available compartments, blood eosinophil count is certainly the most accessible. Absolute blood eosinophil count has become the most used criteria of type-2 disease in asthma, with the minimal cut-off associated with increased risk being around 150/μL and significant risk increase above 300 to 400/μL.[31,47] Elevated blood eosinophils predicts lung function decline[48,49] and response to inhaled corticosteroids (ICS) treatment.[50]

Blood eosinophil count has also been well demonstrated to predict greater response to biologics. Post-hoc analysis of the DREAM and MENSA trials of mepolizumab showed that as baseline blood eosinophil count (BEC) increased, the rate of exacerbations in the placebo group increased but so did the treatment effect, with no significant effect in those with BEC <150/μL, but up to around 60% reduction at ≥500/μL. A similar pattern was seen with change in lung function and symptom scores.[51] Benralizumab showed a similar trend in the SIROCCO and CALIMA trials, with no effectiveness in the group with BEC <150/μL, and up to 35% to 50% reduction in those with BEC ≥300/μL. Again, similar findings were seen with lung function and symptoms.[52] There are less data on reslizumab as the main trials only included subjects with BEC ≥400/μL, but some smaller studies suggest greater improvements in lung function and symptoms in subjects with higher baseline blood eosinophil.[53,54] Dupilumab, despite targeting the IL-4 receptor alpha, showed a marked increase in effectiveness as baseline BEC increased, with no significant reduction in exacerbations in those with BEC <150/μL, but up to 65% in those with BEC ≥300/μL, as well as significant differences in changes in forced expiratory volume in the first second (FEV1) and Asthma Control Questionnaire-5 in LIBERTY ASTHMA QUEST and the dose-ranging trial.[55–57] Interestingly, although tezepelumab showed effectiveness in reducing exacerbations even in the group of subjects with BEC<150/μL (about 40% reduction), there is a clear increase in effect as blood eosinophils increase, with exacerbations reduction reaching around 75% in the group with BEC ≥ 300 to 450/μL in the PATHWAY and NAVIGATOR studies. Finally, omalizumab also followed this trend in the EXTRA study, with no significant reduction in exacerbation in the low BEC group (<260/μL) and a 30% reduction in the group with BEC ≥260/μL.[58] In short, blood eosinophilia predicts both risk of exacerbations and response to treatment across the spectrum of disease severity.

Fractional Exhaled Nitric Oxide

Studies have shown that FeNO is moderately correlated with sputum and blood eosinophils,[59,60] although the principal interest of FeNO is as a marker for the IL-4/IL-13 pathway and type-2 inflammation in the airway. FeNO has the advantage of being easily measurable with a rapid breathing test at minimal cost. This makes it possible to use it in routine clinical work or first-line settings even without laboratory support. The cut-off for elevated FeNO varies in different publications, but the accepted values are generally of low risk of exacerbation under 20 to 25 ppb and elevated risk above 40 to 50 ppb.[61–63]

There is compelling evidence that elevated FeNO is associated with a greater risk of exacerbations and that it predicts response to treatment. Titrating ICS dose to FeNO has been shown to reduce exacerbations, in some cases even with lower overall ICS doses.[14,64] In subjects with difficult to treat asthma, FeNO can be a useful tool to distinguish refractory airway inflammation from inadequate treatment, adherence problem, or inappropriate inhaler technique. Individuals showing a significant suppression of FeNO after a period of monitored high-dose ICS therapy may show improved asthma control simply with optimization of existing treatments.[65]

Looking at the trials of biologics, isolated elevation in FeNO levels (≥25 ppb) was not associated with response to mepolizumab or benralizumab, and anti-IL-5 biologics do not reduce FeNO.[3,66–68] However, elevated FeNO is an independent predictor of the response to dupilumab, with no significant effectiveness in reducing exacerbations in those with FeNO <25 ppb but up to 70% reduction in the group with FeNO ≥50 ppb. Dupilumab treatment is associated with a significant reduction in FeNO, as could be expected from direct blockade of the IL-4/IL-13 pathway.[55–57] Elevated FeNO has also been shown to predict response to tezepelumab, with a 30% to 45% reduction in exacerbations in the group with FeNO <25 ppb and up to around

75% in those with FeNO $\geq$50 ppb.[18,19] Omalizumab also showed no significant reduction in exacerbations in those with FeNO <19.5 ppb but a 53% reduction in those with FeNO $\geq$19.5.[58]

Elevated FeNO has also been associated with accelerated loss of lung function.[69,70] Recent data from the SHAMAL study demonstrated that in individuals successfully treated with a biologic (benralizumab) and high-dose ICS/long-acting beta-agonists (LABA), the dose of ICS can be tapered down without loss of disease control. However, when ICS/LABA is reduced to only as needed, there is a loss of FEV1 correlating with an increase in FeNO. Thus, FeNO can be a marker of persistent lung inflammation despite what appears to be optimal clinical response to anti-IL5 therapy, and this can lead to airway remodeling in absence of clinically evident disease activity.[71]

Serum Immunoglobulin E

The effectiveness of IgE blockade with omalizumab has been mostly demonstrated in patients with atopic asthma. There is some observational and unblinded data on its use in non-atopic asthma, although the evidence in this population is limited.[72,73] Interestingly, although IgE is used for dosing omalizumab, it does not predict response to treatment.[74,75] Dupilumab and tezepelumab but not the anti-IL-5 biologics reduce serum IgE progressively. This may represent a progressive reduction in B-cell isotype switching in the face of IL-4 and 13 blockade. The implications of this are unclear, and studies have shown no obvious difference in response between atopic and non-atopic subjects.[3,19,76–78] As such, although it identifies an underlying phenotype of asthma, its use as a clinical biomarker has progressively lost ground as novel biologic therapies target other inflammatory pathways **Table 1**.

Putting It All Together

A variety of biomarkers can be used to characterize asthmatic disease, but blood eosinophil count, FeNO, and to a lesser extent serum IgE levels are the most useful. Moreover, while IgE is a marker of disease without having a strong association with severity or treatment response, both blood eosinophils and FeNO are reliable, easily measurable biomarkers clearly associated with disease activity and response to treatments. Furthermore, there is a growing body of data from both meta-analysis of trial data and real-world trials showing variable effectiveness of different biologics based on biomarkers.[79–81] There are currently no solid head-to-head data comparing the different options available, but it is likely that as the volume of evidence grows, the use of biomarkers will eventually shift from a minimal cut-off for eligibility toward a larger decision algorithm to match the right biologic treatment to the right patient based on their specific biomarker signature.

As the authors have mentioned earlier, in patients with both increased blood eosinophils and elevated FeNO, the impact on risk of exacerbations in trial data appears to be multiplicative, independent of treatment step, clinical symptoms, and past exacerbation history **Fig. 3**.[31]

Thus, there exists a subgroup of very high-risk individuals who, paradoxically, are also the ones likely to have the best response to biologics. There may be an opportunity to identify these individuals earlier in disease by using biomarkers and establishing their relative risk at initial diagnosis. Further, although current guidelines recommend a minimal cut-off for background treatment and number of exacerbations before starting biologics, trials earlier in disease history are ongoing, and this may allow us to prevent some of the permanent lung remodeling and clinical burden associated with long-standing severe asthma and frequent oral steroid use. It is our hope that we may eliminate much of these by providing effective treatment earlier, similar to how

Table 1
Impact of asthma biologics on biomarkers

Biologic	Omalizumab	Mepolizumab	Benralizumab	Reslizumab	Dupilumab	Tezepelumab
Baseline eosinophil count	↓	↓↓↓	↓↓↓↓	↓↓↓	Initial ↑ then ↓[a]	↓↓
Fraction of exhaled nitric oxide	↓	↔	↔	↔	↓↓	↓
Total serum immunoglobulin (IgE)	↓↓↓ free IgE[b]	↔	↔		↓↓	↓

[a] There is often an initial increase in BEC after the start of dupilumab, followed by a mild reduction from baseline values. Cases of significant eosinophilia have been documented, including symptomatic episodes of likely pre-existent eosinophilic polyangiitis with granulomatosis.

[b] Omalizumab significantly reduces circulating free immunoglobulin (IgE) levels but usually with a marked increase in total serum IgE levels.

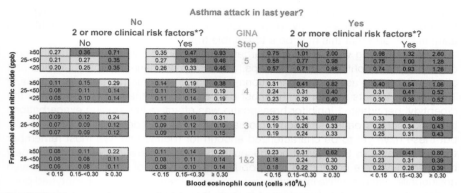

Fig. 3. Prototype asthma attack risk scale derived from data in placebo groups of asthma drug trials. Numbers in each cell are predicted annual asthma attack rates. *Risk factors are defined by the Global Initiative for Asthma guidelines: elevated symptom score (Asthma Control Questionnaire score ≥1.5), poor lung function (forced expiratory volume in the first second [FEV1]<80% predicted), inadequate inhaled steroid use or adherence, reliever over-use (>200 doses of salbutamol/month), previous intubation or intensive care unit admission for asthma, comorbidities (one of chronic rhinosinusitis, obesity, and psychiatric disease) and environmental exposures (one of smoking, allergen, and air pollution). (Couillard S, Laugerud A, Jabeen M, et al., Derivation of a prototype asthma attack risk scale centred on blood eosinophils and exhaled nitric oxide. Thorax 2022;77:199-202.)

the early use of targeted therapies in rheumatology has nearly eradicated the classical presentations of rheumatoid arthritis with ulnar drift and interphalangeal joint deforma-tions and relegated these to the medical textbooks.

Looking Forward

Our current biomarkers provide us with easily measurable targets to identify high-risk individuals and appropriate management strategies for severe asthma, but are partly limited by their non-specific nature. Indeed, blood eosinophils, FeNO, and IgE count can all be elevated independently of significant asthma or because of co-morbid con-ditions, which the clinician must account for when selecting a management strategy. Moreover, as our therapeutic arsenal now directly targets these inflammatory path-ways, we may be dissociating a biomarker from the clinical process it normally re-flects, and our interpretation must allow for this. This is best exemplified by treatment with dupilumab, where even significant transient increases in blood eosin-ophil count are not associated with increased disease activity. Moreover, as touched upon with the SHAMAL data,[71] we have reached a point where we are able to achieve clinical remission, but this does not always reflect complete biological remission as indicated by the biomarkers of elevated FeNO and reduced lung function upon discontinuation of maintenance therapy.

Asthma is a complex disease, and, as in other disease processes such as cancer, it is likely that our therapeutic decisions will have to be based on a variety of different biomarkers that, taken together, give us a better understanding of disease activity in a given individual. Furthermore, although there has been significant progress in the management of type-2 high disease, the same cannot be said of type-2 low dis-ease. Although tezepelumab shows effectiveness here, it remains less impressive than in individuals with type-2 high disease. The macrolide antibiotic azithromycin is also effective, but its mechanism of action is not completely understood, and, in the era of biologics therapy, its use as add-on treatment in this population has not been studied. Nonetheless, there is evidence that infection, especially with non-typable *Haemophilus influenzae*, may drive exacerbations and type-1 inflammation in asthma,[82,83] and that this may be a targetable trait.[84,85]

There is ongoing work in directly targeting neutrophilic inflammation and the production of neutrophil extracellular traps, as these have been implicated in viral and allergen-triggered asthma exacerbations,[86,87] and in chronic neutrophilic asthma.[88] Therapeutic targets remain for the most part elusive, but there is evidence that the dipeptidyl peptidase-1 inhibitor brensocatib was effective in reducing exacerbations in bronchiectasis patients.[89] Some biomarkers have been described in these trials, but these have yet to be characterized enough for routine use. We must remember that initial anti-IL-5 trials failed not because the agents were ineffective, but largely because they were conducted in a population that was not selected for IL5-driven eosinophilic asthma, while later trials in a properly targeted and well-phenotyped population were successful. Therefore, it is likely that identification of more appropriate biomarkers to describe the type-2 low asthma population may be the key in finding effective treatments in this population!

CLINICS CARE POINTS

- Both FeNO and blood eosinophils are easily measurable even in the primary care setting. They should be assessed as early as possible in asthmatic disease as they allow to identification of high-risk individuals.

- Acute and chronic treatment with oral corticosteroids suppresses both FeNO and blood eosinophils. Normal values on treatment should be reassessed at a distance from treatment discontinuation. Measuring biomarkers at the time of exacerbation, but prior to treatment, is often the most indicative.

- In individuals with seasonal allergies and asthma, there can be a similar fluctuation in biomarkers. It is best to assess these at the time of highest symptom burden in the year.

- FeNO is responsive to inhaled corticosteroids. In the presence of uncontrolled disease, it may reflect poor adherence, improper inhaler technique, or insufficient treatment dose, but some individuals will remain with high FeNO despite optimal treatment.

- Macrolides reduce exacerbations and improve symptoms independently of type-2 disease, but the treatment effect is not as great as the one seen with initiation of targeted biologics in the appropriate population.

DISCLOSURE

In the last 5 years, I D. Pavord has received speaker's honoraria for speaking at sponsored meetings from Astra Zeneca, Aerocrine, Almirall, Sanofi/Regeneron, Menarini, and GSK and payments for organizing educational events from AZ, GSK, and Sanofi/Regeneron. He has received honoraria for attending advisory panels with Sanofi/Regeneron, Astra Zeneca, GSK, Merck, Circassia, Chiesi, and Areteia. He has received sponsorship to attend international scientific meetings from GSK, Astra Zeneca, and Sanofi/Regeneron. G. Lavoie has no conflicts of interests to declare regarding this work.

REFERENCES

1. Kips JC, O'Connor B, Fau - Langley SJ, et al. Effect of SCH55700, a humanized anti-human interleukin-5 antibody, in severe persistent asthma: a pilot study. Am J Respir Crit Care Med 2003;167(12):1655–9.

2. Nair P, Pizzichini MMM, Kjarsgaard M, et al. Mepolizumab for prednisone-dependent asthma with sputum eosinophilia. N Engl J Med 2009;360(10):985–93.
3. Pavord ID, Korn S, Howarth P, et al. Mepolizumab for severe eosinophilic asthma (DREAM): a multicentre, double-blind, placebo-controlled trial. Lancet 2012; 380(9842):651–9.
4. Group F-NBW. In: Administration FaD, editor. BEST (biomarkers, EndpointS, and other tools) resource. Silver Spring, MD: National Institutes of Health; 2016.
5. Kay AB. Paul Ehrlich and the early history of granulocytes. Microbiol Spectr 2016;4(4).
6. Huber HL, Koessler KK. The pathology of bronchial asthma. Arch Intern Med 1922;30(6):689–760.
7. Wenzel SE, Schwartz LB, Langmack EL, et al. Evidence that severe asthma can be divided pathologically into two inflammatory subtypes with distinct physiologic and clinical characteristics. Am J Respir Crit Care Med 1999;160(3):1001–8.
8. Zeiger RS, Schatz M, Dalal AA, et al. Blood Eosinophil Count and Outcomes in Severe Uncontrolled Asthma: A Prospective Study. J Allergy Clin Immunol Pract: 2017;5(1):144-153.e8.
9. Gustafsson LE, Leone AM, Persson MG, et al. Endogenous nitric oxide is present in the exhaled air of rabbits, guinea pigs and humans. Biochem Biophys Res Commun 1991;181(2):852–7.
10. Busse WW, Wenzel SE, Casale TB, et al. Baseline FeNO as a prognostic biomarker for subsequent severe asthma exacerbations in patients with uncontrolled, moderate-to-severe asthma receiving placebo in the LIBERTY ASTHMA QUEST study: a post-hoc analysis. Lancet Respir Med 2021;9(10):1165–73.
11. Lehtimäki L, Csonka P, Mäkinen E, et al. Predictive value of exhaled nitric oxide in the management of asthma: a systematic review. Adv Respir Med 2024;92: 36–44.
12. Mogensen IA-O, Alving K, Jacinto TA-O, et al. Simultaneously elevated FeNO and blood eosinophils relate to asthma morbidity in asthmatics from NHANES 2007-12. Clin Exp Allergy 2018;48(8):935–43.
13. Schneider A, Brunn B, Hapfelmeier A, et al. Diagnostic accuracy of FeNO in asthma and predictive value for inhaled corticosteroid responsiveness: A prospective, multicentre study. eClinicalMedicine 2022;50.
14. Kay W, Jan YV, Jason O, et al. Using fractional exhaled nitric oxide to guide step-down treatment decisions in patients with asthma: a systematic review and individual patient data meta-analysis. Eur Respir J 2020;55(5):1902150.
15. Burrows B, Martinez FD, Halonen M, et al. Association of Asthma with Serum IgE Levels and Skin-Test Reactivity to Allergens. N Engl J Med 1989;320(5):271–7.
16. Antoine F, Jonathan M, Stephen RD, et al. Asthma phenotypes and IgE responses. Eur Respir J 2016;47(1):304.
17. Corren J, Parnes JR, Wang L, et al. Tezepelumab in adults with uncontrolled asthma. N Engl J Med 2017;377(10):936–46.
18. Menzies-Gow A, Corren J, Bourdin A, et al. Tezepelumab in adults and adolescents with severe, uncontrolled asthma. N Engl J Med 2021;384(19):1800–9.
19. Corren J, Pham TH, Garcia Gil E, et al. Baseline type 2 biomarker levels and response to tezepelumab in severe asthma. Allergy 2022;77(6):1786–96.
20. Kim H, Ellis AK, Fischer D, et al. Asthma biomarkers in the age of biologics. Allergy Asthma Clin Immunol 2017;13(1):48.
21. Rosenberg HF, Phipps S, Foster PS. Eosinophil trafficking in allergy and asthma. J Allergy Clin Immunol 2007;119(6):1303–10.

22. Sanderson CJ. The biological role of interleukin 5. Int J Cell Cloning 1990;8(Suppl 1):147–53.
23. Wilson SJ, Rigden HM, Ward JA, et al. The relationship between eosinophilia and airway remodelling in mild asthma. Clin Exp Allergy 2013;43(12):1342–50.
24. Perry SF, Purohit AM, Boser S, et al. Bronchial casts of human lungs using negative pressure injection. Exp Lung Res 2000;26(1):27–39.
25. Dunican EA-O, Watchorn DC, Fahy JV. Autopsy and imaging studies of mucus in asthma. lessons learned about disease mechanisms and the role of mucus in airflow obstruction. Ann Am Thorac Soc 2018;15(Suppl 3):S184–91.
26. Scott G, Asrat S, Allinne J, et al. IL-4 and IL-13, not eosinophils, drive type 2 airway inflammation, remodeling and lung function decline. Cytokine 2023;162: 156091.
27. Doran E, Cai F, Holweg CTJ, et al. Interleukin-13 in asthma and other eosinophilic disorders. Front Med (Lausanne) 2017;4.
28. Bonser LR, Erle DA-O. Airway mucus and asthma: the role of MUC5AC and MUC5B. LID. J Clin Med 2017. https://doi.org/10.3390/jcm6120112.
29. Chibana K, Trudeau JB, Mustovitch AT, et al. IL-13 induced increases in nitrite levels are primarily driven by increases in inducible nitric oxide synthase as compared with effects on arginases in human primary bronchial epithelial cells. Clin Exp Allergy 2008;38(6):936–46.
30. Couillard SA-O, Pavord IA-O, Heaney LA-O, et al. Sub-stratification of type-2 high airway disease for therapeutic decision-making: a 'bomb' (blood eosinophils) meets 'magnet' (FeNO) framework. Respirology 2022;27(8):573–7.
31. Couillard SA-O, Laugerud A, Jabeen MA-OX, et al. Derivation of a prototype asthma attack risk scale centred on blood eosinophils and exhaled nitric oxide. Thorax 2022;77(2):199–202.
32. Shrimanker R, Keene O, Hynes G, et al. Prognostic and predictive value of blood eosinophil count, fractional exhaled nitric oxide, and their combination in severe asthma: a *post hoc* analysis. Am J Respir Crit Care Med 2019;200(10):1308–12.
33. McLeod JJ, Baker B, Ryan JJ. Mast cell production and response to IL-4 and IL-13. Cytokine 2015;75(1):57–61.
34. Timothy SCH, Stewart JL, Guy GB. Treatment options in type-2 low asthma. Eur Respir J 2021;57(1):2000528.
35. Bacci E, Cianchetti S, Bartoli M, et al. Low sputum eosinophils predict the lack of response to beclomethasone in symptomatic asthmatic patients. Chest 2006; 129(3):565–72.
36. Green RH, Brightling CE, McKenna S, et al. Asthma exacerbations and sputum eosinophil counts: a randomised controlled trial. Lancet 2002;360(9347): 1715–21.
37. Pavord ID, Brightling CE, Woltmann G, et al. Non-eosinophilic corticosteroid unresponsive asthma. Lancet 1999;353(9171):2213–4.
38. Brusselle GG, Vanderstichele C, Jordens P, et al. Azithromycin for prevention of exacerbations in severe asthma (AZISAST): a multicentre randomised double-blind placebo-controlled trial. Thorax 2013;68(4):322–9.
39. Gibson PG, Yang IA, Upham JW, et al. Effect of azithromycin on asthma exacerbations and quality of life in adults with persistent uncontrolled asthma (AMAZES): a randomised, double-blind, placebo-controlled trial. Lancet 2017; 390(10095):659–68.
40. Wagener AH, de Nijs SB, Lutter R, et al. External validation of blood eosinophils, FE(NO) and serum periostin as surrogates for sputum eosinophils in asthma. Thorax 2015;70(2):115–20.

41. Hastie AT, Moore WC, Li H, et al. Biomarker surrogates do not accurately predict sputum eosinophil and neutrophil percentages in asthmatic subjects. J Allergy Clin Immunol 2013;132(1):72–80.
42. Pizzichini E, Pizzichini MM, Efthimiadis A, et al. Measuring airway inflammation in asthma: Eosinophils and eosinophilic cationic protein in induced sputum compared with peripheral blood. J Allergy Clin Immunol 1997;99(4):539–44.
43. Petsky HL, Li A, Chang AB. Tailored interventions based on sputum eosinophils versus clinical symptoms for asthma in children and adults. Cochrane Database Syst Rev 2017;8(8):CD005603.
44. Aziz-Ur-Rehman A, Dasgupta A, Kjarsgaard M, et al. Sputum cell counts to manage prednisone-dependent asthma: effects on FEV1 and eosinophilic exacerbations. Allergy Asthma Clin Immunol 2017;13(1):17.
45. Ian DP, Roland B, Monica K, et al. Evaluation of sputum eosinophil count as a predictor of treatment response to mepolizumab. ERJ Open Res 2022;8(2):00560–2021.
46. Pavord ID, Pizzichini MM, Pizzichini E, et al. The use of induced sputum to investigate airway inflammation, Thorax, 52 (6), 498–501.
47. Mallah N, Rodriguez-Segade S, Gonzalez-Barcala FA-O, et al. Blood eosinophil count as predictor of asthma exacerbation. a meta-analysis. Pediatr Allergy Immunol 2021;32(3):465–78.
48. Backman H, Lindberg A, Hedman L, et al. FEV_1 decline in relation to blood eosinophils and neutrophils in a population-based asthma cohort. World Allergy Organ J 2020;13(3):100110.
49. Pavord ID, de Prado Gómez L, Brusselle G, et al, QUEST Lung Function Decline Study Group. Biomarkers associated with lung function decline and dupilumab response in patients with asthma. Am J Respir Crit Care Med 2024.
50. Ramadan AA, Gaffin JM, Israel E, et al. Asthma and corticosteroid responses in childhood and adult asthma. Clin Chest Med 2019;40(1):163–77.
51. Ortega HG, Yancey SW, Mayer B, et al. Severe eosinophilic asthma treated with mepolizumab stratified by baseline eosinophil thresholds: a secondary analysis of the DREAM and MENSA studies. Lancet Respir Med 2016;4(7):549–56.
52. Goldman M, Hirsch I, Zangrilli JG, et al. The association between blood eosinophil count and benralizumab efficacy for patients with severe, uncontrolled asthma: subanalyses of the Phase III SIROCCO and CALIMA studies. Curr Med Res Opin 2017;33(9):1605–13.
53. Corren J, Weinstein S, Janka L, et al. Phase 3 study of reslizumab in patients with poorly controlled asthma: effects across a broad range of eosinophil counts. Chest 2016;150(4):799–810.
54. Castro M, Zangrilli J, Wechsler ME, et al. Reslizumab for inadequately controlled asthma with elevated blood eosinophil counts: results from two multicentre, parallel, double-blind, randomised, placebo-controlled, phase 3 trials. Lancet Respir Med 2015;3(5):355–66.
55. Wenzel S, Castro M, Corren J, et al. Dupilumab efficacy and safety in adults with uncontrolled persistent asthma despite use of medium-to-high-dose inhaled corticosteroids plus a long-acting β2 agonist: a randomised double-blind placebo-controlled pivotal phase 2b dose-ranging trial. Lancet 2016;388(10039):31–44.
56. Castro M, Corren J, Pavord ID, et al. Dupilumab Efficacy and Safety in Moderate-to-Severe Uncontrolled Asthma. N Engl J Med 2018;378(26):2486–96.
57. Yang D, Huang T, Liu B, et al. Dupilumab in patients with uncontrolled asthma: type 2 biomarkers might be predictors of therapeutic efficacy. J Asthma 2020;57(1):79–81.

58. Hanania NA, Wenzel S, Rosén K, et al. Exploring the effects of omalizumab in allergic asthma: an analysis of biomarkers in the EXTRA study. Am J Respir Crit Care Med 2013;187(8):804–11.
59. Schleich FN, Seidel L, Sele J, et al. Exhaled nitric oxide thresholds associated with a sputum eosinophil count ≥3% in a cohort of unselected patients with asthma. Thorax 2010;65(12):1039–44.
60. Gao J, Wu F. Association between fractional exhaled nitric oxide, sputum induction and peripheral blood eosinophil in uncontrolled asthma. Allergy Asthma Clin Immunol 2018;14:21.
61. Khatri SB, Iaccarino JM, Barochia A, et al, American Thoracic Society Assembly on Allergy, Immunology, and Inflammation. Use of fractional exhaled nitric oxide to guide the treatment of asthma: an official american thoracic society clinical practice guideline. Am J Respir Crit Care Med 2021;204(10):e97–109.
62. Excellence. NIfHaC. Asthma: diagnosis, monitoring and chronic asthma management 2017;NG80.
63. Global Initiative for Asthma, Global Strategy for Asthma Management and Prevention, 2023. GINA guidelines 2023.
64. Korevaar DA, Damen JA, Heus P, et al. Effectiveness of FeNO-guided treatment in adult asthma patients: a systematic review and meta-analysis. Clin Exp Allergy 2023;53(8):798–808.
65. McNicholl DM, Stevenson M, McGarvey LP, et al. The utility of fractional exhaled nitric oxide suppression in the identification of nonadherence in difficult asthma. Am J Respir Crit Care Med 2012;186(11):1102–8.
66. Shrimanker R, Keene O, Hynes G, et al. Prognostic and predictive value of blood eosinophil count, fractional exhaled nitric oxide, and their combination in severe asthma: a post hoc analysis. Am J Respir Crit Care Med 2019;200(10):1308–12.
67. Hearn AP, Kavanagh J, d'Ancona G, et al. The relationship between Feno and effectiveness of mepolizumab and benralizumab in severe eosinophilic asthma. J Allergy Clin Immunol Pract 2021;9(5):2093–6.e1.
68. Bernstein D, Liu M, Schleich F, et al. The impact of baseline exhaled nitric oxide levels and blood eosinophil count on clinical outcomes in REALITI-A. J Allergy Clin Immunol 2022;149(2):AB189.
69. Yunus Ç, Shoaib A, Jacob Louis M, et al. Type-2 inflammation and lung function decline in chronic airway disease in the general population. Thorax 2024;79(4): 349–58.
70. Nerpin E, Ferreira DS, Weyler J, et al. Bronchodilator response and lung function decline: Associations with exhaled nitric oxide with regard to sex and smoking status. World Allergy Organ J 2021;14(5):100544.
71. Jackson DJ, Heaney LG, Humbert M, et al, SHAMAL Investigators. Reduction of daily maintenance inhaled corticosteroids in patients with severe eosinophilic asthma treated with benralizumab (SHAMAL): a randomised, multicentre, open-label, phase 4 study. Lancet 2024;403(10423):271–81.
72. Ediger D, Günaydın FE, Erbay M, et al. Can omalizumab be an alternative treatment for non-atopic severe asthma? a real-life experience with omalizumab. Tuberk Toraks 2023;71(1):24–33.
73. Atayik E, Aytekin G. The efficacy of omalizumab treatment in patients with nonatopic severe asthma. Allergol Immunopathol (Madr) 2022;50(5):1–6.
74. Bousquet J, Wenzel S, Holgate S, et al. Predicting response to omalizumab, an anti-IgE antibody, in patients with allergic asthma. Chest 2004;125(4):1378–86.
75. Wahn U, Martin C, Freeman P, et al. Relationship between pretreatment specific IgE and the response to omalizumab therapy. Allergy 2009;64(12):1780–7.

76. Jackson DJ, Humbert M, Hirsch I, et al. Ability of serum IgE concentration to predict exacerbation risk and benralizumab efficacy for patients with severe eosinophilic asthma. Adv Ther 2020;37(2):718–29.

77. Lee J, Pollard S, Liu M, et al. Influence of baseline total IgE and history of previous omalizumab use on the impact of mepolizumab in reducing rate of severe asthma exacerbations: results from the real-world REALITI-A study. J Allergy Clin Immunol 2022;149(2):AB191.

78. Corren J, Castro M, O'Riordan T, et al. Dupilumab efficacy in patients with uncontrolled, moderate-to-severe allergic asthma. J Allergy Clin Immunol Pract 2020; 8(2):516–26.

79. Menzies-Gow A, Steenkamp J, Singh S, et al. Tezepelumab compared with other biologics for the treatment of severe asthma: a systematic review and indirect treatment comparison. J Med Econ 2022;25(1):679–90.

80. Tiotiu A, Mendez-Brea P, Ioan I, et al. Real-life effectiveness of benralizumab, mepolizumab and omalizumab in severe allergic asthma associated with nasal polyps. Clin Rev Allergy Immunol 2023;64(2):179–92.

81. Langton DPJ, Collyer TA, Khung SW, et al. Benralizumab and Mepolizumab treatment outcomes in two severe asthma clinics. Respirology 2023.

82. Yang X, Li H, Ma Q, et al. Neutrophilic asthma is associated with increased airway bacterial burden and disordered community composition. Biomed Res Int 2018; 2018:9230234.

83. Ackland JA-O, Barber CA-O, Heinson A, et al. Nontypeable Haemophilus influenzae infection of pulmonary macrophages drives neutrophilic inflammation in severe asthma. Allergy 2022;77(10):2961–73.

84. Jabeen MF, Sanderson ND, Foster D, et al. Identifying bacterial airways infection in stable severe asthma using oxford nanopore sequencing technologies. Microbiol Spectr 2022;10(2):e0227921.

85. Jabeen MF, Nicholas D, Tinè M, et al. Integrated species-level analysis of metagenome and inflammatory mediators reveals dominant and distinct roles of haemophilus influenzae and moraxella catarrhalis in severe asthma. SSRN Preprint 2023.

86. Curren B, Ahmed T, Howard DR, et al. IL-33-induced neutrophilic inflammation and NETosis underlie rhinovirus-triggered exacerbations of asthma. Mucosal Immunol 2023;16(5):671–84.

87. Koga H, Miyahara N, Fau - Fuchimoto Y, et al. Inhibition of neutrophil elastase attenuates airway hyperresponsiveness and inflammation in a mouse model of secondary allergen challenge: neutrophil elastase inhibition attenuates allergic airway responses. Respir Res 2013;14(1):8.

88. Nyenhuis SM, Schwantes EA, Evans MD, Mathur SK. Airway neutrophil inflammatory phenotype in older subjects with asthma. J Allergy Clin Immunol 2010; 125(5):1163–5.

89. Chalmers JD, Haworth CS, Metersky ML, et al, WILLOW Investigators. Phase 2 Trial of the DPP-1 Inhibitor Brensocatib in Bronchiectasis. N Engl J Med 2020; 383(22):2127–37.

Biologics in Asthma
Potential to Achieve Clinical Remission

Orlando Rivera II, MD, Rohit Katial, MD, Flavia C.L. Hoyte, MD*

KEYWORDS

- Asthma ● Remission ● Biologics ● Dupilumab ● Tezepelumab ● Benralizumab
- Mepolizumab

KEY POINTS

- Management of asthma has historically centered around symptomatic therapy, but biologic medications have made asthma remission a more achievable goal.
- Establishing a uniform definition for asthma remission can help set a new standard to effectively compare research outcomes for various asthma therapies, as well as to create precise end goals when managing asthmatics ("treat-to-target").
- Studies on different biologics show varying rates of achieving clinical remission in asthma depending on the criteria incorporated in the definition of clinical remission.
- Although definitions of clinical remission vary among different trials and national guidelines or consensus statements, the core elements of all definitions include symptom control, lack of exacerbations, and no oral corticosteroid use. Optimization and/or stabilization of lung function is also variably included in these definitions, as are biomarkers.

INTRODUCTION

Historically, asthma management has centered on controlling or reducing symptoms in patients with asthma as its primary target. With the advent of novel therapies such as monoclonal antibodies, the approach to asthma management may be shifting toward a new goal: *asthma remission*. Yet despite broad multidisciplinary efforts on an international scale, no consensus has been reached as to what this truly entails due to a lack of well-defined goals. Some chronic inflammatory diseases such as systemic lupus erythematosus, rheumatoid arthritis, and irritable bowel disease have better defined states of disease remission. These conditions have had their definitions for disease remission revised and refined over time and have generally gained widespread acceptance for these definitions, including incorporation into society guidelines. We can learn from this process and apply it toward defining asthma remission. There have been several proposed definitions for clinical remission of

Division of Allergy and Immunology, National Jewish Health, 1400 Jackson Street, Denver, CO 80206, USA
* Corresponding author.
E-mail address: hoytef@njhealth.org

Immunol Allergy Clin N Am 44 (2024) 725–736
https://doi.org/10.1016/j.iac.2024.08.004   **immunology.theclinics.com**

asthma over the years, yet none are universally accepted. Establishing one clear definition for clinical remission could set a new standard in how to effectively compare new asthma therapies, as well as highlight more precise end goals to target when managing patients with asthma in the clinical setting.

WHAT IS REMISSION?

To start, we must first understand some key concepts. The word *remission* as it pertains to pathology generally refers to a state of being, where there is low or absent disease activity (symptoms/findings), which may be spontaneous or due to medical therapy. Disease remission may or may not be a temporary state and could require ongoing medical therapy to maintain. Notably, remission is not the same as *cure* since cure implies eradication of disease and return to the normal state even once therapy is discontinued, whereas remission can be attained on or off therapy and suggests that disease can recur.

Another important distinction is between remission and control. Disease *control* refers to a reduction in severity of symptoms/complications. On the other hand, remission implies *complete disease control* wherein there is minimal or absent disease activity. Anything less than complete disease control should not be considered disease remission. Additionally, some would argue that remission alludes to a more durable absence of disease activity ("*a disease completely controlled for long enough can be considered in remission*"), and indeed "time without symptoms" is a criterion in the proposed definitions for clinical remission in several chronic conditions, including asthma. However, the exact duration of disease control needed to achieve clinical remission can vary depending on the specific disease process in question and the specific criteria for remission being used.

DEFINITIONS OF CLINICAL REMISSION IN ASTHMA

The concept of clinical remission in asthma has historically been limited to that of spontaneous remission, as seen in children and young adults whose asthma remits as part of the natural history of disease in a portion of the population. Spontaneous remission later in adulthood is rare, except in the context of allergic or occupational asthma where the allergic or occupational trigger is removed. Although spontaneous remission is traditionally thought to occur off therapy, clinical remission on treatment has gained more attention in recent years with the advent of modern asthma therapeutics, including both inhaled and biologic therapies, which have made clinical remission a more achievable possibility.

Given the relapsing remitting nature of asthma and the multiple phenotypes of asthma, providing a definition for clinical asthma remission on therapy has proven to be a complex issue. The early definitions of clinical asthma remission were proposed in the context of spontaneous remission and centered around lack of symptoms and lack of asthma medications over the course of 1 to 3 years; however, the ideal definition of clinical remission in asthma would incorporate both objective and subjective measures of disease activity. This more comprehensive definition would include symptom control, lung function measurements, biomarkers of inflammation and potential remodeling, frequency of exacerbations, long-term outcomes, and need for medications, especially systemic/oral corticosteroids (OCS) given their many adverse effects.

Much debate still exists as to what should be considered clinical remission in asthma, and interprofessional cooperation is crucial to these efforts. In 2020, an expert consensus group used a modified Delphi approach to build a framework definition for asthma remission. The criteria proposed by this expert panel are summarized in **Box 1**.[1]

More recently, in 2023, a joint workgroup of the American College of Allergy Asthma and Immunology, Academy of Allergy Asthma and Immunology, and American Thoracic Society published their proposed definition for asthma remission, which can be seen in **Box 2**.[2] This is arguably the most stringent definition of clinical remission thus far as it limits the use of a reliever therapy to no more than once per month and restricts controller medications to low-dose therapy only, in addition to the exacerbation, OCS, symptom control, and lung function criteria used in many of the other recent definitions for clinical remission.

Other international definitions of clinical asthma remission published in 2023 include the Japan Asthma Society guidelines[3] (no exacerbations, no symptoms with asthma control test (ACT) 23 or greater, no OCS use, and no lung function requirement but recommendation to evaluate after clinical remission is reached); the Severe Asthma Network Italy[4] consensus statement (no exacerbations, no symptoms with ACT 20 or greater or ACQ less than 1.5, no OCS use, and lung function stabilization); the J Spanish GEMA 5.3 guideline[5] (no exacerbations, no symptoms, no OCS use, and lung function stabilization and optimization); and the German Respiratory Society S2k guidelines[6] (no exacerbations, no symptoms, no OCS use, and lung function stabilization). Of these, only the Spanish guidelines include a definition of "complete remission," which additionally requires no evidence of airway hyperresponsiveness or bronchial inflammation. The Italian guidelines include a definition for partial clinical remission, which includes 3 of the 4 criteria mentioned earlier, one of which must be no OCS use. While none of these definitions have yet to be widely accepted by the medical community as the "true definition" of clinical asthma remission, they can all serve as examples/templates for future discussions on the matter and allow for critical examination of the merits and limitations of each proposed definition.

Regardless of exact criteria used, most experts tend to agree that clinical remission should encompass at least a 12 month period with no exacerbations, measurable improvement and/or stability of lung function testing, some objective measure of patient's subjective symptoms (ie, questionnaires such as ACQ or ACT), and lack of need for OCS. Despite this, some areas of debate still exist including whether a patient can be in clinical remission if still on maintenance therapy (If so, which controller medications are acceptable? What dose is tolerable?), how best to define improvement/stability in lung function testing (some studies argue for an increase in prebronchodilator forced expiratory volume in 1 second [pre-BD FEV1] $\geq$ 100 mL, while others argue for

---

Box 1
2020 Delphi consensus criteria for clinical remission in asthma

Clinical remission of asthma was defined as 12 months or greater with
- An absence of significant symptoms as measured by a validated clinical instrument
- Lung function optimization/stabilization
- Patient/provider agreement regarding remission
- No use of systemic corticosteroids for exacerbation or long-term control

Complete asthma remission was defined as clinical remission plus
- Objective resolution of asthma-related inflammation
- Negative bronchial hyperresponsiveness test

Andrew Menzies-Gow et al., An expert consensus framework for asthma remission as a treatment goal, Journal of Allergy and Clinical Immunology, 145 (3), 2020, 757-765.

Box 2
American College of Allergy Asthma and Immunology/Academy of Allergy Asthma and Immunology/American Thoracic Society workgroup criteria for on-treatment clinical remission in asthma

All of the following criteria must be met over a 12 month period (on biologic therapy)
1. No exacerbations requiring a physician visit, emergency care, hospitalization, and/or systemic corticosteroid use
2. No missed work or school due to asthma-related symptoms
3. Stable and optimized pulmonary function results on all occasions ($\geq$2 measurements)
4. Continued use of controlled medications (ICS, ICS-LABA, and leukotriene receptor antagonist) only at low–medium dose of ICS, or less, as defined by most recent GINA strategy
5. ACT greater than 20, AIRQ less than 2, ACQ less than 0.75 on all occasions (minimum >2 measurements)
6. Symptoms requiring 1 time reliever therapy (SABA, ICS-SABA, and ICS-LABA) once per month or less

Abbreviations: ACQ, asthma control questionnaire; ACT, asthma control test; AIRQ, asthma impairment and risk questionnaire; GINA, global initiative for asthma; ICS, inhaled corticosteroids; LABA, long-acting beta agonist; SABA, short-acting beta agonist.

Michael Blaiss et al., Consensus of an American College of Allergy, Asthma, and Immunology, American Academy of Allergy, Asthma, and Immunology, and American Thoracic Society workgroup on definition of clinical remission in asthma on treatment, Annals of Allergy, Asthma & Immunology, 131 (6), 2023, 782-785.

---

postbronchodilator [post-BD] FEV1 $\geq$ 80%, and yet others argue for "stability in lung function"), which assessment tool to use (ACT or ACQ? What threshold score should be chosen?), should biomarkers be included (if so, which ones? How reliable are they? What cutoff to use?), and whether absence from school or work due to symptoms should be included within the definition. The 2020 Delphi panel[1] also proposed patient and provider agreement of disease being in remission as one of the possible criteria required for clinical remission, but most other definitions have not included this. With so many details left to adjudicate, multidisciplinary collaboration will be pivotal to better clarify the answers to these questions.

STUDIES LOOKING AT CLINICAL REMISSION OF ASTHMA WITH BIOLOGICS

Our understanding of asthma phenotypes has fundamentally changed the way we approach asthma and has led to more targeted therapies and improvements in clinical outcomes. Asthma remission is now a more attainable goal due to the existence of monoclonal antibodies. Omalizumab was the first biologic agent to be approved for asthma in 2003, but the last 2 decades has seen the rise of multiple other biologics targeting asthma including mepolizumab, reslizumab, benralizumab, dupilumab, and tezepelumab, with several other biologic agents currently being studied (see Lugogo and colleagues' article, "Real-World Studies of Biologics for the Treatment of Moderate-to-Severe Asthma," in this issue). Data concerning clinical asthma remission have been varied across different biologics and across different studies, partly due to a difference in how clinical remission is defined by each of the studies.

A recent observational study by Thomas and colleagues[7] performed secondary analyses of 2 real-world drug registries (the Australian Xolair and Mepolizumab Registries) looking at both omalizumab's and mepolizumab's effectiveness in achieving clinical asthma remission. The definition used for clinical remission in this study included the following criteria: (1) no asthma exacerbations and no need for OCS (maintenance or bursts) during the previous 6 months when evaluated at 12 months and (2) an ACQ-5 less than 1 at 12 months. The study included 453 severe asthmatics, and although it was not included within their definition of clinical remission, the authors also explored optimization/stabilization of the subject's lung function at 12 months. Optimization of lung function was defined as a post-BD FEV1 of 80% or greater predicted. Of the subjects on omalizumab, 22.8% were able to achieve clinical remission at 12 months using the definition provided earlier, but only 19.1% achieved clinical remission and optimization of lung function. On the other hand, 29.3% of subjects on mepolizumab were able to achieve clinical remission, and 25.2% were able to achieve remission and optimization of lung function.

The rate of clinical remission on mepolizumab has also been analyzed in post hoc analyses of the REDES (Real World Effectiveness and Safety of Mepolizumab in a a Multicentric Spanish Cohort of Asthma Patients Stratified by Eosinophils) and REALITI-A (Real-World Oral Corticosteroid-Sparing Effect of Mepolizumab in Severe Asthma) trials. The REDES study[8] was a real-world, multicenter, retrospective, observational study of the safety/efficacy of mepolizumab in which 318 patients aged 18 years or older with severe eosinophilic asthma (many of whom also had chronic rhinosinusitis with nasal polyposis) were administered 100 mg of mepolizumab subcutaneously every 4 weeks for 12 months. In a post hoc analysis of this study,[9] the authors used 2 different definitions for clinical remission: (1) a 3 component definition that included being exacerbation-free for 52 weeks, ACT score of 20 or greater and being OCS free at 52 weeks and (2) a 4 component definition that included the prior 3 criteria plus a % pred post-BD FEV1 of 80% or greater. Of the 318 participants, 37% met the criteria for the 3 component definition of clinical remission versus 30% for the 4 component criteria. Another real-world study, REALITI-A,[10] was a 2 year observational, single-arm, prospective study examining the steroid-sparing effects of mepolizumab in patients aged 18 years or older who were newly prescribed 100 mg of mepolizumab and monitored for 1 to 2 years on the biologic. In a post hoc analysis by Brusselle and colleagues,[11] the authors assessed the proportion of subjects from the REALITI-A study who met their definition of asthma clinical remission at weeks 52 and 104 following mepolizumab therapy. They defined clinical remission of asthma as (1) having no exacerbations, (2) having an ACQ-5 score less than 1.5, and (3) being OCS-free. At 52 weeks, the authors found that 29% of 214 subjects met the 3 component criteria for clinical remission. At 104 weeks, 33% of 184 subjects met these criteria. When including a post-BD FEV1 of 80% or greater of predicted as a fourth criterion, 35% of 74 subjects met the 4 component definition for clinical asthma remission at 52 weeks. At 104 weeks, 37% of 52 subjects met the 4 component criteria.

In similar manner, the ability of benralizumab to help patients achieve clinical remission has been analyzed through post hoc analyses of 4 large trials studying the efficacy and safety of benralizumab. These include the SIROCCO (Efficacy and Safety of Benralizumab for Patients with Severe Asthma Uncontrolled with High-Dosage Inhaled Corticosteroids and Long Acting B2 Agonist), CALIMA (Efficacy and Safety Study of Benralizumab in Adults and Adolescents Inadequately Controlled on Inhaled Corticosteroid Plus Long-acting β2 Agonist), ANDHI (A Study of the Safety and Effectiveness of Benralizumab to Treat Patients With Severe Uncontrolled Asthma.), and XALOC-1 (Benralizumab in Severe Eosinophilic Asthma by Previous Biologic Use and Key Clinical Subgroups) trials. SIROCCO[12] and CALIMA[13] were 2 randomized, double-blind, parallel-group, placebo-controlled, phase 3 studies undertaken in greater than 300 different sites across more than 10 countries. Each study enrolled greater than 2500 patients aged 12 to 75 years with severe asthma despite medium-to-high dosage inhaled corticosteroids and long-acting β_2-agonists (ICS/

LABA), and a history of 2 exacerbations or greater in the last 12 months. In both trials, the subjects were randomized (1:1:1) to receive benralizumab 30 mg every 4 weeks, benralizumab every 8 weeks (with first 3 doses given at 4 week intervals), or placebo for 48 weeks (56 weeks in CALIMA). ANDHI[14] was a similar but smaller study with 656 patients with eosinophilic asthma. In contrast, XALOC-1[15] was a large, multinational, retrospective, observational, real-world analysis of patients with severe eosinophilic asthma at baseline, followed for 12 months or greater after initiating benralizumab. The definitions used for clinical remission in the post hoc analysis of all these trials invariably included a lack of OCS use and asthma exacerbations as part of their criteria. In addition, the SIROCCO/CALIMA and ANDHI trials included an increase in pre-BD FEV1 100 mL or greater, whereas XALOC-1 did not include FEV1 changes as a criterion. While the analysis of SIROCCO/CALIMA was limited to ACQ-6 less than 1.5 (or <0.75 in the more stringent criteria) as a measure of control, XALOC-1 defined symptom control as ACQ-5 less than 1.5 or ACT 16 or greater. Clinical remission in the SIROCCO/CALIMA and ANDHI trials ranged between 26.3% and 28.7%,[14,16] while in the XALOC-1 trial, it was significantly higher ($\sim$43%[15]), likely due to the difference in criteria used.

To compare, in the Liberty Asthma QUEST (Evaluation of Dupilumab in Patients With Persistent Asthma)[17] trial (a randomized, double blind, placebo-controlled, parallel group study) and the TRAVERSE (Long-Term Safety and Efficacy of Dupilumab in Patients with Moderate-to-Severe Asthma)[18] open label extension, researchers examined the safety and efficacy of subcutaneously administered dupilumab 200 or 300 mg every 2 weeks for a total of 52 and 96 weeks, respectively. These studies would both demonstrate that dupilumab not only significantly reduced severe asthma exacerbations in asthmatics, but also had sustained improvement of asthma control and lung function in this population at the end of the follow-up period. A retrospective analysis of these studies[19] used the following definition for clinical remission: (1) no asthma exacerbations for 12 months or greater, (3) an ACQ-5 score total score less than 1.5, (3) no need for OCS use for 12 months or greater, and (4) post-BD FEV1 of 80% or greater at studies' end (OR pre-BD FEV1 $\geq$ 100 mL in TRAVERSE study). From these criteria, approximately 35% and approximately 38.2% of patients treated with dupilumab were able to achieve clinical asthma remission at 52 and 96 weeks. Clinical remission was also sustained from 52 to 96 weeks in 70.2% of patients.

With regards to tezepelumab, NAVIGATOR (Study to Evaluate the Efficacy and Safety of Tezepelumab in Adult Subjects With Inadequately Controlled, Severe Asthma)[20] was a phase 3, multicenter, randomized, double-blind, placebo-controlled trial studying the efficacy and safety of tezepelumab in patients with severe uncontrolled asthma. NAVIGATOR randomized 1056 subjects to receive either tezepelumab or placebo every 4 weeks for a total of 52 weeks. In an exploratory analysis of NAVIGATOR by Castro and colleagues,[21] on-treatment clinical remission of asthma was attributed to those who—by study's end—had (1) no asthma exacerbations, (2) an ACQ-6 score of less than 0.75, (3) no need for OCS, (4) improvement of pre-BD FEV1 greater than 20% OR pre-BD FEV1 of greater than 80%, (5) a Clinical Global Impression of Chance (CGI-C) score of "much improved" or "very much improved," and (6) a Patient Global Impression of Severity (PGI-S) score of "no symptoms" or "minimal symptoms." Depending on the interpretation of the subjective assessment tools (CGI-C and PGI-S), a total of 14% to 28.5% of subjects on tezepelumab were able to achieve on-treatment clinical remission in this trial. A subset of subjects who completed either NAVIGATOR, described earlier, or SOURCE (Study to Evaluate the Efficacy and Safety of Tezepelumab in Reducing Oral Corticosteroid Use in Adults With Oral Corticosteroid Dependent Asthma),[22] an OCS-sparing study of 150 OCS-dependent subjects randomized to either tezepelumab or placebo for 48 weeks (4 weeks induction, 36 weeks steroid-reduction, 8 weeks maintenance), were enrolled into DESTINATION LTE (Long-Term Safety and Efficacy of Tezepelumab in People with Severe, Uncontrolled Asthma Long-Term Extension; 52–104 weeks)[23] and EFU (Extended Follow-Up; 104–140 weeks),[24] with tezepelumab treatment continuing for another year following conclusion of the NAVIGATOR/SOURCE trials and ceasing at week 100. Brightling and colleagues[24] performed a subanalysis of those who had previously achieved on-treatment clinical remission and their ability to achieve *off-treatment clinical remission*, which was defined as (1) no asthma exacerbations or OCS use, (2) an ACQ-6 score of less than 1.5 from week 104 through 140, and (3) a pre-BD FEV1 of greater than 95% of the patient's baseline at week 104 during the EFU. By week 104, 33.5% (127 of 379) of subjects met criteria for *on-treatment clinical remission*. Of those who continued into the EFU, 22.0% (62 of 282) met criteria for *off-treatment remission*.

In CHRONICLE (Observational Study of Characteristics, Treatment and Outcomes With Severe Asthma in the United States),[25] an ongoing noninterventional study of US adults with confirmed severe asthma who on a biologic (either omalizumab, mepolizumab, reslizumab, benralizumab, or dupilumab), the annualized rates of asthma exacerbation were compared 12 months before and every 6 months after biologic treatment initiation. An analysis of this study[26] showed that 318 out of 908 (~35%) have been able to achieve clinical remission (no OCS use; ACT 20 or greater; patient and specialist reported asthma control) in this cohort.

Collaborative efforts have led to the formation of national and international asthma registries, which can serve as some of the most useful sources of data when attempting to analyze clinical asthma remission. An analysis of the Danish Severe Asthma Registry,[27] a nationwide registry including all patients with asthma on biologics, defined *clinical remission* as "*a cessation of exacerbations and maintenance OCS, as well as a normalization of lung function (FEV1>80%) and an ACQ score ≤1.50.*" Among the 274 patients included in their analysis, only 43 (19%) fulfilled this criteria for clinical remission. On an even broader scale, the International Severe Asthma Registry (ISAR),[28] a multinational initiative, has analyzed rates of clinical remission on various biologics. Recently, Perez-de-Llano and colleagues[29] analyzed a group of 3717 patients from ISAR who were treated with anti-immunoglobulin E, anti-interleukin (IL)-5/5R-alpha, or anti-IL-4R-alpha. The authors used the following criteria for clinical remission: greater than 12 months with (1) no asthma exacerbations, (2) no need for OCS, (3) well-controlled (ACQ ≤0.75 or ACT ≥19) or partially controlled symptoms (ACQ >0.75 to <1.5 or ACT >15 to ≤19), (4) post-BD FEV1 greater than 80% predicted, and (5) blood eosinophils less than 300 cells/μL and/or FeNO (fraction of exhaled nitric oxide) less than 50 parts per billion. They reported that 20.3% to 33.5% of patients achieved clinical remission, depending on which specific domains were included in the definition, with 33.5% representing a 3 component definition and 20.3% representing a 4 component definition.[29,30]

As one would imagine and as these studies have demonstrated, the reported clinical remission rate will decrease the more stringent the criteria used to define asthma remission. In a recent cross-sectional study of 39 adult patients with severe asthma on a stable biologic regimen for 6 months or greater, Breslavsky and colleagues[31] looked at the proportion of subjects who were able to achieve specific criteria for clinical remission (**Table 1**). They found that most patients were able to achieve a period of 6 to 12 months without need for SCS (~75%–80%) or exacerbations (~65%) and improvement or stability of lung function (~49%–76%), but symptom control—*measured by validated assessment tools*—was the least commonly fulfilled criteria

Table 1
Subjects achieving specific criteria for remission

Domain	Criteria	N (%)
No systemic corticosteroid use	• For 6 mo • For 12 mo	• 31 (79.5) • 29 (74.4)
No exacerbations	• For 6 mo • For 12 mo	• 26 (66.7) • 25 (64.1)
Lung function	• FEV1 ≥80% pred • FEV1/FVC ≥0.75 • FEV1 improve ≥100 mL • FEV1 improve ≥10%	• 20 (51.3) • 19 (48.7) • 29 (76.3) • 26 (70.3)
Symptom control	• ACT ≥20 • ACQ-6 <1.5 • ACQ-6 ≤0.75	• 20 (51.3) • 21 (53.8) • 15 (38.5)

Abbreviations: ACQ-6, asthma control questionnaire 6; ACT, asthma control test; FEV1, forced expiratory volume in 1 s; FVC, forced vital capacity.

Anna Breslavsky et al., Comparison of clinical remission criteria for severe asthma patients receiving biologic therapy, Respiratory Medicine, 222, 2024, 107528.

(~38%–54%). Depending on the combination of these criteria used, approximately 20% to 41% of participants in the study were reported to have achieved clinical remission of asthma (**Table 2**). As shown in this and several other studies, achieving a few but not all of the criteria is still a worthwhile accomplishment that can make a

Table 2
Proportion of subjects who achieved different composite outcome measures of clinical remission on treatment

				Different Combinations of Criteria—All Include No SCS and No Exacerbations, Plus One Measure of Lung Function and One Measure of Symptom Control			
Specific Criteria According to Domain				6 mo		12 mo	
Domain	Criteria			Composite Criteria	N (%)	Composite Criteria	N (%)
No SCS use	• For 6 mo • For 12 mo			+3a + 4a +3a + 4b	13 (33.3) 12 (30.8)	+3a + 4a +3a + 4b	12 (30.8) 11 (28.2)
No exacerbations	• For 6 mo • For 12 mo			+3a + 4c +3b + 4a	9 (23.1) 10 (25.6)	+3a + 4c +3b + 4a	9 (23.1) 9 (23.1)
Lung function	• 3a FEV1 ≥80% pred • 3b FEV1/FVC ≥0.75 • 3c FEV1 improve ≥100 mL • 3d improve ≥10%			+3b + 4b +3b + 4c +3c + 4a +3c + 4b	9 (23.1) 8 (20.5) 16 (41) 16 (41)	+3b + 4b +3b + 4c +3c + 4a +3c + 4b	8 (20.5) 8 (20.5) 16 (41) 16 (41)
Symptom control	• 4a ACT ≥20 • 4b ACQ-6 <1.5 • 4c ACQ-6 ≤0.75			+3c + 4c +3d + 4a +3d + 4b +3d + 4c	12 (30.8) 14 (35.9) 15 (38.5) 11 (28.2)	+3c + 4c +3d + 4a +3d + 4b +3d + 4c	12 (30.8) 14 (35.9) 15 (38.5) 11 (28.2)

Abbreviations: ACQ, asthma control questionnaire; ACT, asthma control test; FEV1, forced expiratory value in 1 s; SCS, systemic corticosteroids.

Anna Breslavsky et al., Comparison of clinical remission criteria for severe asthma patients receiving biologic therapy, Respiratory Medicine, 222, 2024, 107528.

significant clinical difference for patients. The concept of low disease activity may represent a more attainable goal that is still worthwhile for those who are unable to meet all criteria of clinical remission.

THE FUTURE OF STUDYING ASTHMA

Looking to the future, it is clear that biologics will continue to change the way we manage asthma. Reaching a consensus as a medical community for what clinical asthma remission means would help establish clear treatment goals for physicians and researchers to achieve. Having a standardized metric for measuring clinical remission will make interpretation of research studies pertaining to asthma management easier by allowing for better comparisons of different study outcomes. In the clinical setting, we could better manage patient expectations and have better defined treatment goals.

Researchers continue to make progress on understanding asthma pathogenesis and on developing new methods for asthma management, and the future looks promising for patients with asthma. Asthma genotyping and phenotyping may pave the way to a more personalized approach to asthma treatment and to predicting who is more likely to achieve clinical remission from a certain biologic therapy, yet many questions remain unanswered. Are certain biologics more likely to lead to clinical remission in patients with certain genotypes or phenotypes? Are there any useful biomarkers we can measure that may help us predict which biologic to use in a given patient when striving for clinical remission? Once remission is achieved, is it necessary to continue biologic therapy in order to maintain clinical remission? If not, then how long should the biologic be continued? Striving for a consensus definition of clinical remission in asthma will provide a scaffold for helping to answer these questions and others related to the care of pediatric and adult patients with asthma.

SUMMARY

As the number of biologics available for asthma treatment continues to grow, the ability to target clinical remission becomes an increasingly attainable goal. Ultimately, the aim should be to tailor therapy to high-risk patients earlier in their disease course in order to prevent long-term lung damage and airway remodeling. Aiming for clinical remission early in life could improve overall asthma outcomes and increase the proportion of patients who are able to achieve and maintain clinical remission leading to decreased morbidity and improved quality of life. Establishing a consensus definition thus becomes crucial as it will move us closer to a "treat-to-target" approach that strives for the absence of disease activity and symptoms.

CLINICS CARE POINTS

- Remission is not the same as cure or control. Cure suggests resolution of disease, and control refers to reduction in severity/frequency of symptoms, whereas remission implies that a disease is completely controlled but can recur.

- Incorporating both subjective and objective measures is crucial to defining remission in asthma, although no consensus has been achieved on which specific measures/thresholds to include.

- Biologics have shown potential to help patients with asthma achieve clinical remission given their remarkable ability to reduce asthma exacerbations and OCS use, as well as to improve symptoms and lung function.

DISCLOSURE

R.K. Katial: AstraZeneca: Advisory, speaking; Sanofi/Regeneron: Advisory, speaking; GSK: Advisory. F.C.L. Hoyte: AstraZeneca: Advisory, speaking; GSK: Advisory; Genentech: Advisory; Teva: Advisory; Sanofi: Advisory.

REFERENCES

1. Menzies-Gow A, Bafadhel M, Busse WW, et al. An expert consensus framework for asthma remission as a treatment goal. J Allergy Clin Immunol 2020;145(3): 757–65.
2. Blaiss M, Oppenheimer J, Corbett M, et al. Consensus of an American College of Allergy, asthma, and Immunology, American Academy of Allergy, asthma, and Immunology, and American Thoracic Society Workgroup on definition of clinical remission in asthma on treatment. Ann Allergy Asthma Immunol 2023;131(6): 782–5.
3. Japan Asthma Society (JAS). Practical Guidelines for Asthma Management (PGAM). 2023. Available at: https://jasweb.or.jp/guideline.html. Accessed August 30, 2023.
4. Canonica GW, Blasi F, Carpagnano GE, et al. Severe Asthma Network Italy definition of clinical remission in severe asthma: a Delphi consensus. J Allergy Clin Immunol Pract 2023;11:3629–37.
5. Plaza Moral V, Alobid I, Alvarez Rodriguez C, et al. GEMA 5.3. Spanish guideline on the management of asthma. Open Respir Arch 2023;5:100277.
6. Lommatzsch M, Criee CP, de Jong CCM, et al. Diagnosis and treatment of asthma: a guideline for respiratory specialists 2023 - published by the German Respiratory Society (DGP) e. V. Pneumologie 2023;77:461–543.
7. Thomas D, McDonald VM, Stevens S, et al. Biologics (mepolizumab and omalizumab) induced remission in severe asthma patients. Allergy 2023;79(2):384–92.
8. Arismendi Nunez E, Cisneros C, Blanco-Aparicio M, et al. REDES study: Mepolizumab is effective in patients with severe eosinophilic asthma and Comorbid Nasal Polyps. Airway Pharmacology and Treatment 2022. https://doi.org/10.1183/13993003.congress-2022.2028.
9. Pavord I, Gardiner F, Heaney LG, et al. Remission outcomes in severe eosinophilic asthma with mepolizumab therapy: Analysis of the redes study. Front Immunol 2023;14. https://doi.org/10.3389/fimmu.2023.1150162.
10. Bagnasco D, Lougheed D, Subramanian V, et al. Real-world mepolizumab outcomes in severe asthma: Realiti-A post hoc analysis by exacerbation history. Allerg Immunol (Leipz) 2023. https://doi.org/10.1183/13993003.congress-2023. pa630.
11. Brusselle G, Lougheed MD, Canonica GW, et al. Clinical remission achievement in severe asthma following mepolizumab treatment: results from the Realiti-A study at 2 years. C101. Impact Biologics Asthma Outcomes 2023. https://doi. org/10.1164/ajrccm-conference.2023.207.1_meetingabstracts.a5985.
12. Bleecker ER, FitzGerald JM, Chanez P, et al. Efficacy and safety of benralizumab for patients with severe asthma uncontrolled with high-dosage inhaled corticosteroids and long-acting β2-agonists (SIROCCO): A randomised, multicentre, placebo-controlled phase 3 trial. Lancet 2016;388(10056):2115–27.
13. FitzGerald JM, Bleecker ER, Nair P, et al. Benralizumab, an anti-interleukin-5 receptor α monoclonal antibody, as add-on treatment for patients with severe, uncontrolled, eosinophilic asthma (Calima): a randomised, double-blind, placebo-controlled phase 3 trial. Lancet 2016;388(10056):2128–41.

14. Harrison TW, Chanez P, Menzella F, et al. Exacerbation reduction and early and sustained improvements in SGRQ, lung function, and symptoms of nasal polyposis with benralizumab for severe, eosinophilic asthma: Phase IIIb ANDHI trial. B101. New Biological Treatments for Asthma. 2020. Available at: https://doi.org/10.1164/ajrccm-conference.2020.201.1_meetingabstracts.a4274.
15. Jackson DJ, Pelaia G, Emmanuel B, et al. Benralizumab in severe eosinophilic asthma by previous biologic use and key clinical subgroups: real-world xaloc-1 programme. Eur Respir j 2024;64(1):2301521.
16. Menzies-Gow A, Hoyte FL, Price DB, et al. Clinical remission in severe asthma: a pooled post hoc analysis of the patient journey with benralizumab. Adv Ther 2022. Available at: https://www.ncbi.nlm.nih.gov/pmc/articles/PMC9056458/.
17. Busse WW, Maspero JF, Rabe KF, et al. Liberty asthma quest: phase 3 randomized, double-blind, placebo-controlled, parallel-group study to evaluate dupilumab efficacy/safety in patients with uncontrolled, moderate-to-severe asthma. Adv Ther 2018;35(5):737–48.
18. Wechsler ME, Ford LB, Maspero JF, et al. Long-term safety and efficacy of dupilumab in patients with moderate-to-severe asthma (traverse): an open-label extension study. Lancet Respir Med 2022;10(1):11–25.
19. Pavord ID, Israel E, Szefler SJ, et al. Dupilumab induces clinical remission in patients with uncontrolled, moderate-to-severe, type 2 inflammatory asthma. C101. Impact of Biologics on Asthma Outcomes 2023. https://doi.org/10.1164/ajrccm-conference.2023.207.1_meetingabstracts.a5995.
20. Menzies-Gow A, Colice G, Griffiths JM, et al. NAVIGATOR: a phase 3 multicentre, randomized, double-blind, placebo-controlled, parallel-group trial to evaluate the efficacy and safety of tezepelumab in adults and adolescents with severe, uncontrolled asthma. Respir Res 2020;21(1):266.
21. Castro M, Ambrose CS, Colice G, et al. On-treatment clinical remission with tezepelumab among patients with severe, uncontrolled asthma in the phase 3 navigator study. Eur Respir Soc 2022. Available at: https://erj.ersjournals.com/content/60/suppl_66/2287.
22. Wechsler ME, Colice G, Griffiths JM, et al. Source: a phase 3, multicentre, randomized, double-blind, placebo-controlled, parallel group trial to evaluate the efficacy and safety of tezepelumab in reducing oral corticosteroid use in adults with oral corticosteroid dependent asthma. Respir Res 2020;21(1). https://doi.org/10.1186/s12931-020-01503-z.
23. Menzies-Gow A, Wechsler ME, Brightling CE, et al. Long-term safety and efficacy of tezepelumab in people with severe, uncontrolled asthma (destination): a randomised, placebo-controlled extension study. Lancet Respir Med 2023;11(5):425–38.
24. Brightling CE, Jackson D, Kotalik A, et al. Biomarkers and clinical outcomes after cessation of tezepelumab after 2 years of treatment (destination). Airway Pharmacology and Treatment 2023. https://doi.org/10.1183/13993003.congress-2023.oa1415.
25. Panettieri RA, Lugogo N, Moore WC, et al. Real-world effectiveness of benralizumab in US subspecialist-treated adults with severe asthma: findings from Chronicle. Respir Med 2023;216:107285.
26. Chipps B, Lugogo N, Carr W, et al. Clinical remission with biologic use among US subspecialist-treated patients with severe asthma: results from the Chronicle Study. J Allergy Clin Immunol 2022;149(2). https://doi.org/10.1016/j.jaci.2021.12.494.
27. Hansen S, Von Buelow A, Soendergaard MB, et al. Clinical response and remission in patients with severe asthma treated with biologic treatment: findings from

the nationwide Danish severe asthma registry. Airway Pharmacology and Treatment 2022. https://doi.org/10.1183/13993003.congress-2022.3553.

28. FitzGerald JM, Tran TN, Alacqua M, et al. International severe asthma registry (ISAR): protocol for a global registry. BMC Med Res Methodol 2020;20. https://doi.org/10.1186/s12874-020-01065-0.

29. Perez-de-Llano L, Scelo G, Tran TN, et al. Exploring definitions and predictors of severe asthma clinical remission post-biologic in adults. Am J Respir Crit Care Med 2024. Available at: www.atsjournals.org/doi/abs/10.1164/rccm.202311-2192OC.

30. Pavord ID. Remission in the world of severe asthma. Am J Respir Crit Care Med 2024. https://doi.org/10.1164/rccm.202405-0894ed.

31. Breslavsky A, Al Qaied A, Tsenter P, et al. Comparison of clinical remission criteria for severe asthma patients receiving biologic therapy. Respir Med 2024;222: 107528.

Real-World Studies of Biologics for the Treatment of Moderate-to-Severe Asthma

Mauli Desai, MD[a],*, Adam Haines, MD[b],
John J. Oppenheimer, MD[c]

KEYWORDS

- Severe asthma • Real-world studies • Omalizumab • Mepolizumab • Reslizumab
- Benralizumab • Dupilumab • Tezepelumab

KEY POINTS

- Real-world studies of biologics for asthma confirm their efficacy in heterogeneous populations.
- Biologics used in a real-world setting decrease asthma exacerbations and oral corticosteroid use.
- Biologic therapy can be chosen based on a patient's asthma phenotype and relevant clinical biomarkers.
- Real-world data are emerging for the newest of biologics, which includes a biologic agent approved for use in T2-asthma and non-T2 asthma.

INTRODUCTION

The approval of biologics for use in severe asthma has led to a paradigm shift in the treatment of severe asthma, enabling a more personalized, phenotype-driven approach. Randomized controlled trials (RCTs) are required to establish the efficacy and safety of new and emerging biologics for the treatment of severe asthma and to identify populations most likely to benefit.

As these biologics "hit the market," patients and treating physicians alike are thankful to have non-systemic corticosteroid-based treatment options, especially ones that may also address comorbid conditions, such as chronic rhinosinusitis with nasal

[a] Division of Allergy & Immunology, Department of Medicine, Albert Einstein College of Medicine, Montefiore Medical Center, 111 East 210th Street, Bronx, NY 10467, USA; [b] Division of Allergy & Immunology, Department of Pediatrics, Albert Einstein College of Medicine, Montefiore Medical Center, 111 East 210th Street, Bronx, NY 10467, USA; [c] Division of Allergy& Immunology, Department of Medicine, UMDNJ-Rutgers, 110 Bergen Street Suite 1, Newark, NJ 07103, USA
* Corresponding author.
E-mail address: maudesai@montefiore.org

Immunol Allergy Clin N Am 44 (2024) 737–750
https://doi.org/10.1016/j.iac.2024.07.007
0889-8561/24/© 2024 Elsevier Inc. All rights reserved, including those for text and data mining, AI training, and similar technologies.

polyposis (CRSwNP) and allergic rhinitis. That said, many gaps in our understanding of how best to use biologics in clinical practice remain. More data are needed, particularly when multiple biologic options exist and patients may have overlapping eligibility for more than 1 biologic. Real-world studies can help close these gaps and give insight into whether or not RCT findings are generalizable to the typical asthma population seen in clinical practice.

In this article, the authors will review some of the important real-world studies published for available biologics for moderate-to-severe asthma. Naturally, the least real-world evidence exists for the newest biologics. It is important for clinicians to stay abreast of emerging literature on these therapeutics to utilize them in the most effective manner.

THE IMPORTANCE OF REAL-WORLD STUDIES IN SEVERE ASTHMA

Asthma is a complex and heterogeneous disease, the full scope of which is not captured by phase III RCTs because of necessarily strict inclusion and exclusion criteria for study participation. As such, there exists a disparity between research trial populations and those seen in clinical practice. Due to strict exclusion criteria, RCTs frequently exclude some of the most severe asthmatics. Furthermore, smokers and former smokers are frequently excluded, creating a gap in our knowledge about biologic use in these populations. In a study by Brown T., et al, from the United Kingdom, authors compared characterization data for 342 severe asthma patients in the Wessex Severe Asthma Cohort against comprehensive trial eligibility data for phase IIB and phase III RCTs of biologics for severe asthma published after 2000.[1] For the 37 RCTs of 20 biological therapies that were identified, only 9.8% (range 3.5%–17.5%) of severe asthma patients from the cohort were found to be eligible for enrollment in the phase III trials. A large part of the exclusions was due to stipulations regarding airflow obstruction, bronchodilator reversibility, and smoking history. Notably, authors found that a median of 78.9% (range 73.2%–86.6%) of their patients with severe eosinophilic asthma would have been excluded from phase III trials of anti-interleukin (IL)-5/IL-5R-targeted therapies.

RCTs are conducted in a controlled, idealized setting where parameters such as adherence are closely monitored. Real-world issues such as cost of medication are generally not at play during the treatment of study subjects. As such, real-world studies can deepen our understanding of how best to use biologics in clinical practice, where populations are diverse, have comorbid conditions, and may experience unique barriers to receiving care. Real-world studies are also important for gathering data about switching from one agent to another, achieving clinical remission, as well as long-term safety in a larger and more diverse population.

IMMUNOGLOBULIN E -TARGETED THERAPY

Omalizumab is the first biologic that was approved for the treatment of asthma. It was approved by the Federal Drug Administration (FDA) in 2003 for use in patients aged 12 years and older who have moderate-severe persistent asthma despite the use of inhaled corticosteroids (ICS), and in 2016, this approval was expanded to include children aged 6 years and older.[2] Omalizumab is a recombinant humanized immunoglobulin G1 (IgG1) monoclonal antibody that targets human immunoglobulin E (IgE) by binding to the domain that interacts the high-affinity Fc-epsilon-RI (FCeRI) receptor found on mast cells and basophils.[3]

There are 3 sentinel RCTs for omalizumab (INNOVATE, EXTRA, and EXALT), all published between 2006 and 2011.[4-6] Investigators showed that treatment of poorly controlled asthma with omalizumab significantly reduced asthma exacerbation rates in the treatment arm compared to placebo in the INNOVATE trial (0.68 vs 0.91, RRR = 26%, P = .042) and the EXTRA trial (0.66 vs 0.88, relative risk reduction = 25%, P = .006) over a 48 -week treatment period.

Major RCTs studying omalizumab, such as INNOVATE and EXTRA, were limited by homogenous patient populations, short length of follow-up, and strict regimens for other asthma treatment.[4,5] Real-world studies of omalizumab have provided additional information on optimizing usage of omalizumab, specifically regarding patient selection, biomarker use, and treatment efficacy in a heterogeneous population. Omalizumab has been available for use in the treatment of asthma for the past 20 years; as such, this drug has the most real-world data in the literature.[7]

Real-World Evidence of Omalizumab for Asthma

A United States study published in 2013 reported on real-world outcomes when omalizumab was used as add-on therapy for patients with uncontrolled asthma on combination ICS and long-acting beta-agonist (LABA)[8] In this study, 374 of a total 767 patients were placed on omalizumab in combination with inhaled therapy. Compared to those on inhaler therapy alone, the addition of omalizumab was associated with an adjusted relative risk of 0.57 (95% confidence interal [CI], 0.43–0.78) for hospitalization or ED visits for asthma. Another early, large observational trial published in the same year mined the eXpeRience registry, a multinational registry of patients with allergic asthma that enrolled patients started on omalizumab in the preceding 15 weeks, and then followed them for up to 2 years while on treatment.[9] Primary endpoints included changes in oral corticosteroid (OCS) requirements for maintenance therapy and ICS requirements. At baseline, 28% percent of participants required OCS as part of their maintenance therapy. Marked reductions in maintenance OCS use were seen at months 12 (16.1%) and 24 (14.2%). Investigators also used the Global Evaluation of Treatment Effectiveness (GETE) score to assess treatment response. The global evaluation scale is given to the patient and their physician at the end of the treatment period, at which time they are asked to rate the perceived effectiveness of biologic treatment on a 5-point categorical scale. In this study, 64.2% of the patients had an excellent or good response to omalizumab using the GETE score. The reported percentage of excellent or good responders was similar to the percent reported at 28 weeks (60.5%) in the INNOVATE trial.[4]

One of the first meta-analyses of omalizumab using existing real-world data, published in 2015, identified 25 studies regarding the effectiveness of omalizumab for asthma.[10] The authors found that the use of omalizumab in eligible patients led to multiple short-term and long-term benefits including reductions in severe exacerbations, hospitalizations, and asthma medication use, improved lung function and quality of life, and attainment of asthma control.

The Prospective Observational Study to Evaluate Predictors of Clinical Effectiveness in Response to Omalizumab (PROSPERO) trial was published in 2019 and is a prospective, single-arm, 48-week multicenter study of 806 patients aged 12 and older with allergic asthma who were eligible for omalizumab based on physician-assessed need. The exacerbation rate significantly improved from a mean of 3.00 ± 3.28 in the 12 months before baseline to 0.78 ± 1.37 through month 12 (P<.001) with the addition of omalizumab.[11] After 12 months of treatment with omalizumab, the percentage of patients with 1 or more exacerbations through month 12 was reduced by 81.9% compared to the 12 months prior to the beginning of the study period. While there were significant reductions in fractional expired nitric oxide (FeNO) and peripheral eosinophilia after completing treatment, there were no differences in forced expiratory volume in 1 second (FEV$_1$) at baseline (2.41 L ± 0.81 L) versus at month 12 (2.47 L ± 0.81 L).

In PROSPERO, patients were considered responders to treatment if they met 1 of 3 responder criteria: (1) exhibited an exacerbation rate reduction of 50% or more from baseline, (2) changed from uncontrolled at baseline based on an Asthma Control Test (ACT) score of 19 or less to controlled at the end of the study (ACT ≥20) or who achieved at least a 3-point improvement in ACT score, or (3) achieved at least a 120 mL improvement in FEV$_1$ from baseline to the end of the study.[11] In the responder analysis, 77.8% (n = 495/636) demonstrated an exacerbation reduction of 50% or more, 64.7% (n = 510/788) met criteria for ACT improvement, and 35.9% (226 of 630) demonstrated FEV$_1$ improvement of 120 mL or more. It should be noted that baseline biomarker status was not associated with a clinically relevant difference in response to therapy, which conflicts with the EXTRA trial, which found greater response to therapy in patients with high baseline T2 biomarker levels (FeNO, peripheral eosinophils, and periostin levels).[12]

A more recent, large meta-analysis of omalizumab real world effectiveness that included 86 observational studies published between 2005 and 2018 analyzed data for patients with severe allergic asthma who were treated with omalizumab for ≥16 weeks.[7] The primary outcome assessed by this study was the GETE. Secondary outcomes included mean change in FEV$_1$, annualized rate of severe exacerbations, OCS use, health care resource utilization (HCRU), and work/school absenteeism. The authors found that GETE was good/excellent in 77% patients at 16 weeks (risk difference: 0.77; 95% CI, 0.70–0.84; $P<.01$) and in 82% patients at 12 months (0.82, CI 0.73–0.91; $P<.01$). The authors also found significant improvements in secondary endpoints, including significantly reduced annualized rate of severe asthma exacerbations (risk ratio [RR]: 0.41, 95% CI, 0.30–0.56; I2 = 96%), the proportion of patients receiving OCS (RR: 0.59, 95% CI, 0.47–0.75; I2 = 96%), and unscheduled physician visits, at 12 months versus baseline. Additionally, improvements in mean FEV$_1$ and ACT scores were seen at 16 weeks, 6 months, and 12 months.

ANTI-INTERLEUKIN 5/INTERLEUKIN-5 RECEPTORα THERAPIES

Currently, 3 biologics are available that target and block the IL-5 pathway in asthmatics. Mepolizumab and reslizumab target IL-5. Benralizumab targets the IL-5Rα found on the surface of eosinophils, and via a mechanism called antibody-dependent cell-mediated cytotoxicity, it is felt to result in the apoptosis and rapid depletion of eosinophils.[13] Key RCTs for IL-5 targeted biologics have found that they not only reduce exacerbations in eosinophilic asthma, but that they also have a steroid-sparing effect.

Real-World Effectiveness of Mepolizumab

Retrospective real-world studies have shown that mepolizumab is effective and well-tolerated when used in broad, less homogeneous severe asthma populations than those studied in clinical trials. In a retrospective study of 346 patients, Llanos and colleagues found that mepolizumab treatment led to a 38.4% reduction in all exacerbations (from 2.68 to 1.65 events/patient/year; $P<.001$) and a 72.7% reduction in exacerbations requiring hospitalization (from 0.11 to 0.03 events/patient/year; $P = .004$) compared with baseline.[14] Treatment was also associated with decreased asthma exacerbation-related costs (excluding the cost of therapy) per person and decreased use of oral and inhaled corticosteroids. Multiple studies have shown similar findings with regard to real-world reductions in oral corticosteroid use following mepolizumab therapy.[15–17]

In another large, retrospective study, Casale and colleagues examined claims and diagnosis codes in a health care database as well outcomes data in order to study the efficacy of mepolizumab stratified by common comorbidities. Of the 639 patients, 73.2% had atopic diseases, 55.6% had respiratory infection, and 45.1% had chronic sinusitis as comorbidities.[18] Across comorbidity subgroups, significant reductions in the mean rate of exacerbations were seen during the follow-up year (1.0–1.5 per year) compared with baseline (2.2–2.6 per year). Furthermore, significant reductions in exacerbations requiring hospitalizations were also seen across all groups, except for the nasal polyp group (which authors postulate may be due to a small sample size). The greatest improvements were seen in the nasal polyp subgroup and the lowest in the depression or anxiety subgroup. They also found significant reductions in corticosteroid claims and exacerbation-related health care resource utilization. These findings underscore the differential impact certain comorbidities have on asthma burden. Another retrospective study, evaluating mepolizumab and omalizumab in the real world found them to be efficacious, but noted a poorer biologic response in patients with psychological co-morbidity.[19]

Another retrospective real-world study of mepolizumab examined comorbidities as well as other patient characteristics to identify features of "responders" and "super responders." In this study by Kavanagh JE et al. published in 2020, authors analyzed data from 99 patients receiving at least 16 weeks of treatment with mepolizumab, and classified patients as "responders" or "non-responders" (responders had >50% reduction in exacerbations and >50% reduction in maintenance OCS [mOCS]).[20] They also examined features of "super responders" (those who were exacerbation-free and off mOCS at 1 year). They found that mepolizumab treatment was associated with decreased asthma exacerbations and decreased mOCS dosage compared with baseline (with 57% able to discontinue mOCS completely). In the analysis, 72.7% (95% CI, 63.0–80.7) of the patients were classified as responders, and 28.3% (95% CI, 20.2–38.0) of the patients were classified as super responders. Super-responders were more likely to have concomitant nasal polyposis, a lower body mass index, and lower OCS requirements at baseline. Retrospective studies conducted outside the United States, in Italy, France, Spain, and Japan, also confirm the safety and efficacy profile of mepolizumab in the real-world setting.[16,17,21,22]

REALITI-A is a prospective, observational, real-world (84 centers), international (7 countries) study of 822 patients treated with mepolizumab 100 mg subcutaneous at the physician's discretion.[15] Pilette and colleagues recently published an analysis of the REALITI-A study 1 year after initiation of mepolizumab treatment and found a real-world OCS-sparing effect. They reported that in the 822 patients receiving mepolizumab, the rate of clinically significant exacerbations decreased by 71% between the pre-treatment and 1-year follow-up period (rate ratio 0.29 [0.26–0.32]; $P<.001$). Additionally, median mOCS dose was reduced by 75% in patients receiving baseline mOCS (n = 319). Notably, 64% of the patients had a reduction in mOCS dose of 50% or greater compared with baseline, and 43% were able to discontinue mOCS altogether. A post hoc analysis of this data, published by Liu and colleagues in December 2023, analyzed 1 year outcomes in the presence and absence of comorbidities at enrollment such as chronic rhinosinusitis with nasal polyps (CRSwNP), gastroesophageal reflux disease (GERD), depression/anxiety, and chronic obstructive pulmonary disease (COPD).[23] The proportion of patients in REALITI-A with CRSwNP, GERD, depression/anxiety, and COPD was 39%, 39%, 26%, and 10%, respectively. Clinically significant exacerbations decreased by 63% or more across comorbidity subgroups, and OCS use decreased as well. Patients with versus without CRSwNP showed the greatest treatment response (75% reduction in clinically significant exacerbations). Patients without GERD, anxiety/depression, and COPD had greater improvements than those patients with these comorbidities, highlighting the complexity of treating patients with these conditions and the importance of considering comorbid states when starting treatment and in those that continue to have symptoms despite the use of a biologic agent.

Real-World Effectiveness of Benralizumab

A large real-world study of benralizumab, published in 2021, examined 120 patients who received the biologic for severe eosinophilic asthma at a single center. The authors followed exacerbation rates, OCS use, spirometry, ACT scores, and quality of life (QOL) scores.[24] The primary outcome was "responders to treatment," defined as a >50% reduction in exacerbation rates or mean OCS use in 48 weeks of treatment. Notably, 86% of the patients were found to be responders to treatment and 39% were found to be super-responders, defined as those who had no exacerbations or OCS use after starting treatment. They found 18 patients (13.8%) to be non-responders, of which a subset was found to have evidence of anti-benralizumab antibodies or chronic airway infections. When comparing responders to non-responders, responders were less likely to be of female sex (58% vs 83.3%, $P = .041$), were of older age (53.8 years vs 47.0 years, $P = .57$), and had higher baseline FeNO levels (48 ppb vs 29 ppb, $P = .048$).

The ZEPHYR-1 study, published in 2022, was a retrospective cohort study of a United States insurance claims database that included patients who started benralizumab between November 2017 and November 2018. The study cohort (n = 204) included individuals who were biologic naïve for the 12 months prior to initiation of benralizumab. They found a 55% reduction in exacerbation rate after benralizumab initiation compared to prior to initiation (3.25 vs 1.47 per person-year, $P<.001$) and a 32% reduction in steroid dependence ($P<.001$).[25] ZEPHYR-1 also included a persistent user cohort and a switch-user cohort, which included patients who were treated with mepolizumab or omalizumab during the 12 months prior to starting benralizumab; similar outcomes observed for the patients in the persistent user cohort and for the switch-user cohort.

A larger follow-up retrospective cohort study published by Carstens and colleagues in 2023, titled ZEPHYR-2, aimed to study real-world efficacy of benralizumab in patients with severe asthma phenotypes. They included patients with 2 or more asthma exacerbations in the 12 months prior to benralizumab initiation and stratified patients into 3 non-mutually exclusive cohorts: blood eosinophil counts (<150, ≥150, 150–<300, <300, or ≥300 cells/uL) (n = 429), switch-users (as previously defined in ZEPHYR-1) (n = 349), and individuals with 18 or 24 months of follow-up after index-date (n = 419).[26] In the eosinophil cohort, the authors found a significant reduction in exacerbation rates for all subgroups (52%–54% reduction, $P<.001$). Again, significant reductions in exacerbation rates were found in the switch-user group and among individuals followed for up to 24 months. This study highlights the real world effectiveness of benralizumab in managing severe asthma across a heterogenous population of patients with eosinophilic asthma, and in those inadequately controlled with other biologics.

Real World Effectiveness of Reslizumab

Since the FDA approval of reslizumab for severe eosinophilic asthma in 2016, there have been relatively few studies of its real world effectiveness. A small single-center study published in 2019 included 26 patients with poorly controlled severe eosinophilic asthma.[27] Patients were included if their baseline Asthma Control Questionnaire-6

(ACQ-6) score was greater than 1.5, peripheral eosinophilia measuring >0.4 cells $\times$ 10^9/L while on high-dose ICS, and frequent hospitalizations or persistent ICS requirements. All patients received reslizumab 3 mg/kg intravenously every 4 weeks. ACQ-6, glucocorticoid use, exacerbation history, and FEV_1 were regularly assessed in these patients. The authors found a reduction in ACQ-6 from 3.5 to 1.7 at 1 year and 2.0 at 2 years of treatment ($P = .0001$). Additionally they found a 79% reduction in annual exacerbation frequency at 1 year (mean = 1.74 exacerbations/year) compared to baseline (mean = 8.31 exacerbations/year), and 88% at 2 years (mean = 0.91 exacerbations/year, $P<.00001$).

A larger US study published in 2021 examined clinical outcomes and HCRU among individuals treated with reslizumab in 215 subjects. Outcome data were obtained after at least 7 months of treatment with reslizumab and included exacerbations, OCS use, FEV_1% predicted, and HCRU. When compared to the baseline period prior to initiation, the authors found significant improvements in individual outcomes including reduction in mean number of exacerbations per patient (2.84 ± 2.41 vs 0.94 ± 1.86), improvement in FEV_1% percent predicted ($65.1\% \pm 20.5\%$; vs $73.1\% \pm 23.1\%$; $P<.001$) and ACT scores (13.8 ± 4.2; vs 18.6 ± 4.0; $P<.001$). Cumulative HRCU, which included inpatient admissions, emergency department visits, urgent care visits, and unscheduled outpatient appointments was reduced by 26.5% ($P<.001$).[28]

A meta-analysis of all anti-IL5 therapies pooled 2 real-world studies of reslizumab to better understand its effect on annualized rates of exacerbations, oral steroid use, and peripheral eosinophilia.[29] The authors found a pooled effect of reslizumab in these studies to reduce annualized rates of exacerbations by -6.72 (95% CI -8.47, $-.497$), oral steroids dose reductions by -3.90 mg (95% CI -5.26, -2.54), and peripheral eosinophils by -603.60 cells/uL (95% CI -838.69, -368.51). These pooled effect results represented a mean difference from a random effects meta-analysis model. The authors concluded that the effects of reslizumab in real world studies are similar to those derived in RCTs, confirming the drug's efficacy in typical patients with severe asthma.

ANTI-INTERLEUKIN 4/INTERLEUKIN 13 PATHWAY

Dupilumab is a monoclonal antibody that blocks IL4R alpha, thereby downregulating the IL4 and IL-13 inflammatory pathways. Dupilumab was FDA approved for the treatment of eosinophilic and/or oral steroid-dependent asthma in 2018, and is also approved for use in atopic dermatitis, CRSwNP, eosinophilic esophagitis, and prurigo nodularis. Pivotal RCTs of dupilumab use in the treatment of asthma have demonstrated the effectiveness of dupilumab in decreasing exacerbation rates and improving asthma control, quality of life, and lung function.[30,31] Treatment has been associated with reductions in T2 biomarkers, such as FeNO and serum IgE, while blood eosinophil levels remain unchanged or even increase. In many dupilumab-treated patients, steroid reduction is feasible while still maintaining favorable clinical outcomes.[30]

Real World Effectiveness of Dupilumab

Available real-life studies on dupilumab confirm the treatment efficacy seen in RCTs. In a French multi-center retrospective cohort study of 64 patients, the addition of dupilumab to maximal standard of care for 12 months led to improvements in ACT scores (from 14 [7–16] to 22 [17–24]; [$P<.001$]) and mean FEV_1 from (58% [47–75] to 68% [58–88]; [$P=.001$]), as well as reductions in daily prednisone use (from 20 [10–30] to 5 [0–7] mg/d; [$P<.001$]).[32] The majority of patients required daily oral steroids at baseline during enrollment. Annual exacerbations decreased from (4 [2–7] to 1 [0–2]; [$P<.001$]). Hypereosinophilia $\geq1500/mm^3$ was seen at least once during the follow-up period in 16 patients (25%) on treatment. Hypereosinophilia persisted after 6 months in 8 subjects (14%); notably, blood eosinophil count did not impact clinical response in the study.

The US Advantage study, published in 2023, is a real-world, retrospective study of patients initiated on dupilumab treatment between November 2018 and September 2020, using data from a US electronic medical database (TriNetX Dataworks, Cambridge, MA, USA). In the 2,400 patients evaluated, dupilumab treatment significantly reduced exacerbation rates by 44%, and reduced systemic OCS prescriptions by 48%. Treatment effectiveness was seen independent of exacerbation history, eosinophil levels, or COVID-19 impact.[33] Another real-world study, published by Pelaia and colleagues, found that dupilumab efficacy was rapid in onset (seen after just 4 weeks of add-on therapy) in patients with severe asthma and nasal polyposis.[34] Treatment was associated with improved symptom scores, decreased OCS use, improved lung function, and reduced FeNO levels. Efficacy was seen in both allergic and non-allergic patients with CRSwNP.

ANTI-THYMIC STROMAL LYMPHOPOIETIN

Tezepelumab is a monoclonal antibody directed against thymic stromal lymphopoietin, an upstream signaling molecule secreted by bronchial epithelial cells. It was approved by the FDA in December 2021 for the treatment of severe asthma. There are no specific biomarker requirements for eligibility, making tezepelumab the first biologic available for the treatment of severe, non-T2 type asthma. The NAVIGATOR study, a large-scale phase III RCT of tezepelumab use in patients age 12 to 80 with severe persistent asthma, studied asthma-related outcomes during a treatment period of 52 weeks with an additional 12 weeks of post-treatment follow-up. The authors found that individuals treated with tezepelumab had a 56% reduction in the rates of annualized asthma exacerbations compared to those treated with placebo (0.93 [95% CI 0.80, 1.07] vs 2.10; $P<.001$). When only analyzing patients with peripheral eosinophil counts less than 300 cells/uL, patients treated with tezepelumab had a 41% reduction in rates of annualized exacerbations (1.02 with vs 1.73; $P<.001$).[35]

At present, no large-scale real world studies of tezepelumab have been published. Real-world data are emerging, as evidenced by the recent publication of several abstracts regarding tezepelumab use in the real world.[36–38]

SWITCHING BIOLOGIC THERAPIES

Many real-world studies have been published regarding switching from one biologic agent to another for the treatment of severe refractory asthma. With the increase in available biologic therapies and improved disease phenotyping, there is a need for this kind of research that can improve clinician knowledge regarding when to switch and time to achieve a clinical response after failing prior biologic therapy. While omalizumab was the first approved biologic therapy, many of the existing real-world studies focus on studying successful switching of patients from omalizumab to alternate biologic therapies. The following sections will outline the existing real-world data studying switching to alternate biologics in patients with refractory severe asthma.

Switching to Mepolizumab

One real-world study confirmed the benefit of switching from omalizumab to mepolizumab in patients with uncontrolled severe eosinophilic asthma despite therapy with omalizumab.[39] This would intuitively make sense given the underlying pathologic underpinnings of eosinophilic asthma. That said, there are overlapping severe asthma phenotypes, and patients may meet criteria for multiple biologics. Another study showed that this switch, from omalizumab to mepolizumab, in cases of omalizumab failure led to a reduction in lost work days, annual exacerbations, and adverse events related to OCS. A slight increase in economic costs related to biological treatment was observed, but this was outweighed by the benefits.[40] These data show that mepolizumab provides clinically significant benefits for patients with overlapping allergic and eosinophilic phenotypes (with blood eosinophils >500 cells/μL); the most common comorbidity seen in these patients was nasal polyposis. It suggests that patients with severe asthma with high blood eosinophils and nasal polyps have a better response to anti-IL-5 rather than anti-IgE, regardless of atopy and IgE levels.

Switching to Reslizumab

There are no dedicated real-world studies on switching to reslizumab in patients previously treated with alternate biologics. Rather, the majority of real-world studies focus on switching from anti-IL-5 therapies such as mepolizumab and reslizumab to anti-IL-5Rα therapy with benralizumab. One real-world study of 134 adults included in a Dutch severe asthma registry who were treated with reslizumab for at least 6 months found that patients had significant reductions in annualized rates of asthma exacerbations both in patients who were biologic naïve as well as those who had been previously treated with a biologic therapy.[41] The authors also found significant reductions in the proportion of OCS users after reslizumab treatment.

Switching to Benralizumab

The majority of existing data regarding switching biologic treatment to anti-IL-5Rα therapy is in patients with severe eosinophilic asthma whose symptoms are refractory to prior anti-IL-5 therapy. A multi-center retrospective analysis in Germany was published in 2020, which examined outcomes in patients with severe eosinophilic asthma whose disease was refractory to either mepolizumab or reslizumab.[42] The most common documented reasons for discontinuing prior anti-IL-5 therapy was inadequate treatment response (67%), persistent impairment in physical fitness (43%), and ongoing OCS requirement (40%). Of 665 patients who were treated with anti-IL-5 therapy, 595 were deemed too stable on treatment and excluded, while 70 (10.5%) were deemed uncontrolled and started on benralizumab therapy. When compared to outcomes after 4 months of the previous anti-IL-5 therapy (48 on mepolizumab and 12 on reslizumab), 4 months of benralizumab therapy led to a reduction in the percent of patients requiring OCS (31.7% vs 53.3%, $P<.001$), improvement in forced expiratory volume in 1 second/ forced vital capacity (FEV_1/FVC) (68% vs 61%, $P = .011$), and improvement in ACT scores (19 vs 16, $P<.001$). Annualized exacerbation rates were lower in those treated with anti-IL-5Rα therapy versus anti-IL-5 therapy, but the result was not statistically significant (1.1 ± 3.5 PPY vs 1.88 ± 2.2 PPY; $P=.092$). A smaller study from Spain of 27 patients who were switched to benralizumab from anti-IL-5 therapy found significant reductions in exacerbation rates in this population (-2.12 PPY, 95% CI 0.99–3.24, $P=.002$).[43]

Some patients have biomarkers and disease comorbidities that may make it challenging to choose anti-IgE versus anti-eosinophil targeted therapy as an initial biologic of choice. To date, a real-world study in Italy has evaluated the effectiveness of switching from omalizumab to benralizumab in 20 patients with severe eosinophilic asthma.[44] Patients were considered omalizumab failures if after 12 months of therapy they continued to have recurrent exacerbations or poorly controlled symptoms. Patients were then treated with benralizumab for 12 months. When compared to omalizumab treatment, converting to benralizumab resulted in fewer exacerbations (3 vs 4.6, $P<.01$), reduced mean daily use of rescue inhalers (0.1 vs 1.95, $P<.001$), improved ACT scores (20 vs 15, $P<.05$), and improved FEV_1 (2.18 L vs 1.81 L, $P<.05$). Prior to any biologic treatment, 17 patients (85%) were on regular OCS treatment, which decreased to 14 patients (70%) after omalizumab therapy, and to 4 patients (20%) after benralizumab treatment, showing that the addition of benralizumab allowed for the successful reduction of OCS use in the great majority of their patients.

Switching to Dupilumab

While there are now multiples studies demonstrating the real-world efficacy of dupilumab,[32,33] limited data exist about switching from a previous monoclonal antibody therapy to dupilumab. One real-world study published in 2021 retrospectively analyzed 38 patients with severe asthma who were switched to dupilumab from a previous anti-IgE or anti-IL-5 medication.[45] After 3 to 6 months of therapy with dupilumab, 76% of the patients demonstrated a response to dupilumab. The authors found that these patients had decreased exacerbation rates, improved asthma control, and improved lung function. Patients with increased FeNO (≥ 25 ppb) during previous biologic therapy were more often to respond to dupilumab than patients with lower FeNO (<25 ppb). These findings are consistent with post-hoc analysis of the LIBERTY ASTHMA QUEST phase 3 trial, which found that patients with higher baseline FeNO showed greater reductions in annualized rates of exacerbations and FEV_1 when they received dupilumab compared to placebo.[46] In another retrospective review of 26 patients with severe asthma treated with dupilumab, of which 16 patients had previously been treated with an alternative biologic therapy for their asthma, the authors found that dupilumab treatment significantly reduced the number of annual exacerbations from 3.4 ± 4.1 to 1.6 ± 2.7 PPY ($P<.01$) at the last follow-up regardless of previous biologic use.[47]

DUAL BIOLOGIC THERAPY

For patients who have suboptimal control of asthma on a single biologic, the question arises as to whether or not combining biologics may have an additive, complementary effect on asthma control. Safety data on the use of multiple biologics are lacking, and there is concern about cost. The first RCT of combining approved biologics for severe asthma, the Study of Magnitude and Prediction of Response to Omalizumab and Mepolizumab in Adult Severe Asthma (PREDICTUMAB), is now recruiting subjects. Some real-world experiences have been described, mostly in case series, using 2 biologics for asthma, particularly in those suffering from type 2 comorbidities such as atopic dermatitis and eosinophilic disorders.

There is, however, insufficient data at this time, and currently no guidelines recommend concurrent administration of 2 biologics for the treatment of asthma and T2 comorbidities.[48]

SUMMARY

We have entered a new era of precision medicine for the treatment of severe asthma, with multiple biologics, targeting different pathways, available for use. The growing literature on real-world use of biologics confirms the generalizability of RCT data. Real-world studies have demonstrated that these medications are effective in reducing annual exacerbation rates and OCS use in the heterogeneous populations seen in clinical practice (which includes patients with comorbidities, smoking history, etc, that may have been excluded from RCTs). As the literature grows, and addresses questions such as switching and combining biologics, our understanding of how best to use biologics for specific phenotypes and overlapping phenotypes will become more defined. Taking a closer look at a subset of patients achieving highly well-controlled asthma, namely "super-responders" as well as non-responders, may shed further light on optimal use of biologics, and forthcoming data on clinical remission outcomes in the real world will help define our goals and measures of success in treating severe asthma.

CLINICS CARE POINTS

- Phenotype-driven asthma management in a real-world clinical setting can help identify the biologic agent most likely to have the greatest likelihood of success, as measured by reductions in clinically significant asthma exacerbations and steroid use.

- Clinical biomarkers (such as blood eosinophil count, serum immunoglobulin E (sIgE) level and exhaled nitric oxide (FeNO) can be used to determine a patient's asthma phenotype; elevations in these biomarkers support a diagnosis of T2 asthma.

- Multiple biologic therapy options exist for T2 asthma, the most common type of asthma, with some patients having overlapping eligibility for more than one biologic. Other factors can be considered when choosing a biologic (such as elevation in a specific biomarker, presence of comorbidities, cost, dosing schedules).

- Although most biologics are approved for use in T2-asthma, a newer biologic is available for patients without any elevation in T2 biomarkers

DISCLOSURES

Dr M. Desai does not have any relevant disclosures. Dr J.J. Oppenheimer: DSMB, Adjudication: GSK, Sanofi/Regeneron, AZ, Amgen, Novartis, Consultant: GSK, Amgen, Bryn, ARS, UpToDate, Medscape, Annals of Allergy Asthma Immunology, ABAI.

REFERENCES

1. Brown T, Jones T, Gove K, et al. Randomised controlled trials in severe asthma: Selection by phenotype or stereotype. Eur Respir J 2018;52(6). https://doi.org/10.1183/13993003.01444-2018.
2. Omalizumab, Xolair, label. Available at: https://www.accessdata.fda.gov/drugsatfda_docs/label/2016/103976s5225lbl.pdf. [Accessed 7 December 2023].
3. Kumar C, Zito P. Omalizumab. StatPearls 2023. Available at: https://www.ncbi.nlm.nih.gov/books/NBK545183/. [Accessed 7 December 2023].
4. Humbert M, Beasley R, Ayres J, et al. Benefits of omalizumab as add-on therapy in patients with severe persistent asthma who are inadequately controlled despite best available therapy (GINA 2002 step 4 treatment): INNOVATE. Allergy 2005; 60(3):309–16. https://doi.org/10.1111/j.1398-9995.2004.00772.x.
5. Hanania NA, Alpan O, Hamilos DL, et al. Omalizumab in severe allergic asthma inadequately controlled with standard therapy: a randomized trial. Ann Intern Med 2011;154(9):573–82. https://doi.org/10.7326/0003-4819-154-9-201105030-00002.

6. Bousquet J, Siergiejko Z, Swiebocka E, et al. Persistency of response to omalizumab therapy in severe allergic (IgE-mediated) asthma. Allergy 2011;66(5):671–8. https://doi.org/10.1111/j.1398-9995.2010.02522.x.

7. Bousquet J, Humbert M, Gibson PG, et al. Real-World Effectiveness of Omalizumab in Severe Allergic Asthma: A Meta-Analysis of Observational Studies. J Allergy Clin Immunol Pract 2021;9(7):2702–14. https://doi.org/10.1016/j.jaip.2021.01.011.

8. Grimaldi-Bensouda L, Zureik M, Aubier M, et al. Does omalizumab make a difference to the real-life treatment of asthma exacerbations?: Results from a large cohort of patients with severe uncontrolled asthma. Chest 2013;143(2):398–405. https://doi.org/10.1378/chest.12-1372.

9. Braunstahl GJ, Chlumský J, Peachey G, et al. Reduction in oral corticosteroid use in patients receiving omalizumab for allergic asthma in the real-world setting. Allergy Asthma Clin Immunol 2013;9(1):47. https://doi.org/10.1186/1710-1492-9-47.

10. Alhossan A, Lee CS, MacDonald K, et al. "Real-life" Effectiveness Studies of Omalizumab in Adult Patients with Severe Allergic Asthma: Meta-analysis. J Allergy Clin Immunol Pract 2017;5(5):1362–70.e2. https://doi.org/10.1016/j.jaip.2017.02.002.

11. Casale TB, Luskin AT, Busse W, et al. Omalizumab Effectiveness by Biomarker Status in Patients with Asthma: Evidence From PROSPERO, A Prospective Real-World Study. J Allergy Clin Immunol Pract 2019;7(1):156–64.e1. https://doi.org/10.1016/j.jaip.2018.04.043.

12. Hanania NA, Wenzel S, Rosén K, et al. Exploring the effects of omalizumab in allergic asthma: an analysis of biomarkers in the EXTRA study. Am J Respir Crit Care Med 2013;187(8):804–11. https://doi.org/10.1164/rccm.201208-1414OC.

13. Kolbeck R, Kozhich A, Koike M, et al. MEDI-563, a humanized anti-IL-5 receptor alpha mAb with enhanced antibody-dependent cell-mediated cytotoxicity function. J Allergy Clin Immunol 2010;125(6):1344–53.e2. https://doi.org/10.1016/j.jaci.2010.04.004.

14. Llanos JP, Ortega H, Bogart M, et al. Real-World Effectiveness of Mepolizumab in Patients with Severe Asthma: An Examination of Exacerbations and Costs. J Asthma Allergy 2020;13:77–87. https://doi.org/10.2147/JAA.S236609.

15. Pilette C, Canonica GW, Chaudhuri R, et al. REALITI-A Study: Real-World Oral Corticosteroid-Sparing Effect of Mepolizumab in Severe Asthma. J Allergy Clin Immunol Pract 2022;10(10):2646–56. https://doi.org/10.1016/j.jaip.2022.05.042.

16. Taillé C, Chanez P, Devouassoux G, et al. Mepolizumab in a population with severe eosinophilic asthma and corticosteroid dependence: results from a French early access programme. Eur Respir J 2020;55(6). https://doi.org/10.1183/13993003.02345-2019.

17. Domingo Ribas C, Carrillo Díaz T, Blanco Aparicio M, et al. REal worlD Effectiveness and Safety of Mepolizumab in a Multicentric Spanish Cohort of Asthma Patients Stratified by Eosinophils: The REDES Study. Drugs 2021;81(15):1763–74. https://doi.org/10.1007/s40265-021-01597-9.

18. Casale T, Molfino NA, Silver J, et al. Real-world effectiveness of mepolizumab in patients with severe asthma and associated comorbidities. Ann Allergy Asthma Immunol 2021;127(3):354–62.e2. https://doi.org/10.1016/j.anai.2021.05.021.

19. Fong WCG, Azim A, Knight D, et al. Real-world Omalizumab and Mepolizumab treated difficult asthma phenotypes and their clinical outcomes. Clin Exp Allergy 2021;51(8):1019–32. https://doi.org/10.1111/cea.13882.

20. Kavanagh JE, d'Ancona G, Elstad M, et al. Real-World Effectiveness and the Characteristics of a "Super-Responder" to Mepolizumab in Severe Eosinophilic Asthma. Chest 2020;158(2):491–500. https://doi.org/10.1016/j.chest.2020.03.042.

21. Bagnasco D, Caminati M, Menzella F, et al. One year of mepolizumab. Efficacy and safety in real-life in Italy. Pulm Pharmacol Ther 2019;58:101836. https://doi.org/10.1016/j.pupt.2019.101836.

22. Nagase H, Tamaoki J, Suzuki T, et al. Reduction in asthma exacerbation rate after mepolizumab treatment initiation in patients with severe asthma: A real-world database study in Japan. Pulm Pharmacol Ther 2022;75:102130. https://doi.org/10.1016/j.pupt.2022.102130.

23. Liu MC, Bagnasco D, Matucci A, et al. Mepolizumab in Patients With Severe Asthma and Comorbidities: 1-Year REALITI-A Analysis. J Allergy Clin Immunol Pract 2023;11(12):3650–61.e3. https://doi.org/10.1016/j.jaip.2023.07.024.

24. Kavanagh JE, Hearn AP, Dhariwal J, et al. Real-World Effectiveness of Benralizumab in Severe Eosinophilic Asthma. Chest 2021;159(2):496–506. https://doi.org/10.1016/j.chest.2020.08.2083.

25. Chung Y, Katial R, Mu F, et al. Real-world effectiveness of benralizumab: Results from the ZEPHYR 1 Study. Ann Allergy Asthma Immunol 2022;128(6):669–76.e6. https://doi.org/10.1016/j.anai.2022.02.017.

26. Carstens D, Maselli DJ, Mu F, et al. Real-World Effectiveness Study of Benralizumab for Severe Eosinophilic Asthma: ZEPHYR 2. J Allergy Clin Immunol Pract 2023;11(7):2150–61.e4. https://doi.org/10.1016/j.jaip.2023.04.029.

27. Ibrahim H, O'Sullivan R, Casey D, et al. The effectiveness of Reslizumab in severe asthma treatment: a real-world experience. Respir Res 2019;20(1):289. https://doi.org/10.1186/s12931-019-1251-3.

28. Wechsler ME, Peters SP, Hill TD, et al. Clinical Outcomes and Health-Care Resource Use Associated With Reslizumab Treatment in Adults With Severe Eosinophilic Asthma in Real-World Practice. Chest 2021;159(5):1734–46. https://doi.org/10.1016/j.chest.2020.11.060.

29. Charles D, Shanley J, Temple SN, et al. Real-world efficacy of treatment with benralizumab, dupilumab, mepolizumab and reslizumab for severe asthma: A systematic review and meta-analysis. Clin Exp Allergy 2022;52(5):616–27. https://doi.org/10.1111/cea.14112.

30. Castro M, Corren J, Pavord ID, et al. Dupilumab Efficacy and Safety in Moderate-to-Severe Uncontrolled Asthma. N Engl J Med 2018;378(26):2486–96. https://doi.org/10.1056/NEJMoa1804092.

31. Busse WW, Maspero JF, Rabe KF, et al. Liberty Asthma QUEST: Phase 3 Randomized, Double-Blind, Placebo-Controlled, Parallel-Group Study to Evaluate Dupilumab Efficacy/Safety in Patients with Uncontrolled, Moderate-to-Severe Asthma. Adv Ther 2018;35(5):737–48. https://doi.org/10.1007/s12325-018-0702-4.

32. Dupin C, Belhadi D, Guilleminault L, et al. Effectiveness and safety of dupilumab for the treatment of severe asthma in a real-life French multi-centre adult cohort. Clin Exp Allergy 2020;50(7):789–98. https://doi.org/10.1111/cea.13614.

33. Blaiss M, Bleecker ER, Jacob-Nara J, et al. Real-world effectiveness of dupilumab in patients with asthma: Findings from the US advantage study. Ann Allergy Asthma Immunol 2023. https://doi.org/10.1016/j.anai.2023.11.006.

34. Pelaia C, Lombardo N, Busceti MT, et al. Short-Term Evaluation of Dupilumab Effects in Patients with Severe Asthma and Nasal Polyposis. J Asthma Allergy 2021;14:1165–72. https://doi.org/10.2147/JAA.S328988.

35. Menzies-Gow A, Corren J, Bourdin A, et al. Tezepelumab in Adults and Adolescents with Severe, Uncontrolled Asthma. N Engl J Med 2021;384(19):1800–9. https://doi.org/10.1056/NEJMoa2034975.

36. Gupta M, Harjinder S, Diaz J, et al. Tezepelumab-ekko Improved Asthma Control and Asthma Symptom in Adults with Uncontrolled and Severe Asthma in Real-Life. J Allergy Clin Immunol 2023;151(2 Supplement):AB21.

37. Nopsopon T, Brown A, Akenroye A. The Real-world Effectiveness of Tezepelumab in a Cohort of Patients with Severe Asthma. J Allergy Clin Immunol 2024;153(2 Supplement):AB96.

38. Gomez L. Real-Life Tezepelumab-ekko Study On The Effectiveness Of Asthma Control And Patient Characteristics In Adults And Adolescents With Severe Uncontrolled Asthma. J Allergy Clin Immunol 2024;153(2 Supplement):AB102.

39. Chapman KR, Albers FC, Chipps B, et al. The clinical benefit of mepolizumab replacing omalizumab in uncontrolled severe eosinophilic asthma. Allergy 2019; 74(9):1716–26. https://doi.org/10.1111/all.13850.

40. Carpagnano GE, Resta E, Povero M, et al. Clinical and economic consequences of switching from omalizumab to mepolizumab in uncontrolled severe eosinophilic asthma. Sci Rep 2021;11(1):5453. https://doi.org/10.1038/s41598-021-84895-2.

41. Hashimoto S, Kroes JA, Eger KA, et al. Real-World Effectiveness of Reslizumab in Patients With Severe Eosinophilic Asthma - First Initiators and Switchers. J Allergy Clin Immunol Pract 2022;10(8):2099–108.e6. https://doi.org/10.1016/j.jaip.2022.04.014.

42. Drick N, Milger K, Seeliger B, et al. Switch from IL-5 to IL-5-Receptor α Antibody Treatment in Severe Eosinophilic Asthma. J Asthma Allergy 2020;13:605–14. https://doi.org/10.2147/JAA.S270298.

43. Martínez-Moragón E, García-Moguel I, Nuevo J, et al. Real-world study in severe eosinophilic asthma patients refractory to anti-IL5 biological agents treated with benralizumab in Spain (ORBE study). BMC Pulm Med 2021;21(1):417. https://doi.org/10.1186/s12890-021-01785-z.

44. Pelaia C, Crimi C, Nolasco S, et al. Switch from Omalizumab to Benralizumab in Allergic Patients with Severe Eosinophilic Asthma: A Real-Life Experience from Southern Italy. Biomedicines 2021;9(12). https://doi.org/10.3390/biomedicines 9121822.

45. Mümmler C, Munker D, Barnikel M, et al. Dupilumab Improves Asthma Control and Lung Function in Patients with Insufficient Outcome During Previous Antibody Therapy. J Allergy Clin Immunol Pract 2021;9(3):1177–85.e4. https://doi.org/10.1016/j.jaip.2020.09.014.

46. Pavord ID, Deniz Y, Corren J, et al. Baseline FeNO Independently Predicts the Dupilumab Response in Patients With Moderate-to-Severe Asthma. J Allergy Clin Immunol Pract 2023;11(4):1213–20.e2. https://doi.org/10.1016/j.jaip.2022.11.043.

47. Numata T, Araya J, Miyagawa H, et al. Real-World Effectiveness of Dupilumab for Patients with Severe Asthma: A Retrospective Study. J Asthma Allergy 2022;15:395–405. https://doi.org/10.2147/JAA.S357548.

48. Thomes R, Darveaux J. Combination biologic therapy in severe asthma: a case series. Ann Allergy Asthma Immunol 2018;121(5):S91. https://doi.org/10.1016/j.anai.2018.09.297.

Biologics in Asthma
Emerging Biologics

Brinda Desai, MD[a], Muhammad Adrish, MD, MBA[b],
Arjun Mohan, MD[c], Njira L. Lugogo, MD/MSc[d],*

KEYWORDS

- Asthma • Biologics • Inflammation • Type 2 asthma

KEY POINTS

- Despite the widespread acceptance of biologics in asthma, there remain concerns of residual disease activity given the prevalence of a partial response to therapy, in about half of the patients receiving biologic therapy.
- Newer biologic and nonbiologic therapeutics are needed to improve outcomes, particularly in severe asthma.
- Improved understanding of inflammatory pathways and drug biology with optimized drug delivery, has led to opportunities for additional novel targets for asthma treatment.

INTRODUCTION

We are in an exciting period of discovery with multiple emerging therapies for asthma.

Our understanding of pathophysiology and heterogeneity of the disease has led to multiple targeted therapies that have been discussed extensively in earlier articles in this issue. Approximately one-third of the patients with severe asthma on biologic therapy achieve optimal disease control with minimal to no residual disease activity. For these patients, we envision a future where asthma remission on treatment is a distinct and achievable possibility.[1] For the remainder of our patients, this remarkable response remains elusive, likely related to the inherent complexity (such as redundancies) and variability of inflammatory pathways in asthma.[2]

Technological advances now allow us to target novel inflammatory pathways, downregulate more than one mechanism, and interrupt downstream activation of factors that have the potential to disrupt multiple cytokines concurrently. Understanding pharmacokinetics and drug delivery to the lungs is of critical importance as we evaluate new

[a] Department of Medicine, University of California San Diego, 9500 Gilman Drive, La Jolla, CA 92093, USA; [b] Department of Pulmonary & Critical Care, Baylor College of Medicine, One Baylor Plaza, Houston, TX 77030, USA; [c] Department of Medicine, University of Michigan, 300 North Ingalls Street, Suite 2d21, Ann Arbor, MI 48109, USA; [d] Department of Medicine, University of Michigan, 300 North Ingalls Street, Suite 2c40, Ann Arbor, MI 48109, USA
* Corresponding author.
E-mail address: nlugogo@med.umich.edu

Immunol Allergy Clin N Am 44 (2024) 751–763
https://doi.org/10.1016/j.iac.2024.07.008   immunology.theclinics.com

ways of targeting inflammation in asthma. In this article, we will review emerging therapies (**Table 1**) as well as novel nonbiologic interventions with the goal of providing a more comprehensive understanding of the therapeutic landscape. Finally, we will contextualize future drug development by reviewing the existing challenges and the use of technological advancements to overcome barriers and develop new treatments.

EMERGING THERAPIES
Interleukin-33

Interleukin (IL)-33 is a member of the IL-1 family of cytokines. It is expressed in the endothelial, epithelial, and fibroblast-like cells and has a well-recognized role in cancer immunology and allergic inflammation.[3] Typically, IL-33 is a tightly sequestered protein in the cell nucleus bound to chromatin and is passively released with tissue injury, which can be seen in response to cigarette smoke, pollutants, and viral or bacterial pathogens.[3] These injuries activate the release of IL-33 from airway epithelial cells early during inflammation; hence, it is considered an alarmin[3] (**Fig. 1**). There are 3 key alarmins that are produced following epithelial injury, including thymic stromal lymphopoietin (TSLP), IL-33, and IL-25. Once released, IL-33 binds to a heterodimeric receptor complex, activating immune and structural cells such as bronchial epithelial and airway smooth muscle cells and fibroblasts.[4] IL-33 is an attractive target as this alarmin and its receptor, suppression of tumorigenicity 2 (ST2), are expressed by cell types not exclusive to type 2 (T2)-high inflammation.[5] The demonstrated impact of anti-IL-33 and anti-ST2 antibodies on asthma outcomes has been modest till date, but overall still encouraging.

In asthma, astegolimab, an anti-ST2 antibody resulted in a reduction in annual asthma exacerbation rate in adults with uncontrolled severe asthma with variable levels of eosinophilia including those patients with low (<300 cells/μL) eosinophils.[5] Itepekimab, a human immunoglobulin G4 (IgG4)[P] monoclonal antibody (mAb) against IL-33, demonstrated efficacy in adults with moderate-to-severe asthma on inhaled glucocorticoids plus long-acting beta-agonists. In this novel study design, itepekimab was studied either alone (ie, monotherapy biologic) or in combination with dupilumab and compared to dupilumab alone, or placebo.[6] Itepekimab resulted in a significantly lower incidence of loss of asthma control and a significant increase in prebronchodilator forced expiratory volume in the first second (FEV1) compared to placebo.[6] The study was designed to determine whether itepekimab would confer additive benefits when combined with dupilumab. To our knowledge, this is the first clinical trial evaluating dual biologics in asthma.[6,7] Interestingly, and contrary to expectations, combination therapy was not more efficacious than monotherapy. In fact, this group had a lower impact on asthma control than each monotherapy. Itepekimab did not reduce blood eosinophil counts, and the reduced efficacy of combination itepekimab plus dupilumab, may be a consequence of incomplete inhibition of type 2 inflammation.[6] Other trials with anti-IL-33 antibodies are ongoing. Tozorakimab, a human IgG1 anti-IL-33 antibody that inhibits IL-33 signaling through the ST2 receptor and prevents oxidation of advanced glycation end products/epidermal growth factor receptor (RAGE/EGFR), is being studied in a phase II trial in uncontrolled moderate–severe asthma.[8] Previous studies showed that tozorakimab inhibited ST2-dependent inflammatory responses driven by IL-33 in human epithelial cells and a murine model of epithelial injury.[9]

Dual Interleukin-13/Thymic Stromal Lymphopoietin

IL-13 induces the expression of the nitric oxide synthase enzyme in epithelial cells, which leads to goblet cell hyperplasia, mucus hypersecretion and airway smooth

Table 1
Summary of emerging targets for asthma

Drug	Phase	Population	Key Conclusions
Anti-IL-33			
Astegolimab	Phase II	Adults with uncontrolled severe asthma with variable levels of eosinophilia including those patients with low (<300 cells/µL) eosinophils	Reduction in annual asthma exacerbation rate
Itepekimab	Phase III	Adults with moderate-severe asthma on inhaled glucocorticoids and long-acting beta-agonists	Lower incidence of loss of asthma control Increase in prebronchodilator FEV1 compared to placebo
Tozorakimab	Phase II	Adults with uncontrolled moderate–severe asthma	Pending, study ongoing
CNTO 7160	Phase I	Adults with mild asthma or atopic dermatitis	No apparent clinical benefit
Anti-IL-13/TSLP			
SAR443765	Phase I	Adults with mild-to-moderate asthma with elevated FeNO (≥25 ppb)	Reduction in FeNO and type 2 biomarkers and eosinophils Improvement in FEV1 and reduction in airway resistance
Anti-JAK/STAT			
GDC-0214/RG6151	Phase I	Adults with mild asthma	Dose-dependent reductions in FeNO
Anti-OX40/OX40 ligand			
Amlitelimab	Phase II	Adults with moderate-to-severe asthma	Pending, study ongoing
Anti-IL-6			
Tocilizumab	Phase II	Adults with mild allergic asthma	No clinical benefit
Anti-IL-5			
Depemokimab	Phase III	Adolescents and adults with severe asthma	Reduction in the rate of clinically significant exacerbations over 52 wk

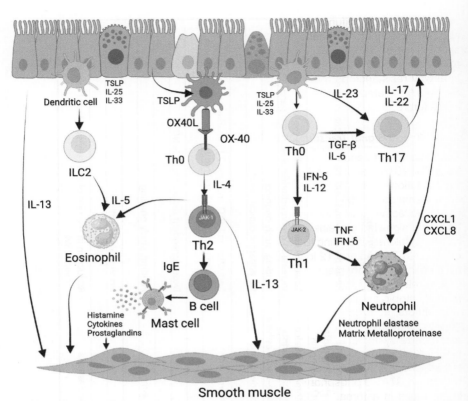

Fig. 1. Pathways for T2 high and T2 low asthma. T2 high pathways lead to increased airway eosinophils, T-helper cell-2 (Th2), and innate lymphoid cell-2 (ILC-2). T2 low inflammation leads to neutrophilic or pauci-granulocytic inflammation. (Created with BioRender.com.)

muscle contraction, causing bronchoconstriction.[10] IL-13 and IL-4 play a significant role in the T2 inflammatory pathway by recruiting eosinophils from the circulation and contributing to chemotaxis into the airway mucosa.[11] Fractional exhaled nitric oxide (FeNO) is a marker of T2 airway inflammation, specifically IL-13. Elevated FeNO is associated with an increased exacerbation risk, lower FEV1, and an accelerated rate of lung function decline.[12,13] While further research is needed in certain subpopulations,[14] anti-IL-13 blockade with lebrikizumab alone did not significantly reduce asthma exacerbation rates.[15] Dupilumab's blockade of IL-4 and IL-13, however, prevents eosinophil migration into lung tissue and is a highly effective therapy with excellent long-term data supporting its safety and efficacy.[16–19] Given the redundancy in inflammatory pathways, there is interest in targeting multiple pathways simultaneously.[20] Technological advances using nanobody technology have provided an opportunity for multiple antibodies to be administered in a single dose. TSLP is a cellular-epithelium-derived mediator and alarmin that is released in response to pollution, viruses, or allergens inducing both T2 and non-T2 cytokine production. This leads to bronchial hyperresponsiveness, mucus hypersecretion, and airway remodeling.[21] Tezepelumab is an anti-TSLP mAb approved for the treatment of severe asthma irrespective of inflammatory phenotype, given its efficacy on T2 and non-T2 inflammation.

SAR443765 is a bifunctional nanobody molecule blocking both TSLP and IL-13. Nanobody technology is described later in this article. Phase I results indicate that a single dose of SAR443765 demonstrated a substantial reduction in FeNO, T2 bio-markers and eosinophils as well as a rapid improvement in FEV1 along with reduction in airway resistance as measured by impedance oscillometry.[22] This suggests that SAR443765 therapy may be a promising new treatment of patients with type 2 asthma in the future.[22]

Janus Kinases/Signal Transducer and Activator of Transcription Proteins

The inhibition of Janus kinases/signal transducer and activator of transcription pro-teins (JAK/STAT) activation is an area of emerging interest given the probability that this inhibition has the potential to downregulate multiple cytokines, resulting in potent anti-inflammatory effects. Although these are small molecule agents rather than bio-logics, selective JAK inhibitors could impact both T2 and non-T2 inflammation. JAKs are signaling proteins associated with the receptor subunits of many asthma-related cytokines, including IL-13, IL-4, IL-5, TSLP, interferon-γ, IL-6, and IL-23, asso-ciated with T2 high and T2 low asthma. These cytokines depend on JAK signaling to elicit an inflammatory response.[23] Traditionally, oral JAK inhibitors have been utilized in the treatment of inflammatory conditions such as rheumatoid arthritis and more recently atopic dermatitis; however, their use in asthma has been limited by potential side effects, specifically opportunistic infections, and risk of cytopenia. The emer-gence of selective JAK inhibitors that can be delivered via inhalation has the potential to minimize systemic side effects while providing maximal therapeutic effects in the airway.[24] It is notable that not all JAK family members participate equally in signal transduction. JAK1 inhibition blocks IL-13-induced STAT6 phosphorylation and IL-6-induced STAT 3 phosphorylation, thus inhibition of JAK1 has potential therapeutic implications in asthma.[25,26] One promising JAK inhibitor progressing through drug development and trials is GDC-0214/RG6151. In patients with mild asthma, a phase I study demonstrated that GDC-0214/RG6151 resulted in dose-dependent reductions in FeNO without systemic side effects.[24]

OX40/OX40 Ligand

The OX40 receptor is preferentially expressed on T cells, and its ligand, OX40 L, is pri-marily expressed on antigen-presenting cells such as dendritic cells. OX40 L expression occurs primarily following activation by TSLP. Thus, OX40 L plays a sentinel role in adaptive responses by promoting Th2 polarization from naïve T-cells, which leads to the production of T2 cytokines even in an environment with low levels of IL-4.[27] OX40/OX40 L are part of the tumor necrosis factor (TNF) family and have been of recent interest as potential therapeutic targets in severe asthma. In addition to T2 polarization, OX40L and CD30L play a role in the development of memory T cells that drive lung inflammation in mice.[28] In animal models, inhibiting interaction between OX40/ OX40 L and CD30/CD30 L effectively reduced the CD4 memory T-cell response to aller-gens and decreased allergic lung inflammation on subsequent allergen challenge.[28] However, these findings have not been substantiated in human models.[29] In a human allergen challenge model, OX40 L blockade neither reduced allergen-induced airway re-sponses nor airway hyperresponsiveness but decreased serum immunoglobulin E (IgE) and airway eosinophils.[29] These findings may have been impacted by the study design, which may have resulted in administration of insufficient doses of the antibody due to a truncated treatment duration.[29] There are currently ongoing phase II studies targeting these pathways including a dose ranging study in moderate-to-severe asthma with amlitelimab (NCT05421598).[30] It is highly likely that the utility of these therapies will come to light in the next several years.

Interleukin-6

IL-6 is a proinflammatory cytokine involved in acute phase reactions and cellular and humoral immune responses.[31] In the lungs, IL-6 is produced by several cells in response to allergens, respiratory viruses, exercise, environmental particles, and inhaled toxic particles, and this causes increased inflammation in those with asthma.[31,32] Thus, IL-6 blockade is an attractive target in asthma management. Tocilizumab is a human IgG1 anti-IL-6 receptor antibody that has been studied as a potential treatment of asthma. Tocilizumab was initially developed for the treatment of rheumatoid arthritis and more recently studied in severe acute respiratory syndrome coronavirus 2 infection (SARS-COV-2).[33] To our knowledge, there are no published large clinical trials of tocilizumab therapy in asthma. A case report of 2 pediatric patients with severe persistent, nonatopic asthma treated with tocilizumab, demonstrated improvement in clinical symptoms.[34] However, in a concurrent randomized controlled trial of 11 patients with asthma, tocilizumab did not improve lung function in comparison to placebo.[35]

While further research is needed to explore the benefit of targeting IL-6 in asthma, particularly in at-risk populations such as obese asthma patients,[36] careful consideration must be given to the safety profile of these agents and broader consequences of IL-6 blockade. For example, anti-IL-6 therapies have been associated with severe infections (such as tuberculosis), increased transaminase levels and cytopenias.[37] Serious drug-induced liver injury, including acute liver failure, hepatitis, and jaundice, has also been observed with tocilizumab.[37]

Interleukin-17

IL-17 has been reported to be significantly involved in neutrophilic (a form of non-T2) asthma. The role of neutrophils in asthma has been studied but the presence of a neutrophilic asthma phenotype remains an area of ongoing debate. Several studies support that neutrophilic inflammation can be associated with severe asthma[38,39] while others argue that the presence of neutrophils may be a consequence of treatment with glucocorticoids.[40] Elevated levels of IL-17 have been reported in bronchoalveolar lavage fluid and airway tissue. IL-17 stimulates airway smooth muscle cells resulting in an increased airway hyperresponsiveness. Brodalumab is a human mAb that binds to IL-17RA. While blockade of this receptor was initially promising for treating asthma, subsequent studies failed to demonstrate therapeutic efficacy with brodalumab.[41] There are no ongoing trials targeting the IL-17 pathway in asthma. IL-23 has been shown to promote IL-17 production and neutrophil recruitment in animal models. However, a phase IIa trial with risankizumab, an anti-IL-23 mAb, did not demonstrate a treatment effect in asthma.[42]

Interleukin-5

Targeting IL-5 or its receptor in severe asthma with biologics such as mepolizumab, benralizumab, and reslizumab has been a safe and successful strategy.[43-45] Current biological agents require administration every 4 to 8 weeks depending on the drug. This dosing frequency can lead to nonadherence as well as an increased resource utilization. Efforts have been made to produce biologics with much longer half-life. GSK3511294, aka depemokimab, is a humanized anti-IL-5 agent, which has been engineered to increase affinity for IL-5 receptor and potentially extend the half-life. This agent acts on the same receptor as mepolizumab, and the in vitro studies have demonstrated 29 fold increase in potency compared to mepolizumab. It is critical to note that the effects of targeting IL-5 go beyond the depletion of eosinophils to include effects on barrier function, airway remodeling and airway hyperresponsiveness.[11] In a phase I clinical study, a single dose of depemokimab was administered at different dosing strengths, and patients were followed for up to 40 weeks.[46] Compared to placebo, depemokimab was associated with greater than 48% reduction in blood eosinophil counts in a dose-dependent manner and was also well tolerated. This agent is now being studied in a phase 3 trial of adults and adolescents with severe eosinophilic asthma (NCT04718103).

CHALLENGES AND BARRIERS IN DRUG DELIVERY TO THE LUNGS

Advances in asthma therapy require technological advances to tackle ongoing challenges in the use of biologic and other anti-inflammatory therapies. There are challenges with regards to the manufacturing and storage of biologics, more targeted drug delivery to the lungs and the short half-life of some of the currently available biologics, all of which can be potentially addressed by technological advances.

An understanding of the biology of current therapies is a crucial first step to speculating future options. Biologics are complex large molecules that typically consist of peptides and proteins, including antibodies.[47] Therapeutic antibodies are glycoproteins belonging to immunoglobulin families with most of the currently approved agents coming from the IgG subclass, which have a half-life of about 10 to 21 days.[48] Typical IgG structure consists of 4 peptide chains of which 2 are light chains and 2 are heavy chains that are connected via a disulfide bond and electrochemical interaction. Their typical molecular weight can reach up to 150,000 Da.[48] Complementarity determining region (CDR) is present on the fragment antigen binding region and involved in binding with the epitope on the target antigen. The heavy chains contain the fragment crystalline (Fc) region, which carries the effector functions via complement cascade enzymes or by the Fc receptor binding. The Fc region also contains the site for the neonatal Fc receptor, which plays an important role in antibody transport. To reduce immunogenicity, antibodies are further engineered to replace murine sequence derived amino acids with human sequence.

Over the years, several noninvasive routes have been investigated for biologic delivery including oral, nasal, transdermal, and inhalational routes.[49–53] Of these routes, inhalational route appears to be of particular interest for respiratory diseases. Due to its large surface area and extensive vascular network, the lungs can enable rapid onset of action for an inhaled agent with minimal systemic effects. Despite these potential benefits, developing inhalational biologics has been a challenge. Inhalational delivery of antibodies into the lung is carried by the generation of aerosol-containing particles with size ranging between 1 and 5 μm (**Fig. 2**). Several factors play a role in determining the location of aerosol particle deposition in the lung. Airway geometry, mucociliary clearance, humidity, pH, and lung lining fluid are some of the important barriers to therapeutic efficacy. Biologics tend to be highly prone to degradation under stress from elevated temperatures, shear forces, light exposure, and extreme pH.[54] Physical degradation of the protein can lead to aggregation, which not only reduces its activity but also can lead to immunogenicity. Biologics with exogenous sequences are at risk of being recognized as nonself by host immune cells, leading to the formation of antidrug antibodies. In addition, the highly branching structure of the lung poses a challenge to depositing an effective dose of inhaled agents in the distal airways. Generally, particles between 1 and 5 μm can reach and deposit into the lower airways. Thickness of airway lining fluid also varies between the central and distal airways. As

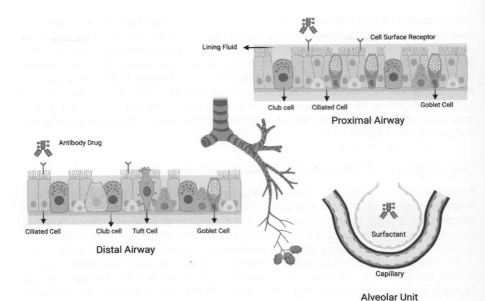

Fig. 2. Biological barriers to inhaled drug delivery in the airways: the lining fluid, mucociliary clearance, and pulmonary surfactant. (Created with BioRender.com.)

inhalational particles must dissolve to release the active drug, optimal site for deposition and pharmacologic action of inhaled biologic agents are not well understood.

Furthermore, successful landing of the inhalational agent on the airway surface may not lead to adequate pulmonary absorption, which relies on a highly complex mechanism. Inhalational biologics can be absorbed by 3 different mechanisms including paracellular diffusion by tight junction, transcytosis, and transcellular diffusion via endocytosis or pinocytosis.[55,56] Large molecules tend to follow the transcellular route, whereas lower weight molecules follow the paracellular route. Peptide transporters assist with the transcytosis of smaller peptides. Mucociliary and surfactant barriers play an important role in drug delivery. The 3 dimensional mesh structure of mucus enables it to trap inhaled particles and move them to the pharynx for expulsion from the airways.[57] Similarly, antibodies may also interact with surfactant components leading to aggregation and removal from the lungs. Pathologic conditions such as asthma, chronic obstructive pulmonary disease, cystic fibrosis can have modified barriers in the form of highly viscous mucus further affecting pulmonary drug delivery. As opposed to the long half-life of systemic biologics, inhaled antibodies tend to be eliminated from lungs within 1 to 2 days after administration.[48] Several proteolytic enzymes can be found in the lung whose expression can be increased in different lung diseases. While protease/antiprotease balance is critical for a healthy lung, antibodies can be particularly sensitive to degradation by proteases. Together these processes pose significant challenge to the development of inhalational biological agents.

COLD CHAIN-RELATED LIMITATIONS OF SUBCUTANEOUS BIOLOGICS

Currently, there are 6 biological agents that are approved for asthma treatments. Except for reslizumab, all the remaining biologic agents are administered subcutaneously. Omalizumab, benralizumab, and mepolizumab are humanized IgG1 antibodies, dupilumab is human IgG4 antibody and tezepelumab is human IgG2 subclass antibody. IgG1 subclass antibodies tend to have stronger effector function and longer half-life.[48]

These biologic agents vary in required storage temperatures, warm up times before administration, and the amount of time they can be stored at room temperature. Omalizumab has the shortest shelf life out of refrigerator of 2 days before it expires, whereas tezepelumab can be kept at room temperature for up to 30 days.[48] For long-term storage, all these agents require storage in a refrigerator between 36°F and 46°F. On the day of drug administration, biologic agents need to be warmed to room temperature 30 to 60 minutes prior to their use.[58] It is critical that patients understand these cold chain requirements for their specific biological agent. Furthermore, the need for cold storage limits the ability of biologics to be used in resource limited settings and introduces complexities and expenses with drug delivery to patients.

TECHNOLOGICAL ADVANCES IN BIOLOGIC DELIVERY

Hamers and colleagues[59] were the first to identify heavy chain antibodies (HCAb) in the blood of *Camelus dromedarius*, a one-humped camel. HCAb consists of 2 heavy chain constant regions (CH2 and CH3), heavy chain variable domain (VHH) and are linked by a hinge region. Subsequent studies showed that VHH can be expressed independently as a single-domain antibody called a nanobody. Nanobodies are small size structures with a molecular weight of below 15 kDa, allowing improved tissue penetration. Its unique structure that contains 4 conservative framework regions (FRs) and 3 complementarity determining regions (CDRs), attributes high antigen binding affinity and specificity. These CDRs provide stability to the nanobodies when exposed to high temperature, whereas the hydrophilic FRs prevent aggregation and allow for their function as monomers.[60] In addition, the extended CDR3 loop enhances the ability of the nanobody to bind with diverse antigens. Combining these benefits with easy production, diverse delivery routes, and high adaptability has led to increased application in biomedical studies.

Nanobodies are not without limitations. Their monovalent forms require modifications to enhance their therapeutic capability. The smaller size of nanobodies can also lead to rapid renal clearance, which usually require conjugation with albumin or polyethylene glycol.[61] Nanobodies also require the use of camelids, which may lead to space constraints for industrial production as opposed to usual monoclonal antibodies, which are generated via immunizing mice. The first nanobody drug, caplacizumab, was approved in 2019 by FDA for the treatment of adults with acquired thrombotic thrombocytopenic purpura.[62] More recently, as mentioned earlier, SAR443765 was studied in 36 patients with mild-to-moderate asthma and elevated FeNO of 25 or greater parts per billion.[22] A single dose of this nanobody reduced FeNO starting at week 1 after administration. This drug is now being studied in a phase 2b study (NCT06102005).[23]

SUMMARY

Emerging biologics that focus on novel targets are enhancing the discovery of new treatments for asthma. The increased understanding of inflammatory mechanisms, coupled with technological advancements, will allow us to tackle asthma heterogeneity and the likely prevalence of multiple upregulated inflammatory pathways in each unique patient. The future of asthma care is exciting, and we expect that many of the therapies currently in development will make it to clinical practice, adding to the armamentarium of clinicians who will be increasingly charged with determining the best approach to selecting and initiating advanced asthma therapies.

CLINICS CARE POINTS

- Asthma is a complex and heterogeneous disease, but advances in our understanding of the underlying disease have led to multiple new biologics, and the pipeline for future therapies is robust.
- It is apparent that clinicians will need to employ strategies to phenotype patients as a basis of identifying potential upregulated pathways as we consider incorporating these future therapies into practice.

DISCLOSURE

N.L. Lugogo received consulting fees from Amgen, AstraZeneca, Avillion, Genentech, GSK, Nioxx, Novartis, Regeneron, Sanofi, and Teva; honoraria for nonspeakers bureau presentations from GSK, TEVA, and Astra Zeneca, United Kingdom; and travel support from AstraZeneca, Sanofi, Teva, Israel, Regeneron, and GSK; her institution received research support from Amgen, United States AstraZeneca, Avillion, Bellus, Evidera, Gossamer Bio, Genentech, United States GSK, Janssen, United States Regeneron, United States Sanofi, United States, Novartis, Switzerland and Teva. She is an honorary faculty member of Observational and Pragmatic Research Institute (OPRI) but does not receive compensation for this role. N.L. Lugogo participated in the draft of the article, provided edits of all versions of the article and provided final approval of the version to be published. I have disclosed all relevant conflict of interests. B. Desai had effort supported by a T32 training grant (T32 grant: NIH T32 AI 007469).

REFERENCES

1. Perez-de-Llano L, Scelo G, Tran TN, et al. Exploring definitions and predictors of severe asthma clinical remission post-biologic in adults. Am J Respir Crit Care Med 2024. https://doi.org/10.1164/rccm.202311-2192OC.
2. Farinha I, Heaney LG. Barriers to clinical remission in severe asthma. Respir Res 2024;25(1):178.
3. Calderon AA, Dimond C, Choy DF, et al. Targeting interleukin-33 and thymic stromal lymphopoietin pathways for novel pulmonary therapeutics in asthma and COPD. Eur Respir Rev 2023. https://doi.org/10.1183/16000617.0144-2022.
4. Saikumar Jayalatha AK, Hesse L, Ketelaar ME, et al. The central role of IL-33/IL-1RL1 pathway in asthma: From pathogenesis to intervention. Pharmacol Ther 2021. https://doi.org/10.1016/j.pharmthera.2021.107847.
5. Schleich F, Bougard N, Moermans C, et al. Cytokine-targeted therapies for asthma and COPD. Eur Respir Rev 2023. https://doi.org/10.1183/16000617.0193-2022.
6. Wechsler ME, Ruddy MK, Pavord ID, et al. Efficacy and safety of itepekimab in patients with moderate-to-severe asthma. N Engl J Med 2021;385(18):1656–68.
7. Castro M, Corren J, Pavord ID, et al. Dupilumab efficacy and safety in moderate-to-severe uncontrolled asthma. N Engl J Med 2018;378(26):2486–96.
8. Study Details | Study to Assess the Efficacy and Safety of MEDI3506 in Adults With Uncontrolled Moderate-to-severe Asthma | ClinicalTrials.gov. Available at: https://clinicaltrials.gov/study/NCT04570657. [Accessed 10 May 2024].
9. England E, Rees DG, Scott IC, et al. Tozorakimab (MEDI3506): an anti-IL-33 antibody that inhibits IL-33 signalling via ST2 and RAGE/EGFR to reduce inflammation and epithelial dysfunction. Sci Rep 2023. https://doi.org/10.1038/s41598-023-36642-y.

10. Rael EL, Lockey RF. Interleukin-13 Signaling and Its Role in Asthma. World Allergy Organization Journal 2011;4(3):54–64.
11. Pelaia C, Heffler E, Crimi C, et al. Interleukins 4 and 13 in asthma: key pathophysiologic cytokines and druggable molecular targets. Front Pharmacol 2022;13: 851940.
12. Loewenthal L, Menzies-Gow A. FeNO in Asthma. Semin Respir Crit Care Med 2022;43(5):635–45.
13. Murugesan N, Saxena D, Dileep A, et al. Update on the Role of FeNO in asthma management. Diagnostics 2023;13(8).
14. Corren J, Szefler SJ, Sher E, et al. Lebrikizumab in uncontrolled asthma: reanalysis in a well-defined type 2 population. J Allergy Clin Immunol Pract 2024;12(5): 1215–24.e3.
15. Hanania NA, Korenblat P, Chapman KR, et al. Efficacy and safety of lebrikizumab in patients with uncontrolled asthma (LAVOLTA I and LAVOLTA II): replicate, phase 3, randomised, double-blind, placebo-controlled trials. Lancet Respir Med 2016;4(10):781–96.
16. Sardon-Prado O, Diaz-Garcia C, Corcuera-Elosegui P, et al. Severe Asthma and Biological Therapies: Now and the Future. J Clin Med 2023;12(18).
17. Peters AT, Sagara H, Corren J, et al. Impact of dupilumab across seasons in patients with type 2, uncontrolled, moderate-to-severe asthma. Ann Allergy Asthma Immunol 2024;132(4):477–84.e4.
18. Agrawal A, Varshney R, Gattani A, et al. Development of hemagglutinin-neuraminidase homologous peptides as novel promising therapeutic agents against peste des petits ruminants virus. Protein J 2023;42(6):685–97.
19. Sher LD, Corren J, Pavord ID, et al. Dupilumab long-term efficacy in patients with non-OCS-dependent asthma with and without evidence of allergic asthma. J Asthma 2023;60(9):1767–74.
20. Holgate ST, Wenzel S, Postma DS, et al. Asthma. Nat Rev Dis Primers 2015;1(1): 15025.
21. Parnes J, Molfino NA, Colice G, et al. Targeting TSLP in Asthma. J Asthma Allergy 2022;15:749–65.
22. Deiteren E, Krupka K, Imberdis N, et al. Targeting of TSLP and IL-13 by the Novel NANOBODY® Molecule SAR443765 Reduces FeNO in Asthma Following Single Dose Exposure (abstract). Am J Respir Crit Care Med 2023;207:A6816.
23. Braithwaite IE, Cai F, Tom JA, et al. Inhaled JAK inhibitor GDC-0214 reduces exhaled nitric oxide in patients with mild asthma: A randomized, controlled, proof-of-activity trial. J Allergy Clin Immunol 2021;148(3):783–9.
24. Nilsson M, Rhedin M, Hendrickx R, et al. Characterization of selective and potent JAK1 inhibitors intended for the inhaled treatment of asthma. Drug Des Dev Ther 2022;16:2901–17.
25. Sohn SJ, Barrett K, Van Abbema A, et al. A Restricted Role for TYK2 catalytic activity in human cytokine responses revealed by novel TYK2-selective inhibitors. J Immunol 2013;191(5):2205–16.
26. Zak M, Hanan EJ, Lupardus P, et al. Discovery of a class of highly potent Janus Kinase 1/2 (JAK1/2) inhibitors demonstrating effective cell-based blockade of IL-13 signaling. Bioorg Med Chem Lett 2019;29(12):1522–31.
27. Kaur D, Brightling C. OX40/OX40 Ligand Interactions in T-Cell Regulation and Asthma. Chest 2012;141(2):494–9.
28. Gracias DT, Sethi GS, Mehta AK, et al. Combination blockade of OX40L and CD30L inhibits allergen-driven memory TH2 cell reactivity and lung inflammation. J Allergy Clin Immunol 2021;147(6):2316–29.

29. Gauvreau GM, Boulet L-P, Cockcroft DW, et al. <scp>OX</scp> 40L blockade and allergen-induced airway responses in subjects with mild asthma. Clin Exp Allergy 2014;44(1):29–37.

30. Dose ranging study of amlitelimab in adult participants with moderate-to-severe asthma - full text view - ClinicalTrials.gov. Available at: https://classic.clinicaltrials.gov/ct2/show/NCT05421598. [Accessed 10 May 2024].

31. Kaur S, Bansal Y, Kumar R, et al. A panoramic review of IL-6: Structure, pathophysiological roles and inhibitors. Bioorg Med Chem 2020. https://doi.org/10.1016/j.bmc.2020.115327.

32. Yokoyama A, Kohno N, Fujino S, et al. Circulating interleukin-6 levels in patients with bronchial asthma. Am J Respir Crit Care Med 1995;151(5):1354–8.

33. Khan FA, Stewart I, Fabbri L, et al. Systematic review and meta-analysis of anakinra, sarilumab, siltuximab and tocilizumab for COVID-19. Thorax 2021. https://doi.org/10.1136/thoraxjnl-2020-215266.

34. Esty B, Harb H, Bartnikas LM, et al. Treatment of severe persistent asthma with il-6 receptor blockade HHS public access. J Allergy Clin Immunol Pract 2019;7(5):1639–42.

35. Revez JA, Bain LM, Watson RM, et al. Effects of interleukin-6 receptor blockade on allergen-induced airway responses in mild asthmatics. Clin Transl Immunology 2019;8(6):e1044.

36. Peters MC, McGrath KW, Hawkins GA, et al. Plasma interleukin-6 concentrations, metabolic dysfunction, and asthma severity: a cross-sectional analysis of two cohorts. Lancet Respir Med 2016;4(7):574–84.

37. Crisafulli S, Isgrò V, La Corte L, et al. Potential Role of Anti-interleukin (IL)-6 Drugs in the Treatment of COVID-19: Rationale, Clinical Evidence and Risks. BioDrugs 2020;34(4):415–22.

38. JATAKANON A, UASUF C, MAZIAK W, et al. Neutrophilic inflammation in severe persistent asthma. Am J Respir Crit Care Med 1999;160(5):1532–9.

39. Gibson PG, Simpson JL, Saltos N. Heterogeneity of airway inflammation in persistent asthma. Chest 2001;119(5):1329–36.

40. Gao H, Ying S, Dai Y. Pathological roles of neutrophil-mediated inflammation in asthma and its potential for therapy as a target. J Immunol Res 2017;2017.

41. Busse WW, Holgate S, Kerwin E, et al. Randomized, double-blind, placebo-controlled study of brodalumab, a human anti-IL-17 receptor monoclonal antibody, in moderate to severe asthma. Am J Respir Crit Care Med 2013;188(11):1294–302.

42. Brightling CE, Nair P, Cousins DJ, et al. Risankizumab in severe asthma — a phase 2a, placebo-controlled trial. N Engl J Med 2021;385(18):1669–79.

43. Deeks ED, Brusselle G. Reslizumab in eosinophilic asthma: a review. Drugs 2017;77(7):777–84.

44. Tian BP, Zhang GS, Lou J, et al. Efficacy and safety of benralizumab for eosinophilic asthma: A systematic review and meta-analysis of randomized controlled trials. J Asthma 2018;55(9):956–65.

45. Morjaria JB, Emma R, Fuochi V, et al. An evaluation of mepolizumab for the treatment of severe asthma. Expet Opin Biol Ther 2019;19(6):491–500.

46. Singh D, Fuhr R, Bird NP, et al. A Phase 1 study of the long-acting anti-IL-5 monoclonal antibody GSK3511294 in patients with asthma. Br J Clin Pharmacol 2022;88(2):702–12.

47. Liang W, Pan HW, Vllasaliu D, et al. Pulmonary delivery of biological drugs. Pharmaceutics 2020;12(11).

48. Sécher T, Heuzé-Vourc'h N. Pulmonary Delivery of Antibody for the Treatment of Respiratory Diseases. In: Lam J, Kwok PCL, editors. Respiratory Delivery of Biologics, Nucleic Acids, and Vaccines. AAPS Introductions in the Pharmaceutical Sciences, vol 8. Springer, Cham. 2023. https://doi.org/10.1007/978-3-031-47567-2_2.
49. Ferrati S, Wu T, Kanapuram SR, et al. Dosing considerations for inhaled biologics. Int J Pharm 2018;549(1–2):58–66.
50. Morales JO, Fathe KR, Brunaugh A, et al. Challenges and future prospects for the delivery of biologics: oral mucosal, pulmonary, and transdermal routes. AAPS 2017. https://doi.org/10.1208/s12248-017-0054-z.
51. Rohrer J, Lupo N, Bernkop-Schnürch A. Advanced formulations for intranasal delivery of biologics. Int J Pharm 2018;553(1–2):8–20.
52. Montenegro-Nicolini M, Morales JO. Overview and future potential of buccal mucoadhesive films as drug delivery systems for biologics. AAPS PharmSciTech 2017;18(1):3–14.
53. Vllasaliu D, Thanou M, Stolnik S, et al. Recent advances in oral delivery of biologics: nanomedicine and physical modes of delivery. Expet Opin Drug Deliv 2018;15(8):759–70.
54. Depreter F, Pilcer G, Amighi K. Inhaled proteins: challenges and perspectives. Int J Pharm 2013;447(1–2):251–80.
55. Wolff RK. Safety of inhaled proteins for therapeutic use. J Aerosol Med 1998; 11(4):197–219.
56. Niven RW. Delivery of biotherapeutics by inhalation aerosol. Crit Rev Ther Drug Carrier Syst 1995;12(2–3):151–231.
57. Sanders N, Rudolph C, Braeckmans K, et al. Extracellular barriers in respiratory gene therapy. Adv Drug Deliv Rev 2009;61(2):115–27.
58. Tan LD, Nguyen N, Alismail A, et al. Management of uncontrolled asthma: a framework for novel and legacy biologic treatments. J Asthma Allergy 2022;15: 875–83.
59. Hamers-Casterman C, Atarhouch T, Muyldermans S, et al. Naturally occurring antibodies devoid of light chains. Nature 1993;363(6428):446–8.
60. Jin BK, Odongo S, Radwanska M, et al. Nanobodies: a review of generation, diagnostics and therapeutics. Int J Mol Sci 2023;24(6).
61. Salvador JP, Vilaplana L, Marco MP. Nanobody: outstanding features for diagnostic and therapeutic applications. Anal Bioanal Chem 2019;411(9):1703–13.
62. Hanlon A, Metjian A. Caplacizumab in adult patients with acquired thrombotic thrombocytopenic purpura. Ther Adv Hematol 2020;11. 2040620720902904.

UNITED STATES POSTAL SERVICE®

Statement of Ownership, Management, and Circulation (All Periodicals Publications Except Requester Publications)

1. Publication Title	2. Publication Number	3. Filing Date
IMMUNOLOGY AND ALLERGY CLINICS OF NORTH AMERICA	006 – 361	9/18/2024

4. Issue Frequency	5. Number of Issues Published Annually	6. Annual Subscription Price
FEB, MAY, AUG, NOV	4	$375.00

7. Complete Mailing Address of Known Office of Publication (Not printer) (Street, city, county, state, and ZIP+4®)

ELSEVIER INC.
230 Park Avenue, Suite 800
New York, NY 10169

Contact Person
Malathi Samayan

Telephone (Include area code)
91-44-4299-4507

8. Complete Mailing Address of Headquarters or General Business Office of Publisher (Not printer)

ELSEVIER INC.
230 Park Avenue, Suite 800
New York, NY 10169

9. Full Names and Complete Mailing Addresses of Publisher, Editor, and Managing Editor (Do not leave blank)

Publisher (Name and complete mailing address)

Dolores Meloni, ELSEVIER INC.
1600 JOHN F KENNEDY BLVD. SUITE 1600
PHILADELPHIA, PA 19103-2899

Editor (Name and complete mailing address)

TAYLOR HAYES, ELSEVIER INC.
1600 JOHN F KENNEDY BLVD. SUITE 1600
PHILADELPHIA, PA 19103-2899

Managing Editor (Name and complete mailing address)

PATRICK MANLEY, ELSEVIER INC.
1600 JOHN F KENNEDY BLVD. SUITE 1600
PHILADELPHIA, PA 19103-2899

10. Owner (Do not leave blank. If the publication is owned by a corporation, give the name and address of the corporation immediately followed by the names and addresses of all stockholders owning or holding 1 percent or more of the total amount of stock. If not owned by a corporation, give the names and addresses of the individual owners. If owned by a partnership or other unincorporated firm, give its name and address as well as those of each individual owner. If the publication is published by a nonprofit organization, give its name and address.)

Full Name	Complete Mailing Address
WHOLLY OWNED SUBSIDIARY OF REED/ELSEVIER, US HOLDINGS	1600 JOHN F KENNEDY BLVD. SUITE 1600 PHILADELPHIA, PA 19103-2899

11. Known Bondholders, Mortgagees, and Other Security Holders Owning or Holding 1 Percent or More of Total Amount of Bonds, Mortgages, or Other Securities. If none, check box ▶ ☐ None

Full Name	Complete Mailing Address
N/A	

12. Tax Status (For completion by nonprofit organizations authorized to mail at nonprofit rates) (Check one)
The purpose, function, and nonprofit status of this organization and the exempt status for federal income tax purposes:
☒ Has Not Changed During Preceding 12 Months
☐ Has Changed During Preceding 12 Months (Publisher must submit explanation of change with this statement)

PS Form 3526, July 2014 [Page 1 of 4 (see instructions page 4)] PSN: 7530-01-000-9931   PRIVACY NOTICE: See our privacy policy on www.usps.com.

13. Publication Title			14. Issue Date for Circulation Data Below
IMMUNOLOGY AND ALLERGY CLINICS OF NORTH AMERICA			AUGUST 2024

15. Extent and Nature of Circulation			Average No. Copies Each Issue During Preceding 12 Months	No. Copies of Single Issue Published Nearest to Filing Date
a. Total Number of Copies (Net press run)			88	78
b. Paid Circulation (By Mail and Outside the Mail)	(1)	Mailed Outside-County Paid Subscriptions Stated on PS Form 3541 (Include paid distribution above nominal rate, advertiser's proof copies, and exchange copies)	57	49
	(2)	Mailed In-County Paid Subscriptions Stated on PS Form 3541 (Include paid distribution above nominal rate, advertiser's proof copies, and exchange copies)	0	0
	(3)	Paid Distribution Outside the Mails Including Sales Through Dealers and Carriers, Street Vendors, Counter Sales, and Other Paid Distribution Outside USPS®	17	16
	(4)	Paid Distribution by Other Classes of Mail Through the USPS (e.g., First-Class Mail®)	12	11
c. Total Paid Distribution (Sum of 15b (1), (2), (3), and (4))			86	76
d. Free or Nominal Rate Distribution (By Mail and Outside the Mail)	(1)	Free or Nominal Rate Outside-County Copies Included on PS Form 3541	1	1
	(2)	Free or Nominal Rate In-County Copies Included on PS Form 3541	0	0
	(3)	Free or Nominal Rate Copies Mailed at Other Classes Through the USPS (e.g., First-Class Mail)	0	0
	(4)	Free or Nominal Rate Distribution Outside the Mail (Carriers or other means)	1	1
e. Total Free or Nominal Rate Distribution (Sum of 15d (1), (2), (3) and (4))			2	2
f. Total Distribution (Sum of 15c and 15e)			88	78
g. Copies not Distributed (See Instructions to Publishers #4 (page 83))			0	0
h. Total (Sum of 15f and g)			88	78
i. Percent Paid (15c divided by 15f times 100)			97.73%	97.44%

* If you are claiming electronic copies, go to line 16 on page 3. If you are not claiming electronic copies, skip to line 17 on page 3.

PS Form 3526, July 2014 (Page 2 of 4)

16. Electronic Copy Circulation	Average No. Copies Each Issue During Preceding 12 Months	No. Copies of Single Issue Published Nearest to Filing Date
a. Paid Electronic Copies		
b. Total Paid Print Copies (Line 15c) + Paid Electronic Copies (Line 16a)		
c. Total Print Distribution (Line 15f) + Paid Electronic Copies (Line 16a)		
d. Percent Paid (Both Print & Electronic Copies) (16b divided by 16c × 100)		

☒ I certify that 50% of all my distributed copies (electronic and print) are paid above a nominal price.

17. Publication of Statement of Ownership

☒ If the publication is a general publication, publication of this statement is required. Will be printed in the NOVEMBER 2024 issue of this publication.
☐ Publication not required.

18. Signature and Title of Editor, Publisher, Business Manager, or Owner

Malathi Samayan

Malathi Samayan - Distribution Controller

Date 9/18/2024

I certify that all information furnished on this form is true and complete. I understand that anyone who furnishes false or misleading information on this form or who omits material or information requested on the form may be subject to criminal sanctions (including fines and imprisonment) and/or civil sanctions (including civil penalties).

PS Form 3526, July 2014 (Page 3 of 4)   PRIVACY NOTICE: See our privacy policy on www.usps.com.

Moving?

Make sure your subscription moves with you!

To notify us of your new address, find your **Clinics Account Number** (located on your mailing label above your name), and contact customer service at:

Email: journalscustomerservice-usa@elsevier.com

800-654-2452 (subscribers in the U.S. & Canada)
314-447-8871 (subscribers outside of the U.S. & Canada)

Fax number: 314-447-8029

Elsevier Health Sciences Division
Subscription Customer Service
3251 Riverport Lane
Maryland Heights, MO 63043

*To ensure uninterrupted delivery of your subscription, please notify us at least 4 weeks in advance of move.

Printed and bound by CPI Group (UK) Ltd, Croydon, CR0 4YY

12/05/2025

01869426-0001